"*How Healing Works* is the most comprehensive and comprehensible book on how and why people heal. It is a masterful survey of the research on the physical, psychological, and spiritual factors that help us regain and retain our health. Dr. Wayne Jonas is one of America's top docs, a true leader in medicine, who deeply understands the ins and outs of getting well. After reading *How Healing Works*, share it with your physician."
—Larry Dossey, MD Author, *One Mind*

"In the polarized, nonintegrative era twenty-five years ago—the earliest days of introducing natural health and integrative practices into regular care—the arrival on the scene of a healer advocate for a more balanced medicine, who happened to be both army officer and medical doctor, was a great gift. What some of us did not yet know was that Wayne Jonas, then an emerging leader at the National Institutes of Health and in federal policy, incorporated healing practices and traditions from across the globe into his work to understand, bridge, and transform."
—John Weeks Editor in Chief, *The Journal of Alternative and Complementary Medicine*; Publisher, *The Integrator Blog*

"Wayne Jonas distills a lifetime of research, teaching, caring for patients, emotional growth, and inquiry into this wise, generous, and useful offering. He asks the toughest questions and responds in clear, accessible language. He invites us with him on an intimate journey as he presents with candor and courage his own evolution and the remarkable stories of those who have taught him so much about the mysteries of healing, hidden in plain sight. This is required reading for everyone interested in understanding and unleashing our untapped healing potential."
—Joseph Bobrow, Roshi, PhD Author, *Waking Up from War*

"Wayne Jonas is a scientist, physician, teacher, storyteller, and, ultimately, a healer. His book uses a wide lens to examine how healing is not only pharmaceuticals and surgery but involves environmental, behavioral, social/emotional, and cognitive/spiritual dimensions. *How Healing Works* is provocative, engaging, and informative and encourages the reader in their own healing."
—Ted Kaptchuk Professor of Medicine, Harvard Medical School

how healing works

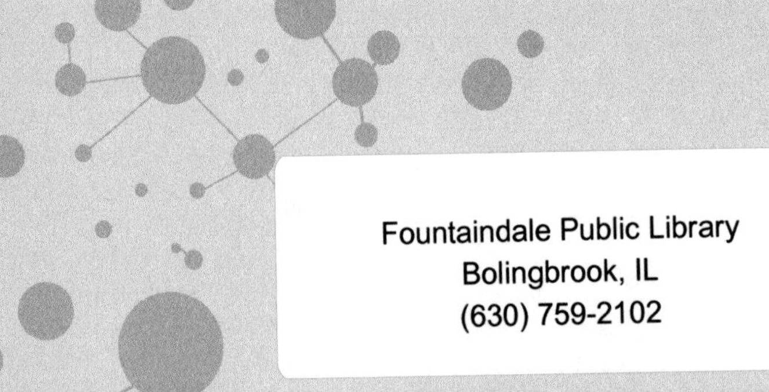

how healing works

GET WELL AND STAY WELL
using your hidden power to heal

WAYNE JONAS, MD

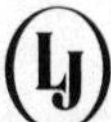

LORENA JONES BOOKS
An imprint of TEN SPEED PRESS
California | New York

Over the past three decades, the author has seen hundreds of patients. Throughout this book, he has drawn on the stories they have generously shared to illustrate the vast range of treatment experiences. Many of the case histories you will read are composites. When the author has based examples on particular patients, he has changed their names and distinguishing features in order to protect their identity. Any resulting resemblance to persons alive or dead is entirely unintentional and coincidental.

In addition, the information and advice presented in this book are not meant to substitute for the advice of your family physician or other trained health-care professionals. You are advised to consult with health-care professionals with regard to all matters pertaining to you and your family's health and well-being.

Published in the United States by Lorena Jones Books, an imprint of the
Crown Publishing Group, a division of Penguin Random House LLC, New York.
www.crownpublishing.com
www.tenspeed.com

Library of Congress Cataloging-in-Publication Data
Names: Jonas, Wayne B., author.
Title: How healing works : get well and stay well using your hidden power to
heal / Wayne Jonas, MD.
Description: California : Ten Speed Press, [2018] | "Lorena Jones books." |
Includes bibliographical references and index.
Identifiers: LCCN 2017022019 (print) | LCCN 2017031344 (ebook)
Subjects: LCSH: Healing. | Nature, Healing power of. | Mind and body. |
BISAC: HEALTH & FITNESS / Healing. | HEALTH & FITNESS / Healthy Living. |
HEALTH & FITNESS / Health Care Issues.
Classification: LCC RZ999 (ebook) | LCC RZ999 .J66 2018 (print) | DDC
615.8/528—dc23
LC record available at https://lccn.loc.gov/2017022019

Hardcover ISBN: 978-0-399-57924-0
eBook ISBN: 978-0-399-57925-7

Design by Margaux Keres and Lisa Ferkel

Illustrations by Six Half Dozen Design Studio

Printed in the United States

10 9 8 7 6 5 4 3 2 1

First Edition

Contents

INTRODUCTION

THE NEED FOR A NEW UNDERSTANDING OF HEALING

Most of the treatments we think produce healing do not work when exposed to rigorous scientific scrutiny. Yet people often get better. Why? How?

This book argues that the vast majority of healing comes from a few basic principles that can be used effectively by any system—ancient or modern, conventional or alternative, proven or unproven—and by both doctors and patients in their daily lives. The secret: to elicit a meaningful response in the person who requires healing.

My approach is based on almost forty years of seeing patients as a mainstream family doctor, as a trained scientist, and as an explorer of many medical systems. I discovered how healing happens through my work with patients, as director of the Office of Alternative Medicine at the National Institutes of Health (NIH), and as a research scientist at the World Health Organization (WHO), Walter Reed Army Institute of Research, and Samueli Institute.

In this book, I'm going to give you a simple, systematic approach to real healing. Drawing on the most rigorous scientific evidence available as well as wisdom from ancient healing traditions, I will show you that:

• Only 20% of healing comes from the "treatment agent" that the doctor applies to you—whether that is surgery, drugs, acupuncture needles, herbs and supplements, diet, or anything else external to you.

• A full 80% of healing comes from constructing a meaningful treatment response, unique to you, which is internal and highly personal, using simple principles and components.

• You can activate your own inherent healing processes and get your physician and others on board to help accelerate your healing journey, making any approach more effective, safer, and less expensive. And these processes can prevent the majority of chronic diseases in the future.

I am not arguing, as some others do, that you can simply think yourself into healing. And I am well aware that understanding what stimulates healing or prevents disease will not fix a broken bone, cure cancer, or stop a heart attack. However, the top ten reasons for seeing a doctor, according to a study by the Mayo Clinic, include pain (especially back pain), fatigue, cognitive dysfunction, hypertension, diabetes, obesity, chronic heart or lung problems, or brain diseases such as Alzheimer's, Parkinson's, or depression. Almost all of these conditions accelerate and increase as we age, so even if you feel healthy now, chances are if you live long enough, you will get more than one of these conditions, unless you seek out ways to prevent them.

If you understand how healing really works for the most common chronic conditions, you can take greater control of your own recovery, increase the likelihood that any specific treatment will be effective, prevent many of the diseases of aging, and radically reduce your dependence on the medical industry. *How Healing Works* provides a way for merging curing and healing—producing true integrative health. Now I invite you to travel with me to see how I discovered this.

section 1

RETHINKING HEALING

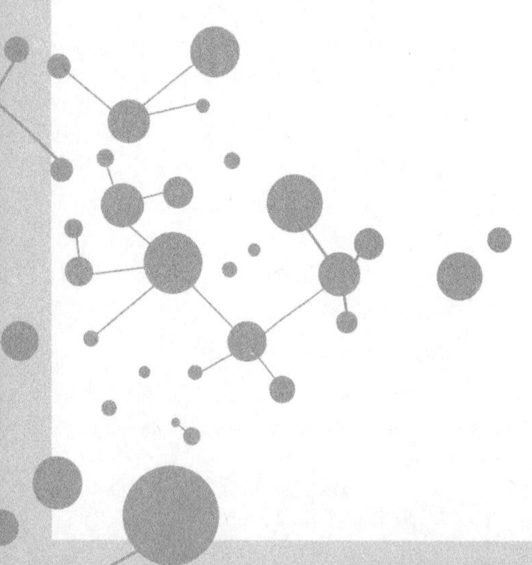

CHAPTER 1

The Paradox of Healing

What we think heals often doesn't, but almost anything can heal.

Most of what we think produces health actually does not. But there is an inherent healing capacity within us all that, when properly released, can produce remarkable recovery, health, and happiness. The healing process is understood and applied in many wisdom traditions and by wise physicians today, but has been obscured by modern medicine's obsession with small parts, and the technologies, techniques, and chemicals that manipulate them. While many of these technologies are extremely valuable, this hyperfocus and the economic rewards driving them has largely squeezed out the essence of what medicine is all about—how to guide a person to healing, wholeness, and well-being.

Let's take a closer look at how we heal.

HIEN

We were miles into the jungle, and my best buddy, Hien, was injured. I was scared. How would we get him out? Although we spoke hardly a word of each other's language—his, Vietnamese, and mine, English—our communication was clear. How would he get back? Would he die out here? There was a war going on, wasn't there? Hien's ankle was markedly swollen. Large amounts of blood collected under the skin. He could barely stand, much less walk on it. Maybe I could run out of the jungle, find my dad, and see if he could call in one of those American military helicopters. I tried to say that to Hien's father, who was the scout master, but he looked unconcerned. We would camp there that night, he said in Vietnamese, and continue hiking in the morning. Then he turned to me and said in broken English, "Hien be okay, Wen. No worry." But I didn't see how he would be okay.

Hien and I were both nine years old, and I was his only American friend, which was not surprising, given that I was the only nine-year-old American boy in Nha Trang, Vietnam, in early 1964. My father was a chaplain in the military, assigned to serve the spiritual needs of American service men and women in Vietnam. At the time, America was not engaged in active combat, and military advisors could bring families there. My father had asked us to come. So, with four kids, ages two to twelve, in tow, my mother packed us up and we moved to Nha Trang, a lovely coastal village in the center of the country. We lived near the beach, in a four-bedroom French "villa," on a fenced-off half-acre lot complete with biting red ants, large gecko lizards often found in the house, and pigs running through the yard. The weather was hot. My mother was occupied with volunteer activities and taking care of my two younger siblings; my older brother was off at boarding school. I was largely free to roam the town. "Just be back before dark," my mom would instruct. Trust and faith seemed to be part of both my parents' natures. A bicycle allowed me to get around the town at will to explore. My father spent most of the week ministering to soldiers in far-off posts and would return on weekends to execute his church duties, visit people in the hospital, and hold services on the base.

I met Hien at the Vietnamese school run by French missionaries that we attended every morning. We became friends while playing marbles. He was a great long-range shooter, and I was good close-up, so when we played team marbles on the playground, we were tough to beat. We won a lot of trading cards—the marble game betting currency of the schoolchildren. After Vietnamese school, I rode my bike across town to do Calvert tutoring lessons in order to keep up with American schools back home. One day while en route, I saw Hien going into a building with his great-grandmother. She was clearly ill, being carried in by her family. Curious, I rode my bike around the back and climbed up a short stone wall to see what was inside. It was a Vietnamese hospital, staffed with traditional practitioners and lots of sick patients, many of them lying outside in the yard.

This traditional Vietnamese hospital was fascinating. It was not at all like the American military hospital a few miles away, with its clean sheets, IVs, and electronic monitors. In the American hospital, nurses and doctors in white uniforms attended to patients, clergy visited on Saturdays, and a few volunteers—like my mother—would open mail and give back massages. Otherwise, the patients were left alone. In the Vietnamese hospital, however, most patients were cared for by their families. Families brought food, cleaned them, and administered herbal medicines, applied hot and cold packs, and gave other types of treatments. There were always people around the patients. The traditional doctors used mostly acupuncture and herbs—and cupping and *moxa*, a curious treatment in which an herb was burned while resting on an acupuncture point, and then was knocked off before actually burning the patient. The contrast in resources to the American hospital—but more important, to their approaches—was startling. I spent hours looking over the wall, watching people come and go, wondering what medical conditions they had and what the doctors and families were doing.

One day I saw Hien and his family with his great-grandmother. Like many other patients who were outside because there weren't enough beds inside the Vietnamese hospital, Hien's grandmother was lying on a mat on the hard ground—weak, frail, and near death's door. My friend was dutifully taking care of her, bringing her soup and feeding it to her one spoonful at a time, and cleaning her up when she had accidents. Despite her weakness, she would lift her head periodically and smile, and they would converse in Vietnamese. The doctors would come out, put needles in different parts of her body, do curious twisting motions with her legs and arms, and occasionally place a poultice of herbal concoctions on her abdomen or forehead. The family was constantly there, with Hien's mother coming for long periods to take care of her. Hien's great-grandmother seemed quite happy and comfortable. One day I rode my bike down and climbed up to look over the wall, and they were gone. I learned later that she had died peacefully, her family around her.

Hien and I joined a Boy Scouts troop, and that's how we ended up together on that backpacking trip when he sprained his ankle. Again, it looked pretty bad to me, very swollen and with blood under the skin just below the leg bone. He couldn't walk on it, and I figured we would have to carry him out the next day. I had brought along a small first aid kit I'd gotten from the American hospital; the treatments for a sprained ankle consisted of tape, Ace bandages, and some aspirin. But that evening, Hien's father pulled out a powder of green herbs and mixed it with water into a paste. He applied the paste to Hien's ankle and put two acupuncture needles in his leg above the sprain. He removed the needles after one hour and left the poultice on overnight. The next day, Hien's ankle was almost normal again, and we resumed the hike. He seemed to have no pain.

How had this happened? At age nine, I had not yet thought of becoming a doctor, but I wondered how these two different approaches to healing—the low-tech acupuncture/herbal/family care approach from traditional Vietnamese practices on the one hand, and the high-tech surgery/drugs/professionals approach of the Americans—could both work. I had seen American medicine work, but now I had seen a completely different system bring comfort to a terminally ill great-grandmother as she died, and also rapidly resolve an ankle sprain without aspirin, ice, or an Ace bandage. How could healing be happening with two such completely different approaches? Later in life, I had pretty much forgotten Hien and his great-grandmother. During medical school, I was taught that those acupuncture needles and herbs were ineffective and unscientific. Modern approaches were considered better—more effective, safer, and faster. I learned to rely on "gold standard" science, especially evidence from randomized, double-blind, placebo-controlled trials. I threw myself fully into modern medicine and science, determined to use the most rigorous evidence to separate what worked from what didn't.

Then Norma came along.

NORMA

"You are such a sweet boy," Norma would say at the start of every visit. "You are the best doctor ever." I blushed. She knew how to handle me. Norma was seventy-nine, with multiple chronic health problems. She loved having a family doctor—a "one-stop shop," she said—to know her and take care of most of her ills. The one problem that affected her most was her osteoarthritis, the joint disease that now impacts one in every five American adults and more than half of those her age. She didn't complain about the pain. What bothered her most was her decreasing ability to volunteer at the hospital. This was one of the greatest sources of joy and meaning in her life. I would see her frequently in the hospital halls, pushing around the free-book cart for patients and guests. She got to know the regular visitors who were the most chronically ill and brought them specific books she thought they would like. The arthritis mostly affected her hands and knees, which made it difficult to handle the books and hand them out.

Norma came to see me often and loved to have me "practice" on her, but all I had to offer her were painkillers and recommendations for heat and stretching. Those didn't help much, and her disease progressed. Her volunteer visits declined and she became sad. Then I read about something that might help—niacinamide, a form of vitamin B_3. I had found an old book about it in my medical school's discard pile. It was written by a doctor named William Kaufman and published in 1949. Dr. Kaufman had given niacinamide in high doses to thousands of patients with arthritis over long periods of time. What was unusual for a doctor in private practice was that he had carefully measured and documented the pain, strength, and range of motion in every patient who took it. He reported that the patients' pain diminished and their strength, range of motion, and moods improved considerably and steadily when taking niacinamide. It seemed perfect for Norma. The one problem was that niacinamide had never been tested scientifically—in a randomized, double-blind, placebo-controlled trial. It did not have the kind of evidence I needed to prescribe or recommend it. So I decided to do such a study myself with Norma and arthritis patients like her.

When I opened enrollment for the study, Norma joined immediately and was an enthusiastic participant. She did all the baseline measurements and agreed to be randomly assigned to get either niacinamide or an identical-looking placebo pill. Neither she nor I would know which one she was getting until after the study was completed. She started her treatment, which involved taking two pills, three times a day. Within a week and then continuing for the three months of the study, she and her arthritis got steadily better in all ways. She began telling everyone that they should sign up for the study; she became my best unofficial recruiter. Soon she stopped using her cane, resumed her daily volunteer book rounds at the hospital, and reported better mood and sleep. Others observed that her normally stiff muscles moved more easily. Her daughter came in at one visit to personally thank me for helping her mother. Norma was smiling more, she said. She was happy. And I was happy. I had found a cure for arthritis! I would be famous! Or so I thought.

When the study was over, I broke the blinding code to find out what she was taking—niacinamide or the placebo pill. Norma had been taking the placebo pill. I was stunned! I thought something was wrong with the label made by the pharmacologist. I checked and double-checked the shipping labels, randomization codes, and the pharmacist's process for dispensing the pills. Nothing was wrong. Norma had gotten remarkably better, perhaps 80% overall, as she took a completely inert pill.

Niacinamide did work—a little. When we statistically analyzed the differences in response between those on the niacinamide and those on the placebo, the niacinamide did work better than the placebo, but by only a small amount. On average, those on the vitamin improved by 29%, compared to a 10% worsening in those on the placebo. While this was statistically significant in favor of the vitamin, the overall difference was small—and the placebo had fewer side effects. High-dose niacinamide can cause liver problems in some people. I was disappointed. I had not found a cure for arthritis after all. But I continued to wonder why Norma had gotten so much better. Something had triggered her healing. Was she just an unusual patient—an aberration? Did I just pick the wrong patients to include in the study? Did I do the study wrong? Pick the wrong treatment?

It was not an aberration. When examined through rigorous science, using randomization, double-blinding, and placebo controls with adequate numbers of patients, most treatments for the most common chronic conditions either do not work or work only 20% to 30% of the time. Most of the drugs prescribed for pain, mental health, ulcers, hypertension, diabetes, Parkinson's disease, and many other conditions show little benefit, with improvement in a minority of those studied. Even surgery, the king of modern medicine, works very little for chronic diseases (especially pain) when studied in a rigorous manner. For example, in a pooled analysis of over eighteen thousand patients, drawn from studies where half the patients got sham (fake) acupuncture (needles are put in the wrong points or not inserted into the skin at all) and the other half got real acupuncture, the groups getting the fake acupuncture had a healing rate of over 80% of that experienced by the those getting real acupuncture. While this rate of improvement from a fake treatment may seem stunning to many readers, it is actually a rather routine finding and also occurs with modern, scientifically developed treatments. For example, studies in which sham (fake) surgery (an imitation of surgery without the actual tissue manipulation) is "performed" on half of a patient test group with chronic pain, it produces 87% as much improvement as seen in those who receive the real surgery. In some studies, the fake surgery worked better than the real surgery and produced fewer side effects. In fact, this type of improvement with fake treatments is found in many areas of modern medicine. The majority of improvement for many treatments occurs with the fake or placebo treatment, whether the placebo is mimicking a drug, herb, needle, or knife. Can treatments still heal even when science has proven them wrong? Impossible, I thought. It took another patient to teach me that this was not impossible at all.

SERGEANT MARTIN

Sergeant Martin crawled from the tangled web of steel that had been his truck, bleeding from every orifice. Although dazed, he got to his buddy, who was lying unconscious and exposed in the middle of the road, and pulled him to safety. Sergeant Martin had suffered an insidious and incapacitating brain injury. Unfortunately, he is one of many: nearly three hundred thousand American service members are living with traumatic brain injury (TBI) suffered while fighting in Afghanistan or Iraq. Rather than penetrate the brain like a bullet, an improvised explosive device (IED) usually produces a close-range shock wave that impacts the brain as a whole. Damage and bleeding in the brain is often global, with small areas of injury spread throughout. Often the extent of the injury is not fully evident for months and gets worse until it stabilizes. The victim is left with multiple functional problems, from memory loss to language problems, mood swings, sleep disturbances, and chronic pain, especially headaches.

Sergeant Martin had all these problems. He would duck at the sound of a door slamming. He avoided social gatherings, worried that something bad might happen. He had almost daily headaches and was constantly on painkillers. He would wake at night in a panic, sure that someone was breaking into the "green zone." He was emotionally labile—sometimes acting like a loving kid, other times screaming at his wife to lock the doors. One morning his wife found a loaded handgun under his pillow. She told him to get rid of it. He said he needed it to sleep at night. They argued. Finally, he agreed to make sure it was not loaded. She threw the ammunition away but worried how this might end. He told her and everybody else that he was not suicidal. He said he had seen what happened to people who said they were; they were locked up in a mental ward.

There is no cure for this type of brain injury. I juggled drugs for Sergeant Martin's headaches, anxiety, sleep disturbances, and other symptoms. I sent him to physical therapy, group therapy, individual psychological counseling, and music therapy. Of those, the only one he really liked was music therapy. He especially loved to listen to Beethoven's Ninth Symphony.

I asked him to rest and work with several specialists in brain injury and PTSD. Over time he improved—but only incrementally and marginally. Soon he settled into chronic dysfunction and left the service with a permanent disability. From then on, all I could do for him was palliation, tweaking his medicines to minimize the side effects and providing him with slightly more relief. It was a discouraging practice. When I told him I had nothing new left to offer him, he dismissed me as his doctor. "I won't accept that," he said on his last visit with me. "You are keeping me stuck in Beethoven's first movement. I know there is more." He paused. "Friend," he said (he had never called me that before), "when I was in Iraq and we hit that roadside bomb, I don't recall pulling my buddy to safety from the road. Others told me I did that. The only thing I remember after the bomb is waking up in the hospital in a daze. I am still in that daze; and I need to wake up again." He made no more appointments. Just like on the battlefield, Sergeant Martin was not going to give up. He was determined to win this battle, too. I only hoped he would eventually win the war going on inside himself.

Doctors don't like to give patients what they call "false hope." The idea is that, when there are no effective treatments for a condition, it is better for patients to learn to cope with reality than seek ineffective and possibly harmful treatments that are unlikely to work. Science helps us determine what works and what does not—and so, we believe, distinguishes true hope from false hope. Sometimes patients interpret this to mean *no* hope and either fall into despair or, like Sergeant Martin, reject the suggestion that they must live with their condition.

Before Sergeant Martin, I thought I knew how to determine true from false hope for my patients using science. Sergeant Martin, however, taught me that it was more complicated than I thought. Distinguishing true from false hope was not just a matter of science—it had to be done jointly by physician and patient together. Neither one alone had a lock on how to handle hope.

Here is what happened: Several months later, I saw Sergeant Martin in the hallway of the hospital, and I hardly recognized him. He had improved remarkably. He said he had fewer headaches, better sleep, and less pain. He spoke more clearly. He was off most of the drugs I had prescribed. He was going back to school, had a part-time job, and was getting along with his family. What had he done, I asked?

"Hyperbaric oxygen," he answered.

"Really?" I asked in disbelief.

"Yep," he continued. "Got forty treatments, and it cured me." He was not cured, but he was clearly much better than I had ever seen him. *It couldn't be from that treatment*, I thought to myself. I had studied hyperbaric oxygen (HBO) therapy and rejected it, as had most scientists, because the research evidence showed that it did not work.

But Sergeant Martin did not care what I said about the science. He had done the impossible when he rescued his buddy after the bomb went off. He would face the impossible now and try to rescue himself. My opinion did not stop him. He had heard from his buddies that HBO might help brain injury, so he had done forty HBO treatments.

I asked him to come in and tell me more about what he had done. He explained that it was his father who found the HBO center and agreed to pay for the treatment sessions, which were not covered by insurance. These sessions involved going into a special HBO center and entering a large chamber where ten patients were treated at once. At the HBO center, Sergeant Martin met a physician, an HBO specialist, who described the treatment and the expected effects and evaluated patients for their baseline symptoms and function. Sergeant Martin went every day (except weekends) and would sit in the chamber with a group of other patients for an hour while breathing 100% oxygen through a mask. He often saw the same patients there each day, several of whom also had a brain injury. The air pressure in the chamber was turned up, which he could feel in his ears, sort of like when you dive down below the surface in a swimming pool.

The technicians explained to him what HBO would do. The theory was that pressurized oxygen diffused into the brain and stimulated healing in damaged areas that had only been "stunned" by the bomb blast and were dormant. The extra oxygen was said to "wake up" the stunned brain and speed it on the road to healing. I didn't buy that explanation, but Sergeant Martin did. And there he stood before me—largely healed. He had reached the final movement of his symphony. He had sung his "Ode to Joy."

He was not the only one. The advocates of HBO presented case after case of apparently miraculous healing. They convinced the United States Congress to authorize federal funding and test whether it truly worked, using rigorous scientific methods. The study conducted by the U.S. military cost more than $30 million. It compared three groups: real HBO; "fake" HBO subjects, who were told they got high oxygen but really got room air; and the usual treatment without either real or fake HBO. The study found that HBO did not work any better than a fake version of the treatment using room air instead of 100% oxygen. That didn't satisfy the advocates of HBO, who said they knew it worked. They claimed they saw improvements in patients with brain injury every day. They also alleged that the study had been done poorly by skeptics who biased the results. At that point, the military asked an independent organization—Samueli Institute, which I directed at the time—to analyze all the studies on HBO (within and outside the military) and, with the help of a panel of experts, including both advocates and skeptics of HBO, to make a final determination on its effectiveness.

The data was clear. The review confirmed that HBO did not work any better than a fake version, which involved sitting in a slightly pressurized chamber breathing room air for forty sessions. But the study revealed something few others had noticed: patients with brain injuries who received either real HBO or the fake HBO treatment did much better than those who got standard treatment alone—the kind of treatment I had provided Sergeant Martin. And the benefit was not small. Those who sat in the chamber for the full forty sessions had more than twice the improvement of those who received only drugs and other therapies. Adding oxygen did not increase that improvement, but going through the treatment helped. There was something about the ritual and delivery of the treatment that produced a dramatic healing effect. Perhaps it was the patients' and physicians' beliefs, perhaps it was the social engagement during the treatment, or perhaps it was some other factor. But it was not the oxygen. The military rejected the treatment after the HBO theory was disproved. But Sergeant Martin was right—he had hope, and he was better. I was happy for him, but confused. Was this another glimpse of a sleeping giant in modern medical research—the placebo effect—that I was to come to know well later in my career? What was I supposed to recommend to the next patient with a brain injury who came into my office? How could I trust my own judgment in medical practice to use the best treatment? And not to give false hope?

CHARLEY

As it turns out, many other physicians were also beginning to doubt their own experience—and with good reason. From the 1960s to the 1990s, a series of scholars using rigorous scientific methods showed repeatedly that many widely used treatments—even those considered "standard of care"—were not only ineffective but actually harmful. Medical opinion should be distrusted, they said, and in its place, a careful and structured process for summarizing clinical research, called "systematic reviews," should be used. This was the approach Samueli Institute used to examine the effect of HBO on brain injury. While I believed in good evidence, the importance of this did not hit me until I inadvertently contributed to the death of a patient by using the standard of care. It still feels like a punch in the gut—and it's no consolation knowing that medical errors are the third leading cause of death in the United States.

Charley was a sixty-six-year-old former Marine whom I hospitalized with a suspected heart attack in 1985. It was a routine admission and management. He had chest pain and nausea that sounded like a possible heart attack; his EKG showed signs of possible heart ischemia (low oxygen) and irregular heartbeats. In 1985, it was routine to hospitalize someone with these symptoms and treat them with bed rest, morphine to ease the pain, nitrates to expand their coronary vessels, beta blockers to slow their heart rate and lower their blood pressure, and antiarrhythmic drugs to prevent the heartbeat from becoming irregular. Most patients improved and were discharged a few days later. Some went on to have further complications.

Charley looked stable when I checked up on him before I went home that evening; he seemed perfectly comfortable. Blood tests indicated he had had a mild heart attack and would likely recover quickly. "See you in the morning," I said.

But that night, I was catching up on my medical journal reading and came across a study that showed I might be harming Charley with the antiarrhythmic drugs. The study randomized patients like Charley to receive either antiarrhythmic drugs or a placebo. Those who received this routine care and got the drugs actually died at a higher rate than those who did not. I put the article aside and decided I would bring it up in morning report. Had anyone else seen this article, I wondered? Should we stop giving these drugs?

I didn't get the chance to discuss it with my colleagues. At about 4 A.M. I got an urgent call from the hospital, telling me that Charley had died. His heart had gone into a fatal rhythm that could not be reversed. I rushed to the hospital to find his wife in his room weeping. What had happened? she asked. I didn't know what to say. Did his heart attack spread and cause the fatal arrhythmia? An autopsy later showed no evidence of that. Had I killed him by giving him the antiarrhythmic drug, as the new study implied? That was the most likely explanation.

The routine use of antiarrhythmics was stopped after the study I had read was confirmed. All in all, it was estimated that at the peak of antiarrhythmic drug use for suspected heart attacks, the medical profession was killing up to fifty thousand people a year. Expert clinical experience was harming patients. Only a placebo-controlled study revealed that.

For thousands of years, medical treatments have been selected and passed down using clinical experience as the best approach to truth. But could accumulated medical wisdom, both from ancient practices like acupuncture and modern drugs like the one given to Charley, be wrong? If so, how could we explain healing?

PARADOX

Since 1991, I have had the good fortune to have jobs that allow me to explore these questions. First, as the director of the Medical Research Fellowship at Walter Reed Army Institute of Research, it was my job to teach the research fellows how to think critically about medical science and apply rigorous methods in their research. Each year we had five or six fellows who were taught in-depth research methods and learned critical evaluation skills. Each fellow did research on a cutting-edge medical topic and carried the study through from start to finish. I adopted evidence-based teaching methods that emerged from Oxford and McMaster universities to teach physicians how to counter the errors of clinical experience. The NIH later adopted some of those teaching methods in their courses on clinical research. Did these same principles apply to ancient healing methods and alternative healing approaches used by most people in the world? I had the opportunity to examine that when I took over as the director of the Office of Alternative Medicine at the NIH and a WHO Traditional Medicine Center of Excellence in 1996 and 1998, respectively. Later, when I was CEO of Samueli Institute, a nonprofit organization dedicated to exploring the science of healing, my team had the chance to do scientific deep dives into ancient and modern healing practices.

This series of jobs allowed me to work with physicians, healers, patients, and researchers around the world to examine three main questions: First, to what extent do the health care practices from diverse traditions actually work when rigorously studied using gold-standard science? Second, what degree of improvement is found from these health care practices when used in regular clinical practice? And, third, are there any common characteristics that cut across all these traditions, ancient or modern, that can explain how their healing happens?

I call what has emerged from this exploration the "paradox of healing." When rigorously studied, ancient traditional practices such as acupuncture and herbal remedies, as well as more recent complementary and alternative treatments such as homeopathy, dietary supplements, and manual therapies, show disappointing results and only small effects. Likewise, data on most of our modern conventional treatments show the same thing. Most drugs for pain, mental health, ulcers, hypertension, and diabetes, for example, show little benefit—often only 20% to 30%. Furthermore, the more carefully the studies are done, the smaller the effects. Even more startling, only about one-third of well-done studies—executed in the laboratory or in the clinic—can be independently replicated. Thus our confidence that even a 20% improvement can be repeatedly obtained is low. Even surgery (when not simply changing anatomy, like fixing a leg or removing a tumor) works minimally. And when these treatments do work, it is often not for the reasons scientists think they do.

Yet the paradox is that all these approaches can work, if applied properly. When we looked at the rate of improvement in patients who received very different types of treatments from around the world, we found that 70% to 80% of people will get better. Later in this book, I will describe Parkinson's patients who get better with treatments as different as ancient Ayurvedic medicine and electrical stimulation of the brain, soldiers with PTSD who get better with yoga or psychotherapy, patients with pain who get better with acupuncture or opioids, and patients whose health improves when under the care of a homeopath or surgeon, even when rigorous studies show little if any effect from these treatments. We need to understand *why* they get better.

CHAPTER 2

How We Heal

Placebo research reveals what most medical science conceals.

There is a sleeping giant in modern medical research that has yet to awaken and reveal itself fully. When it does, it will lay waste to what we think we know about healing. It plays no favorites and so is equally devastating to ancient healing claims, complementary medicine, and mainstream health care. It is called the "placebo response." Failure to understand the importance of the placebo response led me (and all of biomedicine) down the path that contributed to the deaths of patients like Charley. Likewise, failure to use the placebo response causes us to throw out powerful treatments like the ritual used by Sergeant Martin, which could markedly help other soldiers with brain injury. This giant can subvert the good intentions behind how we deliver healing with patients every day. By failing to acknowledge the negative aspects of placebo—called the "*nocebo* response"—we often inadvertently harm with our treatments. Knowing how the placebo response works opens a door to healing that few in medicine enter. But you don't have to wait. In this chapter, I will summarize what we know about the placebo response (and its underlying causes) and how you and your doctor can use it for healing. You will get an inside view of what is coming before our understanding of placebo in medicine has fully awakened.

NORMA

How was I going to tell Norma, my patient with debilitating arthritis, that she had been taking the placebo? She had gotten remarkably better in almost all ways. She remarked to me many times during the study on how well the vitamin was working. She had less pain, was more active, and had returned to her volunteer job at the hospital. She was happier. Others noticed and commented on her improved mood and ability to move. Now I had to tell her. I worried about what would happen when I did. Would she be devastated? Embarrassed? Angry? I worried she would regress to her former state of pain and limited mobility. But I was required both ethically and legally to inform her about what she had been taking.

Norma was a tall, thin woman with long gray hair who still had the sparkle of a young woman in her eye. She reminded me of a reed, easily blown about by the wind. Her psychological nature fit her physical stature to a T. She was gentle and empathetic. She was always willing to follow my suggestions. She was one of my most compliant patients. My fear that she would regress in her healing was based on two longheld assumptions in medicine: first, that her improvement had all been based on her own "belief" that she was getting active treatment; second, that she was a good "placebo responder," usually thought of as someone who is "suggestible" and easily influenced by the opinions of others—especially authorities, like me, her doctor. The premise that some people are suggestible in this way has a long history in medical science. After Anton Mesmer, a German physician in the seventeenth century, claimed he could heal using "animal magnetism," in 1797, his claim was tested by a team that included Benjamin Franklin. They used one of the first double-blind testing methods, in which patients did not know if they were getting the real treatment or a fake version and physicians did not know which patients received the real treatment. One method was placing a blanket or curtain between the therapist and the patient. Patients were told that they were being treated at times when they were not. Other patients were blindfolded so they could not see the therapist or what he was doing. Franklin reported that patients would respond to the suggestion of treatment and this response occurred even when no treatment was given.

This idea that belief and suggestibility were key factors in many patients' healing eventually led to the use of blinded tests of other therapies to see if their efficacy was real. Double-blind methods were first applied to "alternative" treatments like homeopathy by a skeptical medical profession. Eventually these blinding approaches were used for conventional treatments, too, especially new drugs. Soon the double-blind method became accepted as the gold standard for determining whether a treatment worked. All treatment effects had to be separated from the effects of belief to be considered effective.

Both Norma and I had believed she was on the real treatment. Would I harm her if I undermined that belief by telling her she was on the placebo? I thought I would, which would violate my oath to "do no harm," as a physician. But I had to tell the truth.

I waited several weeks to inform her, hoping she would enjoy her good results for a little longer. Fortunately, during that time a way out of this dilemma emerged. The statistician who analyzed the study came back with the overall results. The vitamin had proved to be effective. When comparing the overall improvement in the group taking the niacinamide compared with those taking the placebo pill, the niacinamide group improved about 8% more than the placebo group. This was considered a significant effect; that is, it had a p-value of less than 0.05 in the statistical tests. A p-value of less than 0.05 means that if we did one hundred more studies like the one Norma was in, there would be a 95% chance we would still get at least an 8% or more improvement in the niacinamide group compared with the placebo group. It does not mean the effect of the vitamin was large (it wasn't), only that the small effect we saw was probably real. Probably, but not for certain. To know for sure, most scientists would suggest that the study be repeated a few more times to see if the effect persists. But, at least for this study, the probability was considered high enough by scientific convention for me to tell Norma I had found a viable treatment for her. So several weeks later, when I sat down with Norma to let her know that she was taking the placebo, I could immediately tell her that the study had found the vitamin to be effective and that, if she wanted, we could switch her to the real treatment. In other words, I tried to gloss over the fact that she had gotten better because of her belief, focusing on the prospect of even greater improvement. Fortunately, she was happy with that and continued to do well on the niacinamide. I was off the hook. I chalked up the experience to Norma's suggestibility and assumed that she was an exception rather than the rule. That is, until I met Bill.

BILL

Bill arrived in my office to seek help for his chronic back pain. He came in only at the urging of his wife, as he was skeptical that any doctor could fix him. He had been to many doctors. Finally, he agreed to come in after the pain was so bad that he had to cancel a car trip to see his grandchildren. He told me that his Korean-born wife urged him to see an acupuncturist because acupuncture is used to treat back pain in Korea. So, reluctantly, he came to see me, not because I was an acupuncturist but because he wanted to know if acupuncture could help him or if, as he said, it is "all just placebo."

Bill is the opposite of suggestible. In fact, he doesn't believe that any doctors or treatment can help at all. I could tell by his opinions, his body, and his body language that it is hard to influence him. He has husky round shoulders and a thick belly. He lumbers more than walks into the room and has a limp favoring his right side, which is where he feels most of his back pain.

He sat down slowly in a chair facing me and crossed his arms in front of him. He had that kind of look that says, *Go ahead and try to help—I have already been through it all.*

Nevertheless, he'd come in to see me. He said he did so mainly to "get his wife off of his back" and because I am a physician who practices in the military. He had been in the military and figured I won't make money off any treatment I recommend, so I'm less likely to push something on him. I had about twenty minutes to answer his questions and see if I could help him.

I started by saying there is no easy answer, which he already knew. But then it hit me that I was saying that because he was completely different from Norma, and I, too, didn't actually expect him to get better. I looked over the list of treatments he had tried. These included analgesics; nonsteroidal anti-inflammatory drugs (NSAIDS), such as aspirin or ibuprofen; muscle relaxants; antidepressants; chiropractic manipulation; and injections. At one point he was told to go to bed and rest. Later, he was told to get up and be more active. He was given exercises and physical therapy. He went to a chiropractor. Fortunately, he had not been given traction (which *is* harmful for patients with back pain), but a couple of decades earlier he would have been given that as well. What really put him off about doctors was that he had been told to see a psychiatrist because it was "all in his head." The psychiatrist treated him for depression (which he was sure he did not have) and then finally told Bill not to come back until he really wanted to get well. "The gall of that guy," he told me. "Like I *want* to have this!"

Patients with chronic musculoskeletal pain like Bill are very common; in fact, musculoskeletal conditions are the number-one cause of suffering and the number-one chronic condition that spurs people to visit a doctor, making up over 8% of all visits per year. Back pain is the most common of those musculoskeletal conditions, affecting over 70% of all adults sometime during their life, and is the leading cause of limited activity in the world. It costs the United States over $100 billion per year. There is no measure of how much meaningful life is lost, typified by Bill's inability to see his grandchildren. It is common for patients like Bill with chronic back pain to have undergone multiple treatments. It is common for physicians to prescribe a variety of treatments. Bill came to me because his wife made him ask me about acupuncture, but he didn't believe in it.

"Doc," he asked, "should I try acupuncture? Is it effective or a waste of time? I have to pay for it, because this is not going to be reimbursed by my insurance; should I spend the time, the effort, and the expense? Do I have to believe in it?"

It was a reasonable question, for which I owed him a reasonable answer. I was not sure I had one.

Acupuncture can stimulate natural painkillers in the brain, called endogenous opioids—even in animals. This makes us think the effects are real and not due to the placebo effect. Comparisons of acupuncture treatment for back pain with other treatments, such as drugs, physical therapy, and education, show that it works well. But so does sham acupuncture. This makes the effects seem largely due to the placebo effect. So even though the treatment seemed to be mostly placebo, similar to the vitamin I had tested on Norma, the downside—other than the cost and time spent on treatment—was small. So I suggested to Bill that he try it, but with a limited number of treatments, and then determine if it was working for him. I tried to keep a neutral and objective tone, trying not imply that there was not much hope for it to work. More like a personal experiment. Bill seemed to like that tone and was glad I was not an advocate for the treatment, like his wife, and that I could be objective.

I sent him to an acupuncturist I knew and trusted. After eight sessions, his pain was not much better, and he and I decided it was not worth continuing. While we gave up on the acupuncture, I didn't want to give up on Bill. I asked him if he would like to explore other treatments, and he said he would, but there were not many he hadn't already tried.

His X-rays showed a narrowing of the disk space in his lower spine from arthritis, so I suggested he see a surgeon. Bill was his usual skeptical self. He didn't want to be cut on, and he had friends who had undergone surgery with little benefit. Some were even worse. But Bill had already done almost every treatment available, including intensive physical therapy. So, reluctantly, and with little belief that it would help, he had the surgical procedure. The procedure involved injection of a cementlike substance into his collapsing disk. He thought this seemed less invasive than opening his back up and fusing the disk with rods. The effects were dramatically positive. Three weeks after the procedure, his pain was the lowest it had been in years. He and his wife promptly got in the car and drove ten hours to see their grandchildren. They were very happy. Because Bill was not a suggestible person and did not believe in this treatment, I decided that this confirmed my opinion that "real" treatments were those that worked in those who did not believe. For the suggestible, placebo treatments might be more appropriate.

THE PLACEBO EFFECT

I was wrong. In 1995, I brought together a small group of investigators at the NIH who were studying why placebo seemed to work in some people and not in others. We were interested in understanding why an inert or inactive substance, such as a sugar or salt solution or distilled water with no known pharmacological value, could be effective and how often this happened. This question was popularized in a 1955 article on placebo by Henry Beecher, MD, in the *Journal of the American Medical Association*. Beecher reported that about one-third of all effects seen in medicine were due to the placebo response. This became medical gospel for decades, even though several studies after that reported an approximate 70% response rate to treatments that were later shown to be inert. At the meeting in 1995, Professor Dan Moerman, an anthropologist from the University of Michigan, showed findings that floored the audience. He had collected data from around the world that completely undermined the placebo gospel of Henry Beecher, the belief of most of the medical profession, and my belief that Norma and Bill had each improved for different reasons—one because of suggestibility and belief and the other because of the treatment.

Professor Moerman revealed that the healing effect from fake treatments could vary from 0% to 100%—*even for the same disease and same treatment—depending on the context and cultural meaning* in which they were delivered. One review, for example, studied 117 placebo-controlled trials of a drug treatment for stomach ulcers done across multiple countries. These studies showed objectively that the same inert treatment (a sugar pill) had a wide range of effects from country to country. The healing rate in Germany, for example, was very high, but in the Netherlands and Denmark it was low. In Brazil, hardly any patients with ulcers healed when given placebo. The dramatically varying results were influenced by country, context, delivery, and the patient's interpretation of that delivery. In other words, the cultural context influenced the meaning, which in turn influenced the biology, the pathology, and the outcome. The effects were very specific. For example, in Germany, the placebo healing rates of patients with high blood pressure were low, not high as for ulcers. In fact, the meaning and context surrounding how a treatment was delivered had a much greater impact on healing than the treatment modalities themselves. Inert treatments for pain like Bill's, for example, worked better if you gave them by needle rather than pill; gave them in the hospital rather than at home, applied them more often rather than less frequently, charged more for them rather than less, and delivered them with a positive and confident message rather than a neutral or skeptical message. Acupuncture was found to be more effective the closer the study was conducted to China, where acupuncture was developed and is widespread. I suspect surgery works better in the West, though no one has studied that. It seemed that the magnitude of a person's healing depended less on the suggestibility and belief of the individual patient than on the collective belief of the culture and the ritual created to deliver that belief.

Professor Ted J. Kaptchuk, director of the Center for Placebo Studies at Harvard Medical School, is one of the world's most respected researchers on the placebo response. In a recent analysis, he sheds light on the variability of these effects by comparing three types of healing encounters: Navajo ceremonial chants, acupuncture treatment in the Western world, and the biomedical provision of health care. He describes each encounter as being surrounded by beliefs, narratives, "multi-sensory dramas," and culturally defined influences, all of which can be described as rituals in the treatment of illness. Depending on the setting and the practitioner, such rituals may take the form of communal chanting and practices led by a medicine man; the insertion of needles that takes place in an office redolent with representations of Asian culture; or authoritative white-coated clinicians presiding over complex biomedical testing and treatment technology. Looking at this research, I began to wonder: did my patient Bill get better from surgery not because it was "real," but because surgery was more culturally meaningful to him than the other treatments he had undergone? I was skeptical of this explanation. Bill had been through many treatments and should have benefited even if they were from placebo effects. But two studies conducted after I had seen Bill seemed to contradict this assumption. In those studies, patients were randomly assigned to get either the cement or balloon injections into collapsing disks (like Bill had received) or a fake procedure that mimicked the real injections but did not manipulate the spinal disk in any way. In both studies, patients who underwent the fake procedure did just as well as those who got the real procedure.

I still found this hard to believe. Bill was resistant to treatments and was not in any way suggestible. Could it be that, at least for pain, the meaning and context of a treatment produced much of the healing, even in patients who were not suggestible? Even when "hard" procedures were used, such as surgery, that manipulated tissues and corrected anatomy? To test this assumption, my team and I did a meta-analysis of all surgery studies of chronic pain, whether in the back, knees, abdomen, or heart. We selected studies that compared real surgery to sham surgery, in which patients and doctors went through the ritual of surgery but no real correction of anatomy was done. We were able to determine the quality of the studies and then combine results into a single estimate of the contribution to healing pain from "true" surgery. The final analysis showed equally good improvement of any pain condition when the ritual of surgery was applied to the patient but no actual surgery was done. These sham surgery studies showed that, at least for pain treatments, healing occurs from something else. Could it be that the millions of surgeries done every year to treat pain produce healing because they are powerful types of ritual placebos? Could it be that the healing that occurred in Norma and Bill were not so different after all? As different as they were, could it be that they both had tapped into their own inherent healing capacity in different ways, and that healing was connected to their beliefs and behavior and to those around them more than the specific treatment they received?

Professor Kaptchuk has done two studies exploring to what extent the effect of treatment depends on collective belief verses individual belief. In one study, all patients with a painful abdominal condition (irritable bowel syndrome, or IBS) were given a fake treatment—sham acupuncture. However, the social ritual was varied between groups to enhance the dose of collective belief. In one group, the practitioner came in and said very little and delivered the treatment. In a second group, the practitioner explained how the treatment works and set the expectation that the treatment will work. In the third group, a prominent physician from a prominent medical school delivered the treatment with a full explanation and a story about the good results others had obtained with the treatment. All the patients held about the same amount of individual belief in acupuncture at the beginning of the study. But the greater the social meaning produced by the ritual, the better the effect. In the third group, the benefit the patients experience is greater than that achieved by the best drugs approved for treatment of IBS.

In a second study by Kaptchuk, patients were actually told ahead of time that the treatment was fake. One group was given placebo pills with this description: "Placebo pills made of an inert substance, like sugar pills, that have been shown in clinical studies to produce significant improvement in IBS symptoms through mind-body, self-healing processes." This statement created an expectation that even these placebos have an effect. A second group of IBS patients was given no treatment but with the same quality of interaction with providers. The group given the placebo (and who knew it was placebo) had significantly better pain reduction and improved quality of life.

No matter what form the ritual takes, says Kaptchuk, these can have powerful influences on the healing process. "We cannot explain the effects of rituals using placebo treatments simply by belief and expectation," Kaptchuk explains. "While belief may contribute some to the outcome in these studies, the effects produced by healing rituals are much larger than can be explained by what the patient believes about the treatment. The main reasons these effects occur is still a mystery." Research suggests that healing rituals are associated with modulations of symptoms through neurobiological mechanisms, just like we see from drugs. They can not only affect pain, but change the immune system, alter organ function, shift brain processing, and even influence specific cell receptors and genes. One study, done by renowned placebo researcher Professor Fabrizio Benedetti of the University of Turin, Italy, demonstrated that if you link a placebo treatment ritual to a painkiller, you can continue to get pain relief with the placebo after withdrawing the painkiller. And even more remarkably, the placebo will work using the same cellular mechanism of the painkiller to which it was linked. The body not only can learn to heal, it can be taught which specific mechanism in the body to use to produce the effect. Placebo effects, writes Kaptchuk, are often described as "nonspecific." He suggests instead that they should be considered—and further researched—as the "specific" effects of healing rituals.

THE 80% EFFECT

The giant is stirring. Sugar pills and fake needles or sham surgeries do not heal. Healing comes from the meaning and context in which these various treatment agents get deployed. Modern medicine uses placebo in research not to optimize healing but to separate the effects of belief and meaning from those of the drug or technique itself. According to current convention in science, it is the drug or technique that is the "real" effect. Yet by turning the microscope around and looking at what causes healing when no real treatment is used, science has begun to uncover the underlying mechanisms of how we heal that span all modalities—ancient and modern, alternative or mainstream. Since that NIH meeting in 1995, research on the placebo response has exploded and is dissecting the underlying processes and magnitude of our capacity to heal. This research is now being collated and accelerated by the Society for Interdisciplinary Placebo Science (SIPS). Started in 2015, SIPS has become a forum for looking at how healing works by investigating the underlying mechanisms of the placebo response.

And that healing capacity is large, providing close to 80% of the effects we see in medicine. Since the 1950s, when Henry Beecher first put forth his idea that placebo heals, major placebo responses have been reported in over forty conditions with more being added each year. And the magnitude of those effects is often 60%, 70%, and even 80% for many common conditions. These effects can be produced by any agent—including needles, pills, radiation, chants and prayers, touch, surgery, and talk—provided those treatments are delivered in a way

TREATMENT VERSUS MEANING

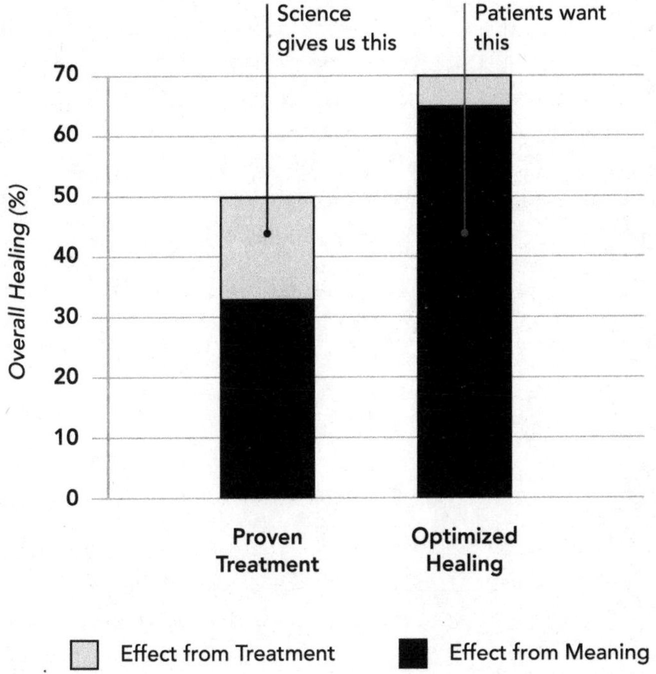

that fits the patient and their expectations and is done using a ritual their culture finds meaningful. For many of these conditions, the effect of the social ritual and the meaning it creates for a patient produces a larger rate of healing than the treatment itself. In many cases, the color of pills, their shape, and the way they are delivered determines their effectiveness as much as—or more than—the medicine they contain. In fact, if you optimized all the factors that produce healing in the "placebo" group of a study, it is possible to push the improvements patients get up to a level that often dwarfs the benefit from the "real" treatment.

From the perspective of science and good evidence, a proven treatment needs to show that it works better than the placebo arms of a study and—preferably—for the reasons the scientists think it works. This is called the "specific effect" and is what good science gives us. From a patient's perspective, however, optimized effects are preferred—whether they are called placebo, "non-specific," or ritual-based. Of course, ideally these treatment rituals are not unsafe, too expensive, or too difficult to do. The effect is like the treatment you see on the right side of the illustration. But when the placebo and ritual effects are enhanced, it becomes very difficult to prove the agent used in these rituals adds much to the effect. So in the context of an optimized treatment, the supposed "real" treatment cannot be proven.

The work of Kaptchuk, Moerman, Benedetti, and others explained why my proven treatments were not working as well as the ones my patients had found. My proven treatments were not optimized or meaningful for them. My evidence-based medicine was coming into conflict with person-centered care.

THE COMMON THREAD

I now began to understand how Norma, Bill, Sergeant Martin, and many other patients I had treated got better, sometimes because of me, often despite me. When Sergeant Martin described the details of his hyperbaric oxygen (HBO) treatment for brain injury, he was describing how, after going against my recommendations, he had entered a ritual that induced underlying mechanisms of healing. How did he do that? First, he expected it to work. It was not just a matter of his own expectation, however; his father, who encouraged and paid for the treatment, was enthusiastic. Second, the nurses, technicians, doctors, and other patients created a milieu that infused that belief with social meaning. The group that underwent treatment each week shared their stories, experiences, and lives, building cultural meaning into the ritual. They became friends and mutual supporters in healing. Finally, the experience of healing—in his case, breathing what he understood to be lifesaving oxygen—was repeated, reinforced, and conditioned in his experience and his physiology. The treatment agent—oxygen—had no therapeutic value in itself for a damaged brain, but it gave him a feeling that something was happening and a sense of well-being, reinforced each week. In the same way pain drugs were "educated" to work in the study by Professor Fabrizio (page 25), Sergeant Martin's brain was taught how to heal each week through social and classical conditioning. Researchers at SIPS have now shown that three main mechanisms—belief and expectation, meaningful social learning, and reinforcement or conditioning—are the underlying mechanisms of the placebo response, and the likely explanation for the majority of human healing in any system or from any treatment.

MAKING MEANING

In an article that Professor Moerman and I wrote several years ago, we suggested that the so-called placebo response can occur and result in healing, whether a proven or unproven substance is used. Every physician and every medical practitioner wants to try to enhance the therapeutic effects of their treatments. I certainly wanted to. I had been sobered by the death of Charley. And I was sobered further when I saw patients get better, often despite my recommendations. However, my greatest worry was whether the approach to science I was using prevented me from optimizing healing. Whether a treatment is labeled as placebo or not is more of an academic and economic question than the primary concern of the clinician and patient. The question for a patient was not whether a treatment was better than placebo, but the likelihood that a patient would get better after the treatment. I realized that in order to maximize the effect of any treatment I offered, I needed to maximize the response from the context and meaning of the treatment for the patient and culture. Research on placebo was making that process visible in a way I had never seen before. Moerman and I suggested that physicians replace the term "placebo effect" with the words "meaning, context, and learning response" or simply the "meaning response." We redefined placebo effect as the physiological, psychological, and clinical effects of meaning when a placebo (or inert treatment) is used. That response is really about healing, and the use of placebos or inert substances in research were of value only to help us understand *how* to heal, not what to heal with. I was beginning to suspect that what health care was mostly about was learning how to heal through meaning. Could it be that many of the thousands of treatments being pushed by practitioners all over the world were just the tools to induce healing by manipulating belief, social meaning, and conditioning through ritual? Was the process of healing being obscured by our constant search for "good evidence" in medicine in which the only "real" treatments are those that can be separated from meaning and context? Was the majority of healing due to the agency of the patient rather that the agent used? The giant was stirring.

BILL FINDS HIS WAY

About eleven months after his surgery, Bill came lumbering back into my office again. He was limping, favoring the right, as before. His wife was not with him this time, but the look of "I have done this before" was. He sat down carefully; I could tell he was in pain. He told me what had happened. After the surgery, he'd felt great. Within three weeks, he had the least amount of pain he'd had in over a decade. So naturally, he became more active, which, he said, "was the whole point." He and his wife drove several times to see the grandchildren. He could play with them, even sitting on the floor for short periods, something he could not do before. About six months after the surgery, he noticed a slight twinge in his back while he was mowing the lawn. At first it seemed minor. Still, he rested for a bit and did some of the physical therapy stretches he knew. Then, at nine months to the day after his surgery, he was reaching over to pick up a toy from the ground and felt a "pop" in the right side of his back. He couldn't stand up straight. The pain was excruciating. He went back to the surgeon. X-rays and CT scans showed "nothing different," and the surgeon did not recommend another surgery. "Give it some time," he was told. But the pain was back, and continued to worsen. Now it was just as bad as before the surgery. He was back on medications and doing physical therapy—and not driving to see the grandchildren anymore. It had been two more months since he felt his back "pop."

"So why have you come back to see me?" I asked. Bill paused and took a deep breath sort of like he was letting go of something he had held on to for a long time. He leaned forward and put his hands on his knees.

"When I was in here last time, asking about acupuncture and asking you did you think it would help my pain, you asked me some questions that I thought were strange. Questions like, did I have any stress and how did I manage it, how did I sleep, and what my diet was like, and did I have any friends. Things like that."

"Yes," I said, "I recall."

Bill took another breath. "Why did you ask those questions? What did that have to do with my pain?"

"Well," I said, "I have learned that a path toward healing often involves things not related to the main conditions people come in to see me for—the pain, for example. I was trying to see how open you were to exploring other aspects of your life that might help you feel well, or if you were just seeking another treatment for your back pain. At the time, it seemed you were just seeking another treatment."

Bill leaned back again but did not cross his arms this time. "I was," he said. "My wife wanted me to try acupuncture, and I came to see if there was any science behind it. You said there was a little bit, so we tried it."

"Yes," I replied. "We tried it, and it didn't work, so we went on to see the surgeon, and it helped." I was not sure where he was going with the discussion, but then he came out with it.

"Dr. Jonas," he said, leaning forward again, "how much science is there to support surgery?"

Now I was a bit worried. Was he angry? Was he looking for ammunition against the surgeon? Or me?

"Well," I said, "about 75% of people get better after surgery and, as it turns out, so do many of those who get fake surgery. So it seems that the ritual of going through surgery has a lot to do with people getting better. They seem to do other things—like being more mentally positive and physically active. That is likely a large part of the healing."

Bill took this in. "Just like acupuncture?" he asked.

I thought for a moment. “Yes,” I said, “just like with acupuncture.”

After Bill’s pain had returned, he had begun to look back at all the treatments he had done, almost a dozen of them. He had noticed that most of them helped for a while but then the pain would return. Some, like surgery, were dramatic but not long lasting; others, like acupuncture were gradual or did not work at all. What Bill wanted to know was if his continued search for “cures” for this pain was the right approach. He had been thinking about the questions I had asked—about stress, sleep, diet, friends, and life balance—and the role it might play in his healing. “The most important thing in life for me is to be available to my kids and grandkids, to be active with them, and to be able to do things with my wife—like traveling once in a while. But I spend so much time dealing with the back pain or going to get treatments for it, I have not been able to do that. When you asked those questions about my life, it started me thinking that I needed to focus more on those rather than all the pain treatments. I want you to help me do that.”

Remarkably, Bill, the “fix me” guy, was starting to realize from his personal experience what I was also coming to from my professional and research experience. That healing and curing, though connected, were not the same. Curing involved what he had been going through—getting a diagnosis and trying out various treatments based on the scientific evidence. That evidence was gathered from research and reviews of research comparing one treatment to another treatment, or to no treatment or to a placebo or sham treatment, to see if it was “real.” These studies examined whether the collective response of a group to a treatment was better than the collective response in another group that was given placebo, no treatment, or another treatment. If the treatment group had acceptable side effects and costs, the treatment was said to have “worked” and was recommended to patients. These studies averaged out the effects in groups. But no individual is average.

Healing, on the other hand, was a more subtle and individual process. It involved finding out what gave a person a sense of well-being. Doing what was most meaningful to them. It involved more than seeking a treatment for a specific symptom or condition; it involved finding and engaging in activities that brought joy and satisfaction. It had more to do with caring for one's deeper self than with getting health care for the body. It involved paying attention to the "meaning and context" of a behavior—the very factors that the research of professors Moerman, Kaptchuk, and Benedetti, and I had found produced the placebo response. It was this meaning and context that my questions to Bill where meant to get at.

"I would be happy to help you do that, Bill," I replied, "if you will help me understand what processes are most helpful for you in getting well. Can we make it a partnership of learning together—finding out how healing happens in your case?"

Bill agreed. So we started to build a healing ritual unique to him.

THE HEALING JOURNEY

Bill became one of the first of many patients to work with me to traverse a healing rather than a cure-focused journey and to learn a process that would help others unlock their inherent healing capacity: the capacity that placebo research indicated contributed up to 80% of the benefit from many treatments and in many conditions. We started by looking at the scientific evidence for the treatments Bill had done over the past fifteen years and for any treatment or self-care method he might be interested in using. We were especially interested in these questions:

- What was the overall improvement from doing the ritual of the treatment, as measured in the placebo group of a study?
- Was the treatment better than no treatment at all?
- Was it better than other treatments for the same condition?
- What were the side effects and harms?
- How complicated was it and what did it cost?

EFFECTIVENESS OF BILL'S LOWER BACK PAIN TREATMENTS

TREATMENT	BETTER THAN PLACEBO?	BETTER THAN NO TREATMENT?	EQUAL OR BETTER THAN A PROVEN TREATMENT?
Acupuncture	No	Possibly	Possibly
* Advice to stay active	Unknown	Unknown	Unknown
* Analgesies	Unknown	Possibly	No
* Antidepressants	Possibly	Unknown	Unknown
* Bed rest	Unknown	No	No
Biofeedback	Possibly	Unknown	Possibly
* Exercises	Unknown	Possibly	Possibly
Injections *(facet joint and trigger point)*	Possibly	Unknown	Unknown
* Manipulation	Possibly	Possibly	Possibly
* Muscle relaxants	Unknown	Unknown	No
* Nonsteroidal anti-inflammatory drugs	Yes	Yes	Yes
* Physical therapies	Unknown	Unknown	Unknown
Traction	No	No	Unknown

KEY

- UNKNOWN
- POSSIBLY
- NO
- YES

** Already used by the patient prior to the first visit*

We placed all this information in a chart. What immediately emerged is that very few treatments—conventional or alternative—had good evidence that they worked in the long run. Most had never been compared to a placebo ritual, and when they had been, almost all of them added only a small amount to the overall outcome—often less than 20%. Some worked slightly better than others, but most treatments had not been compared to each other directly, so it was rare that we could determine whether one treatment was better than another. Almost all of them were better than doing nothing. It appeared that you needed to do *something* to get the most benefit out of the healing ritual, but the specifics of that something was less important than we thought.

While the overall response rate between treatments varied little, the adverse side effects, on the other hand, varied considerably. Major interventions, such as surgery and medication, produced unwanted side effects in more patients than benefited from them. Often 50% to 60% of patients would experience a side effect. Gentler treatments, such as yoga or music, had fewer and less severe side effects—but they were not without problems. Often the research did not even bother to measure side effects, which created a gap in information about them.

When we stepped back and looked at our handiwork, we both immediately saw a pattern emerge. Most treatments did not work better than the ritual and so were not thought to be "real" and were not offered or encouraged by doctors, including me. But looked at another way, almost all the treatment rituals actually helped people get better—often producing improvements in 60%, 70%, or even 80% of patients in the group—just as seen in the placebo literature. Bill commented, "So instead of not having any treatments that work, it looks like I have a wealth of options. I just need to decide which ones I like, can do, and [can] afford." His insight was profound. Bill had gone from a cycle of "Fix me or let me try another treatment I don't like" to a smorgasbord of options. He now had to decide only which ones were the most meaningful to him—that is, the ones he could and wanted to do to achieve his goal of playing with the grandkids. Freed from a mind-set that was looking to the next magic cure for his pain, he could go about building a pathway to well-being based on what was meaningful for him.

To help find and select the most meaningful treatments, Bill started by keeping a journal in which he wrote down observations about what made him feel well and what did not. The "strange" questions I had asked him on his first visit to me became the basis for these observations. They did not have to be linked to his pain. It could be anything he observed that helped him feel better about himself—helped him feel happy and well. After two months of keeping this journal, Bill came back with several insights.

First, his back felt the worst when he did not get enough sleep. He was in a habit of overeating into the evening, usually accompanied by several drinks and reading the stock market on his cell phone before going to bed. He snored a lot and woke up frequently. His doctor had put him on a night breathing treatment called CPAP but he did not like the apparatus. He never took naps. His doctor had also told him he was overweight and needed to lose fifty pounds or he would become diabetic like his father had been. He was already prediabetic. The dietitian he went to gave him a calorie-restricted diet and told him to stop drinking.

Second, he found that he was constantly on the go all day. About what, he wasn't sure, but things just seemed to always be required of him—mostly by his wife, who wanted him to help keep the house repaired and to run errands. While he and his wife had always had a good relationship, after the journaling, he realized that he really didn't talk with her—or anyone else for that matter—about his experiences or worries. For example, when his father had died a few years before, he had done all that was needed for the funeral and burial. His father was an alcoholic, and they had not had been close. He had not engaged much with Bill and his brother, except to yell at them and occasionally hit them. Bill never talked about his relationship with his father with anyone, including his wife, and did not discuss his feelings about his father's death with anyone.

OPENING UP

As we continued to explore questions on healing and Bill continued his journaling, he noted that he did a number of things that made him feel better. A hot shower followed by putting pressure on his back lessened the pain. Stretching had always helped, but he found it difficult to make himself do it because it was painful. Before the pain, he had enjoyed hunting and spending long hours in the woods. Being outdoors in his backyard, watching the birds, now soothed him. In one journal entry Bill wrote the following: "Good night's sleep last night, woke up rested and serene. Katie [his four-year-old grandchild, who was visiting] came in to play; sat for an hour on the floor with a tea set and dolls. No pain. She is such a joy." This triggered a memory for Bill from his childhood. He was about five years old and came running home from school excited about a clay ashtray he had made for this father. His father had come home early with a headache and had been drinking for several hours. On reaching the house, Bill burst into the living room and ran up to his father to show him the ashtray. Startled from his stupor, his father grabbed the ashtray and hurled it across the room, smashing it against the wall. Bill ran to his room and shut the door. He remembers crying for hours. From that day forward, he would tiptoe around his father, uncertain as to how he would react to any situation. He never cried again.

"I don't know why I remembered that episode," Bill said, "There were many others. Maybe being with Katie reminded me of my childhood. I made sure I was not that way with my kids, but I never recall him just sitting on the ground playing tea." He took a deep breath. "I don't know why I told you that story. I have never told anyone that story."

Little did Bill know that opening up to difficult traumas and telling them to someone or writing them down is one of the most effective self-healing behaviors. Extensive research has shown that as little as a single episode of deep self-engagement, usually around a trauma or hurt, can have prolonged healing effects. Research by social psychologist Professor James Pennebaker and others has documented psychological, physiological, and immunological changes from such episodes in well-conducted randomized controlled trials—the gold standard of science. Others have shown that these meaningful engagements can improve pain relief in arthritis, lung function in asthmatics, and immune function in the elderly. They also reduce the need for medical care and lower costs. By giving himself space to observe and map his own healing path, Bill had discovered this for himself.

BILL'S BODY STARTS TO RESPOND

Bill's healing had begun, not from psychotherapy (he would never submit to that) but by observing what he valued most in life, what made things worse, and what made things better. By finding meaning and linking it to the behavior and treatments he wanted, he was building his own self-care rituals. We mapped out a plan. He decided to tackle sleep first. When rested, he felt better all around. He agreed to limit his drinks to two a night; before bed, he would take a hot shower and listen to an audio recording of nature sounds to help him relax. He stopped all electronic reading from bed and darkened his room with blackout curtains, covering up any electronic clocks. We put him on a small amount of the herb valerian (proven in randomized placebo-controlled studies to help people go to sleep) and low-dose, slow-release melatonin (not yet proven in randomized controlled studies), just for a month to assist in conditioning a deep relaxation and help him get into that habit at night. He also took his pain medications as needed. For one month, we did nothing specifically for Bill's pain or back. For the first time in years, it was not the focus of his visits to my clinic or of his daily routine. Yet he reported feeling better. He still had pain, but it did not bother him as much. He was moving more. He was taking less medication.

We then began to work on Bill's body. Pressure helped, so he thought he would like a selective use of massage. It just so happens my group had done a good meta-analysis of massage that showed effectiveness for chronic musculoskeletal pain like Bill's—especially compared to doing nothing, but even a little bit better when compared to sham massage, which involved very light touch. He also found stretching useful but had tried physical therapy and did not want that again. Also, he said he didn't want to keep coming into the hospital or clinic to receive treatment "with all those sick people." Bill was starting to no longer identify as a patient. We chose yoga instead.

There happens to be good research evidence that yoga is effective for easing back pain. The year before, my organization had conducted a comprehensive systematic review of nondrug approaches to pain. Yoga had emerged as one of the best. Recently, the American College of Physicians, the top group of internal medicine doctors in the United States, added yoga and massage to their guidelines for managing back pain. But someone like Bill, with long-term chronic pain, needs to do yoga carefully. Bill could easily set off spasms and fall into a downward spiral if his stretching was not done right. He had injured himself with stretching before. We decided to combine a periodic massage with gentle restorative yoga done slowly and under professional guidance. Soon, he learned how to control the stretches himself and was doing them three times a week—twice a week at home. After about four weeks, he found that when he did the massage/yoga combination, he didn't need his nighttime pain medication, and the yoga alone allowed him to cut his daily medication in half.

Eventually, Bill began to ask about the role of food for his weight and prediabetes. He wanted to explore how he could connect better with this wife and friends. By the time he was ready to explore those issues, however, his back pain was 80% better. Perhaps more important, he knew how to take charge of his own healing. He now knew how to use various agents to enhance his own healing agency.

THE PAIN POINT

Worldwide, chronic pain affects over one in five adults. Primary care settings in Asia, Africa, Europe, and the Americas report persistent pain in 10% to 25% of adults. Worldwide costs from all this pain total in the hundreds of billions per year. But the true costs of pain cannot be measured in money. Chronic pain, like most chronic illnesses, is a multifactorial, multidimensional condition that affects not just the body, but also the mind, the spirit, and the social environment.

Sometimes, a specific cause can be found and fixed. For acute disease, trauma, most infections, and an a few chronic diseases, a specific cure is possible. But for chronic pain and many chronic illnesses, there are no single cures. Bill spent fifteen years looking for a pain cure. What he needed was healing. He needed to become aware of those factors in this life that helped him feel better in general and get well. And he needed assistance in incorporating those into his life. He needed someone to help coach him in the process of self-care.

Most treatment approaches for chronic pain cannot be proven using the gold standard of research—the double-blind, randomized, placebo-controlled trial. Even when studied using this method, the contribution of proven therapies adds only a small amount (on average about 20%) to improvement compared to improvement that comes from meaning and context. The meaning factors produce the other 80% of improvement. Was the impact of the meaning response true for other chronic conditions? Was science missing the cause of improvement in areas other than pain?

CHAPTER 3

How Science Misses Healing

The science of the small and particular.

Is preventing two deaths from heart disease worth the cost to the ninety-eight people who will not get any benefit and the twenty people who will suffer major complications from a treatment? This is an ongoing debate in medicine about a real drug. To put the question bluntly: is preventing death in a few worth producing suffering in many? These are not easy questions to answer and are at their core not scientific questions. They are questions about values. Yet the way we do science obscures this discussion of values. Rarely are the details of the full risks and benefits of a treatment discussed with patients. Doctors and regulators just accept these questions as academic debates. And then plow through with their recommendations. Yet the uncertainty in bioscience is huge. If a patient is at high risk for heart disease, their likelihood of benefit outweighing harm goes up. If they are at low risk—like most of us—their likelihood of being more harmed than helped goes up. And we can't tell ahead of time which category a person falls into. This dilemma confronts us not because the science is bad; rather, it's because of the way we do science—seeking specific effects for particular biological targets that contribute to a disease and then using this information to treat complex, whole people who respond only partially in ways we want, and frequently in ways we don't want. The problem, I discovered, is in the science of the small and particular. The very type of science that benefits us so well for acute disease now harms us when treating chronic disease. This is the consequence of a reductionist science that started with the invention of the microscope and continues with even smaller units of analysis, like single molecules in our genes. For all the power of this type of science, we have not appreciated the limitations and harm it also produces. In this chapter, I will explain how patients who found holistic paths to healing eviscerated my arrogance about the certainty of reductionist science and opened up my mind to discover how healing works.

AADI

Aadi had been tremor-free for more than a year—again. This was the third time he had been "cured." A prominent businessman from Bangalore, India, Aadi had built a highly successful export business that made him quite wealthy. But at age fifty he developed Parkinson's disease. Parkinson's is a chronic and progressive disease in which vital nerve cells in the brain malfunction and die. Over time, the Parkinson's sufferer is unable to control body movements. Aadi's disease progressed rapidly, striking fear in him as he experienced the increasingly severe tremors and rigidity. Darkness descended over his life. He could imagine, he told me when I interviewed him later, all he had built—his business, his family of five girls and one boy, his prominent home and community life—all crumbling before him. He had to "fix it," he said. So he channeled all the drive he had used to build his business into finding a cure. He made trips to the top Parkinson's specialty centers in New Delhi, Bangalore, London, and finally the United States. They confirmed the diagnosis, and he ended up on two drugs designed to boost the chemical dopamine in his brain, along with an antidepressant that he didn't like because he said it made it harder to think. These were all the therapies that have been proven to help in Parkinson's. But Aadi experienced only moderate benefit from the treatment, reducing but not stopping the tremors and doing little for his advancing rigidity and sunken mood. Since he had the means, he looked even wider for possible cures, but all he found were some experimental treatments, such as implanting dopamine-producing cells or electrical devices into his brain. He was desperate enough to consider these therapies.

His wife intervened at this point. Seeing how the disease was ruining her husband and destroying their family, she was desperate, too, but she took a different approach to finding a solution. "You are Indian," she would scold him. "You should go see an Ayurvedic doctor. It is the oldest medical system in the world—developed right here in this country. Why do you fly all over the world seeking a cure when the answer might be right under your nose?"

As a man stern in both business and family life, Aadi resisted. "I don't want that quackery," he said. He tried to ignore her. But he continued to deteriorate. So Aadi's wife visited a local Ayurvedic hospital to inquire if they could treat Parkinson's. They said they could help.

Ayurveda, a word that means "life-knowledge" in Sanskrit, is an ancient traditional Indian medical system—as Aadi's wife had said, one of the oldest medical systems in the world—and is still being practiced widely in India today. It is a prescientific system. Although its origins are likely more than five thousand years old, there has been very little research to verify its claims of healing. Like most traditional health care practices, it is widely used throughout India but less so by the educated and well-off like Aadi. It has been practiced on billions of people for thousands of years but has not been subjected to modern scientific evaluation. Aadi was skeptical when his wife suggested he try it, especially when the first step involved reading his astrological chart to help discern the "spiritual" forces contributing to his Parkinson's. Aadi did not believe in any of that stuff, but his wife continued to insist that he go to an Ayurvedic hospital outside Bangalore and at least try it for a month. After all, she pointed out, he had exhausted all other options and had only gotten worse. Reluctantly, he agreed. That was six years ago.

When I met Aadi, he was about to be discharged from the Ayurvedic hospital for the third time. The hospital is a large complex with rooms and buildings over a number of acres in rural India, about five hours from Bangalore. In addition to simple rooms for patients to stay in overnight, it has temples, massage rooms, group yoga rooms, a large herbal garden and manufacturing facility, and a bath house where hydrotherapy and oil treatments were administered. In the last six years, Aadi had come to the hospital three times, staying four to six weeks each time. The first time he went begrudgingly. The second time, skeptically. This time, enthusiastically. Each time he had walked out largely symptom-free; his tremors were 90% improved, his rigidity gone, his energy improved, and his mood lifted. After each visit he could again focus on his business and family. This time, he had spent five weeks at the Ayurvedic hospital engaging in daily intensive treatments that touched all aspects of his mind, body, and spirit.

Aadi told me that each time he visited the hospital, the treatments largely eliminated his symptoms. The first time, the improvement lasted almost two years. Gradually he had gotten busy and not returned to the doctor. He began to drop off the program of meditation, special diets, herbs, and oil massages that had been prescribed for him to follow. Slowly his symptoms returned. This time, he volunteered to come back for a "booster" treatment. Although he admitted that he was not cured—the tremor was not completely gone—nevertheless he was now fully functional and ready to return home. And he was off all other medications. "Magic," he said, with a smile and a shrug. He still didn't believe in magic, but he knew this worked.

Aadi let me examine him. A full neurological exam showed only a minor tremor that came out with certain tests, and minor dysfunction in his reflexes. Everything else was normal. Had I seen him in my office, I would not have diagnosed him with Parkinson's. Aadi said he went back to the Ayurvedic hospital every twelve to eighteen months for a month of intensive treatment. "What kind of treatment do they provide?" I asked. "Well," said Aadi, "you must ask Dr. Manu about that; he is the head doctor here. I do a lot of things, but most of it seems to be directed toward getting my head back on straight; helping me see what is important in life. In the business of my normal life when I forget who I really am, that is when I get sick. I come here to find out why I was born. They also do a lot of 'cleansing' of my body—with cathartics, oil massages, herbs, and things. I have stopped asking the details. I just know it works. Dr. Manu can explain it better, I am sure," he shrugged. "Go talk to him."

MANU

Dr. Manu Padimadi—or Dr. Manu, as they called him at the Ayurvedic hospital—is a tall, confident man. When he speaks to you, he looks at you intensely, as if he is peering into your soul. It is a bit unsettling. He had managed the hospital for seven years, after fourteen years of study. His father and grandfather had run the hospital before him. His English was an impeccable high British, which, I learned later, he perfected while studying chemistry and molecular biology at Oxford. I didn't know that the first time we met. I was at his hospital in southern India as part of my job as director of a WHO Collaborating Center for Traditional Medicine, seeking to further the scientific understanding of traditional healing systems like Ayurveda. Dr. Manu had set up a process for collecting data on Ayurvedic treatments and was eager to advance research on it. He explained the basic philosophy and approach of ayurveda to me. The primary goal of Ayurveda, he said, was to help the mind experience "universal consciousness." Once that was experienced, he explained, healing arises "because you have found your true self." Aadi, he said, had lost the purpose of his life, pursuing business at the expense of his family, his community, and even his own personal health and growth. Ayurveda began with a spiritual exploration for why he had fallen away from his divine purpose and then designed practices to help bring both his mind and body into better alignment with that purpose. It did this by evaluating the balance of a person's *doshas*. Doshas, Manu explained, are a combination of constitutional characteristics that define each individual. Made up of characteristics of body type and a person's mental and emotional nature, they serve as guides for "personalizing" each patient's path to wellness. In Ayurveda, he explained, there is no distinction between mind and body. Physiology and spiritual elements are all interacting parts of a whole person. In addition, the person needs to be "nudged" toward healing by using small stresses, such as cathartics and herbs. Slightly toxic substances were given infrequently. Fasting and exercise—especially yoga—were also part of the healing regime.

The goal of these treatments, Manu went on, was to "wake up" a person's inherent healing processes—to create mental and physical disturbances that, when applied in the context of life's purpose and direction, helped the person reorder himself or herself, become more whole, and heal. When people had the right elements around them to nourish their bodies, minds, and spirits, and those elements were stimulated to heal in this manner, he explained, patients recover and find new levels of balance and health. "Once wholeness is achieved, it can only be maintained if they continue to connect their actions—including their treatments—to the core meaning in their life," Manu said. "This is what increases the probability that they remain well." Profound stuff, I thought, but what did it mean in daily life?

Each morning, Aadi would get up early and go through a series of rituals and prayers to help him center and become more mindful. He was on a special diet, designed to help balance his dosha energy, and took various herbs and exercises designed to relax and cleanse the body and mind. Breathing and meditation, yoga and fasting were all part of the program. After a month of such a routine, his body would have come back into "balance" and heal itself. Aadi had experienced this now three times. And his Parkinson's had all but resolved each time.

While Dr. Manu's explanation of creating the right meaning and context made sense from my experiences with Norma, Bill, Sergeant Martin, and other patients, the description of doshas, the use of cathartics and small doses of toxins, and especially the role of astrology in guiding treatments seemed like superstition and nonsense. I told Dr. Manu that. Had any of these treatments been rigorously studied or proven in randomized, controlled trials? Had ayurvedic physicians shown that any of them actually caused the healing and recovery they claimed? Was there proof that doshas existed? Could they be measured and manipulated? We knew that Parkinson's disease was caused by low dopamine production in a specific part of the brain—the substantia nigra. Had any of the treatments been shown to increase dopamine in that part of the brain, I asked?

No, Manu admitted, they had not measured the production of dopamine in the brain produced by Ayurvedic treatments. He was open to that. In fact, he said, if there was a noninvasive way to track the biochemical markers of disease improvement for the conditions they treated, he imagined this would markedly help them improve and personalize this ancient system more—and make it more scientific. But, he warned, simply focusing on what produced a rise of dopamine in one area of the brain over a short period of time would be misguided. What was needed to properly study Ayurveda, he explained, was a research approach to monitoring the response of the whole person. More objective ways of tracking that response would be welcome as long as they were not used in ways that interfered with the ability of the whole person to respond as a complex, adaptive system. "Looking at only one small part of a person's disease and treating only that is harmful. First, do no harm," he said with a flash of irony, repeating part of the Hippocratic oath that all Western doctors repeat when they get their degrees.

I was skeptical and a bit annoyed to receive a lecture on the science and ethics of Western medicine from a non-Western doctor in the middle of rural India. Surely, I thought, some of what Aadi was being subjected to was harmful. I had seen studies of toxic heavy metals in Ayurvedic herbs and couldn't imagine how inducing diarrhea and vomiting with cathartics could be good for you. I pointed this out to him.

"Look," said Manu with a slight sigh, "forget the doshas and the astrology and the cathartics for a minute." He went to a whiteboard on the wall of his office and began drawing. "Every major healing system, including modern Western medicine, acknowledges that a person is more than just their body and biochemistry; that to truly treat the whole person, we must acknowledge that they are physical, social, mental, and spiritual." He drew a series of concentric circles on the whiteboard. "Well-being and healing arise when a person is both treated and experiences themselves as a whole person. Our job as physicians is to assist them to understand and make those connections—to find out what is deeply meaningful for them—and then nudge their body and mind with treatments to help them respond in a way that restores balance and wholeness."

MANU'S DRAWING OF THE AYURVEDIC MODEL OF A PERSON

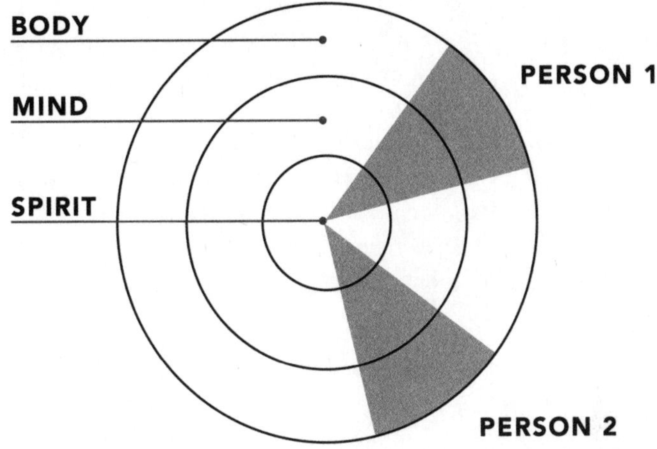

Manu drew a line from the outside circle—the one representing the body—down through the other layers of a person to the spiritual level and then back again. "When this connection is made, wholeness and healing happen. After all, the word *heal* comes from the Old English word *haelan,* from which we also get the words *whole* and *holy*."

I was again struck by the irony that an Indian doctor in an ancient healing center in rural India was giving me an English lesson.

"When Aadi leaves the hospital tomorrow," he continued, "he will leave experiencing that sense of wholeness, balance, and well-being. He will be 90% better in the symptoms of his Parkinson's disease also. Even if I could show you that one of the herbs he takes increases dopamine in the substantia nigra of his brain by 100%, I would still need to deliver that therapy within the context of his whole life to make it work well. His challenge, when he leaves, will be to try and maintain meaning, wholeness, balance, and even holiness in his daily life and reinforce it with behaviors such as periodic fasting and yoga to keep those healing processes active."

XIAO AND MR. COUSINS

I had to admit that some of what Manu said made sense. We are not just bags of chemicals; at any rate, we cannot treat ourselves that way without causing harm. But Manu was proposing a universal process for healing, not requiring knowledge of the specific effect of a treatment on a biological mechanism or outcome. Whatever the explanation for Aadi's remarkable improvement, one thing was clear: he had tapped into it repeatedly, and he was much better than before he engaged in this ancient healing system. Although I was glad to see Aadi's improvement from an otherwise incurable disease, I was distressed at Manu's explanation of how it happened.

Clearly, Dr. Manu was well educated in Western science and medicine as well as ancient Ayurvedic practices. He was one of those rare individuals fully trained in two entirely different systems.

While Manu's explanation made intuitive sense, what bothered me was that I could find practically no evidence to support that his treatments improved Parkinson's disease. And that I could not accept. One of the hallmarks of good scientific evidence in medicine is being able to isolate and prove that a specific treatment produces a specific effect through a specific mechanism. If you looked at all the interventions and treatments Aadi underwent, there were no clinical studies or even basic science studies indicating that those treatments influenced the core biological problem in Parkinson's—the level of dopamine in the substantia nigra part of the brain. Instead, the treatments appeared to be for general wellness enhancement or to stress his system and induce a reactive response not specific to Parkinson's. A review of his interventions revealed that only one had been shown to produce dopamine in the brain. This was a dietary intervention using lentils as part of his meals. A small clinical study found that this food improved dopamine production, but not to a sufficient extent to explain Aadi's remarkable improvement. In addition, dopamine production can be produced by many things, including placebo interventions, as long as the patient expects them to work. There was no reason to think that the herb was any more effective than any other treatments Aadi had done, provided he believed—and the culture believed—that they were going to help him. From what I could tell, Aadi had gotten better because he had some basic health and wellness support (nutrition, exercise, rest), a physiological stress or two to get his system changing (fasting, cathartics, toxins), and manipulation of his belief by a bunch of placebos.

This pattern was not isolated to Ayurvedic. But how common was it? To find out, I set up a program to travel around the world and explore a variety of healing systems. As director of both a WHO Center for Traditional Medicine and the NIH Office of Alternative Medicine, I was specifically interested in examining these systems for their impact on patient outcomes and the scientific foundation they might have. The pattern I saw at the Ayurvedic clinic with Aadi turned out to be quite common within other systems, each of which had its own unique framework, set of interventions, explanations, and rituals. Yet all seemed to follow a basic pattern.

An example was a visit to the Great Wall Hospital outside of Beijing, China, which specializes in treating a disease called ankylosing spondylitis (AK). AK is a progressive autoimmune disease that causes erosion, fibrosis, sclerosis, and freezing of the joints, especially of the spine. It is a genetic disease that affects males more than females, reducing strong, energetic boys and men to invalids in a matter of a few years. In AK, there is a general weakening of the person with an increase in inflammation and pain and a decrease in motion and function. There are no effective treatments. Readers may recall seeing a story by the writer Norman Cousins, who claimed to have cured himself of ankylosing spondylitis with high doses of vitamin C and laughter therapy, neither of which had been proven to reverse the disease. At the Great Wall Hospital, they provided several treatments, but the primary one was a flat-needled microsurgery technique that broke up the fibrosis around the spine. The technique looked very painful, as long, flat acupuncture needles were placed along the spine and wiggled until they broke up the connective tissue. This "microsurgery" was repeated weekly, providing a rather strong nudge—more like a jolt—to the body from which it had to recover and repair itself. These microsurgeries were delivered, however, within a context very similar to what I had seen at Aadi's Ayurvedic Clinic. Families were present everywhere, providing food and care for the patients, supporting and encouraging them as they underwent the therapy. Physical manipulation called *tui na*—a type of body massage (very different from the massages Aadi had undergone)—was also provided. Daily exercise in the form of tai chi was prescribed, along with long periods of rest and sleep between treatments. The herbal medicines given were mixtures said to encourage a proper "balance of chi" or "life energy" and to calm the immune system after the needle treatments. All this was guided by determining how each patient's life energy was impacted by the environment, the seasons, his family, and the stars. Each of these factors was said to guide the chi and to reorder, balance, and heal the patient.

I remember following a young man of twenty-four named Xiao who had progressive and advancing AK. As an only boy in China's one-child policy system, he was prized and doted on by his entire extended family. Quite a gifted athlete, he had joined the track and field team at school and at one point was even being considered for the Olympic team in pole vaulting. But at eighteen-years-old he noticed an increasing pain in his pelvis and back. When heat and physical therapy did not help, his parents took him to the Beijing hospital. X-rays of the spine revealed the characteristic cloudiness of AK between spinal disks and the pelvis. A blood test confirmed that he had HLA-27, a gene associated with 25% of those with the disease—and usually the more severe type. By age twenty-four, Xiao had progressed further, now with more stiffness (called a bamboo spine in medical circles), fatigue, inflammation in the eye (also a rare symptom of AK), and some early cardiac symptoms. When we first met, Xiao joked, "I used to bend the pole in track and field—now I am the pole."

Xiao's mother saw my uncertainty in how to react to this statement. Was he being sarcastic? She put me at ease. "Typical Xiao," she said with a smile, "always joking. Even with advancing disease, he has kept his humor."

"I was lucky to be born into this family," he would say. "I may not be able to vault my body any more to new heights, but I can still vault my spirit."

When Xiao first arrived at the Great Wall Hospital, his family said he was in a wheelchair and unable to walk. He could not turn from right to left or bend forward more than twenty degrees. He was totally dependent on their care. When I examined him, six weeks after he came to the Great Wall Hospital, he was up on his own feet and walking with a cane. He could now turn almost forty-five degrees from side to side. He said he was much better: happier, with more energy, and significantly less pain. He would be there about two more months undergoing other traditional Chinese medicine treatments. Dr. Yu Chen, the hospital director, told me that they got about 60% excellent improvement in patients with ankylosing spondylitis after one to three months of treatment. When I followed Xiao around, the parallels to other medical approaches that produced healing were uncanny: teams of caregivers, including doctors and family members, and specialists in spiritual therapy (Chinese medicine has no psychotherapy as we know it in the West, but uses astrology as in India). Special diets high in spices were prescribed, and combinations of Chinese herbs, some of which contained toxic materials (as do some Ayurvedic treatments), were given. And there was a lot of exercise in the form of tai chi, exposure to the natural environment, and rest and sleep. Xiao and his family were overjoyed at the improvement he had sustained. Dr. Chen said that about half the patients maintain these good effects for several years, but others regress. He had no data to back up any of his claims and had done no clinical trials to demonstrate that this overall procedure worked. A few of the spices and herbal products had been studied in the laboratory for their immune modulation ability, but none of them had been studied in clinical trials with AK patients.

After seeing Xiao I reflected on what Norman Cousins wrote about his own treatment of ankylosing spondylitis. Unable to find an integrative center in the United States, he essentially created his own treatment plan—visiting specialists at UCLA and "alternative" practitioners separately, and then putting together a general health enhancement program involving high-dose vitamin C and laughter over a period of several months. The laughter involved watching old comedy movies such as those of Charlie Chaplin, followed by significant rest and sleep. Strangely, it seemed that both Xiao and Norman Cousins came to laughter as a treatment for their disease. They had other things in common. Cousins was also surrounded by family and friends and mentioned the importance of immersing himself in a natural environment that induced calm—a relaxation response—during what was otherwise a very stressful time. Xiao would take daily walks and do his tai chi in the woods—often with one of his aunts or hospital friends.

Like the Great Wall Hospital's healing environment, the one Norman Cousins produced for himself also had no research to back it up. Subsequent studies of high-dose vitamin C demonstrated very small to negligible effects on the disease. Cousins didn't know it at the time, but when given at the doses he was taking, vitamin C is a toxin—an oxidant rather than an antioxidant—and so produced repeated stress on his body. As for laughter and the immune system, only a small amount of research had been done. Yet Cousins reported that with these treatments, he improved almost to the point of a complete cure.

HOW COMMON?

I wondered: how common is this pattern—support, stimulus, and belief—in healing? To find out, my team and I conducted a series of field investigations on a variety of practices in several countries. Our goal was to analyze what the practices did and what kind of results they were getting. We visited and performed in-depth evaluations of more than thirty centers around the world. And we saw this same pattern in all of them. Under the right conditions, results like that those experienced by Norma, Bill, Sergeant Martin, Aadi, Xiao, and Mr. Cousins were common. These centers and clinics often produced marked clinical effects. And like the others, they lacked scientific proof. We saw that healing was, in fact, possible and could be induced for many chronic diseases. But when we sought to isolate any one treatment component from the rest and measure its contribution on one outcome—as is required by good science to prove them—the effects diminished, disappeared, or at most contributed only 20% to 30% to a patient's improvement. The process and ritual of treatment produced the rest. Was this a common pattern when science was applied to healing no matter the treatment—be it herbs, diet, or drugs?

The more I deeply dove into the science, the weaker what I thought I knew from medical training became. I'd seen Norma, Bill, Sergeant Martin, and other patients flounder under my care, while I was using the best evidence—and then get markedly better after using nonscientific methods, despite my skepticism. Seeing patients like Aadi and Xiao, whose diseases are presumed to be incurable, resolve their symptoms using ancient systems of healing, based on no real science, caused my world to fray around the edges.

There was no good evidence that prayer or astrology, massage, cathartics, or herbs cured Parkinson's disease. Similarly, there was no scientific basis for the belief that needles and tai chi could cure ankylosing spondylitis, or that vitamins cured arthritis, or surgery reversed back pain, or oxygen treated brain injury. How widespread were these phenomena? How often did healing occur? How often did science miss it? And why? Was this simply from lack of research on healing treatments, or was there something in the way we tried to prove healing that interfered with our seeing it? It seemed that the secret to 80% of healing was right under my nose. But how could we test it if we could not even see it? Then I remembered Sarah.

SARAH

Sarah and her baby were not supposed to be in Germany. Her husband, an Army truck mechanic working for an engineering battalion, was on a one-year tour without family. But she came anyway. As a twenty-one-year-old, newly married and a new mother, she did not want to be away from him. So she moved to the town of Dexheim, Germany. I was the physician responsible for the military unit in Dexheim—a small American outpost. Sarah and her husband were both from Kansas, and now Sarah was depressed. This was not surprising, given her environment. She lived off post in a rundown apartment. She hadn't graduated from high school and didn't speak any German. She had a new baby. And she was far away from home. When her husband would come home from days in the field, he would often find the house in a mess and his wife sleeping or crying in her bed with the baby. They came to me for help.

I diagnosed Sarah with postpartum depression, began some counseling, and started her on an antidepressant medication, a type of medication called a selective serotonin reuptake inhibitor, or SSRI. About a month later, she came back in and said she had stopped the medication. Since starting it, she had lost all interest in sex or intimacy, which before the baby had been a major part of life for her and her husband. She was sure it was the medication, since the drop-off in interest had occurred right after she started taking it.

"Doctor," she said, "while my moods are somewhat better, it is making our marriage worse. My husband is understanding, but don't you have anything better?"

I doubted that her decrease in desire for intimacy was due to the medication. More likely, it was a continuing symptom of her postpartum depression. But to counter her opinion would be counterproductive. I asked them to come in together the following week so we could talk about it and I could do a bit more counseling.

Later that week, I was at a medical meeting and consulted one of my colleagues about what to do. The small clinic I ran was in a remote section of Germany, and German doctors did our emergency transport service when we had car accidents or drug overdoses on the post—something that happened about once a month. I spoke German from living in Germany as a child and knew many of the local doctors. On this occasion, I asked one of my closest German colleagues about Sarah's case. "Oh yes," he said, "I've seen many women like this—far from home and homesick. Young and without a social support network, they now have the full responsibilities of a baby and the demands of a husband."

This doctor suggested two things. "First, give her the homeopathic remedy *Gelsemium* and then add the herb *Hypericum*," he said. "Its common name is St. John's wort. It works just as well as the antidepressants, but doesn't have the side effects that you describe. Make sure you explain what it is for and what it should do."

I had never heard of these treatments. I went back to my office and looked for any research on them. *Gelsemium* was a homeopathic remedy that not been studied but, from what I could tell from its very low dose, had to be a placebo. The homeopathic books said it was good for homesickness and described cases similar to Sarah's—but with no testing or proof. St. John's wort, on the other hand, had been studied several times for depression and was slightly better than placebo in randomized controlled trials. It had a good safety profile.

It seemed that there was little downside to these treatments, so I made note of these two additional tools for when I met with Sarah and her husband.

Because her husband had described how their home was quite cluttered and dirty because of her depression, I suggested that we have someone come in and provide household help. I also asked if they would be willing to have someone come watch the baby a couple times a week so Sarah could go to events on the post; she agreed. I then told them about the two remedies that my German colleague had recommended.

I read to her the indications from the book about *Gelsemium* (good for homesickness) and translated the description of St. John's wort from a German flyer. It was "an ancient herb with a beautiful yellow flower—like a ray of sunshine in a plant." Not only did studies show that it lifted mood, but it would be less likely to produce a decline in sexual interest. After hearing that these didn't have the side effects Sarah thought were produced by the antidepressant, they both said, "Absolutely, Doc, we want to try that."

The two medications were not in the military pharmacy, so I told them to go to their local German apothecary to pick them up. I asked them to come back in three weeks.

When she returned, Sarah reported feeling much better. Her husband was out on another a field exercise, but she had not been crying as much and had gone to several of the women's support sessions on base. "I met another woman from Kansas," she said. "She grew up a couple hours from where I did. We meet for coffee now between the women's meetings. And get this," she said, with more animation than I had ever heard from her before. "She is three months pregnant!"

Sarah made a plan to clean up the house with a friend while her husband was gone. I asked her to continue the medicines and come back again in another three weeks, this time with her husband. Three weeks later—now six weeks after the change in environment and treatment—they came in, both smiling.

"Doc," said her husband, "that St. Germ's wort really works! She is feeling much better. Thank you so much."

I never found out how their love life was going, but I assumed a bit better. I followed them for another six months before they returned to the United States, and Sarah continued to do well and the baby began to thrive. I found out on one of the last visits before they left to go home that she had stopped taking both *Gelsemium* and St. John's wort but had continued to function and cope.

Certainly, something had helped Sarah. Perhaps it was the change in the physical environment in her house after someone came in to clean it. Perhaps it was the friend she had made. Perhaps it was because their sex life had improved. Perhaps it was the homeopathic *Gelsemium* (most likely a placebo) or the herb St. John's wort (a mild antidepressant). I wondered, though: was it really the St. John's wort? Her improvement was quite dramatic.

When I looked at the research literature, the evidence indicated that the herb did help with mild to moderate depression, but the effect was small—not much larger than what you'd see with placebo. Was it the herb, the friend, the clean house, or the presumed intimacy that healed her? Why had it worked when the drug did not?

ST. JOHN'S WORT

A few years later, I had the great fortune to test this question directly by helping to design and fund a large clinical study of the same herb and drug for depression that I had given Sarah. It was an unusual type of study, more rigorous than most drug tests. Normally, new drugs are tested in two-armed studies in which patients are randomly assigned to the active treatment (drug or herb, for example) or an identical-looking placebo. These types of clinical studies are expensive, so before a drug gets to such a test, a series of laboratory studies are usually done to show the drug is absorbed into the brain and affects the chemicals thought to be involved in depression. If these first studies are not done, a clinical study comparing a drug to placebo is usually not done. The scientific community was skeptical about St. John's wort's effectiveness because these types of preliminary studies either had not been done or did not show direct effects in the brain. While antidepressants could be explained because of the known effect they had on certain chemicals in the brain—SSRIs, for example, impacted a neurotransmitter called serotonin—there was no specific chemical in a sufficient amount in St. John's wort to affect any known brain chemical related to depression. The herb contained small amounts of several chemicals, and one in particular, called hypericin, seemed to impact the brain in a variety of ways, but the amounts of hypericin in the herb—including the amount I gave to Sarah—were too low to reasonably explain these effects. Most scientists in the United States thought the studies done in Germany, which were funded by the herbal companies who made them, were probably biased, and that the data showing benefit was wrong. Even though I offered to fund the study from my budget at the NIH, the other NIH institutes were hesitant to undertake the test.

Finally, Dr. Bob Temple, one of the most respected researchers at the FDA, had a solution. We should do a three-armed study in which patients were randomly assigned to the herb, a placebo, or a proven FDA-approved antidepressant drug: sertraline (brand name Zoloft), one of the SSRIs with a known mechanism of action and clinical effects, which I had prescribed for Sarah. With this design, the director of the National Institute of Mental Health at NIH agreed to conduct the study. He had always wanted to have his institute run an independent drug study on depression (most were done by pharmaceutical companies), and a direct comparison with the herb and placebo had never been done. We found one of the most respected mental health researchers in the country to do it—Dr. Jonathan Davidson from Duke University. I had known Dr. Davidson for years. A wonderful psychiatrist, originally from England, he was not only a great researcher but also a compassionate and careful physician, the type of psychiatrist who listens carefully to you and spends the time needed to understand you. Like Dr. Manu, he possessed an unusual presence—a healing presence—and his British accent lent an air of sophistication and authority to any encounter.

Dr. Davidson carefully constructed a study designed to separate the placebo and his own healing effects from those of the herb and drug. However, when we approached the companies to supply the herbs and drug—standard procedure even for government-run studies—the drug company balked. They did not want to participate in the study. They made more than a billion dollars a year on the sale of sertraline. When I offered to make public their noncooperation, they relented and agreed to supply the drug. However, before the NIH study began they launched their own, two-armed study, comparing the herb to placebo—exactly the type of study not recommended by the FDA, because it did not have a positive (proven drug) control group. In that study, they selected patients who had worse depression than we planned to test—worse than Sarah had and worse than the subjects of the German studies. Those patients were less likely to respond to the herb. By spending a great deal of money, they sped the trial to completion in an attempt to beat the NIH and show that St. John's wort did not work. And they did, publishing a negative study—St. John's wort and placebo had equivalent effects—a full year before the NIH study was done. The conclusions of this study—that St. John's wort did not work—spread widely. Sales of the herb dropped.

Unlike the public, my colleagues held out for the results of the more rigorous, three-armed study by Dr. Davidson. His study picked the right types of patients; gave them the right doses; did proper blinding with placebo, so no one knew who was getting the herb, drug, or placebo; and included a large enough number of patients to rule out chance. What would it show? Would the herb beat the drug? Likely not, I thought. Would it beat placebo? It should. Would it have fewer side effects than the drug? If Sarah's experience was any indication, it would.

When the data was analyzed and they had broken the blinding code to see the effect in each group, I waited with anticipation. It had been nearly ten years since I had treated Sarah with both the drug and the herb, and it took three years to complete the study. My bet was that the drug and herb would work better than placebo but the herb would not work as well as the drug—but with fewer side effects.

Turns out I was wrong. All three groups—whether they were taking the herb, drug, or placebo—got better at the same rate. There was no difference in the rate or degree of improvement in depression. The herb and placebo had fewer side effects than the drug, however, confirming what I had seen with Sarah.

I was flummoxed. When the study was published in the prestigious *Journal of the American Medical Association* (*JAMA*), the news headlines around the world reported that a major NIH study had shown that St. John's wort did not work. Sales of the herb dropped further. What few people picked up on, however, was that *the proven drug had also not worked any better than placebo*. This was the most important finding of the study, and it was totally missed. The healing effect of the ritual—of just getting treated and seen in the placebo group—was as powerful as both the drug and the herb.

Knowing Dr. Davidson and his bedside manner, I was not surprised that many of the patients got better, including the ones on placebo. I had seen it in my own studies and with patients such as Norma. But the scientists and the public were so focused on whether the herb or drug added more than placebo—by even a small amount—that the actual reasons for healing were completely overlooked. Something about the way we were going about our science—always attempting to reduce it to the smallest, most specific focus—was causing us to miss out on healing.

THE DECLINE EFFECT

The publicity around the *JAMA*-reported study implied that drug treatment was more effective than St. John's wort, and it heightened the likelihood that the drug and not the herb would be prescribed by other physicians. I interpreted it quite differently—as did many of my FDA colleagues. To me, it was further evidence that something other than the agent produced healing. Previous research had demonstrated that between 70% and 80% of the improvement seen in clinical studies with both St. John's wort and antidepressants was also seen in those taking placebo. The single study by Dr. Davidson had simply confirmed this. And this, as it turns out, is more often the rule than the exception. The more rigorously one looks at almost any treatment, the smaller and smaller the effect size becomes compared to placebo; as the science gets better, the difference between placebo and the real treatment diminishes.

This is known as the "decline effect." We see it over and over again in clinical research. The more rigorous and larger a study, the smaller the actual contribution of the active treatment. Early studies, especially smaller pilot studies, frequently show large effects, which encourage physicians and patients to use the treatment. Usually those smaller studies are not enough for FDA approval or to be accepted by the mainstream community as standard of care; therefore, additional and larger studies follow. As those larger and more rigorous studies are done, the effects diminish. When you combine the results of those studies in a method called meta-analysis, frequently the effects became so small as to become irrelevant for use in practice.

What's more, the effects of even proven treatments frequently cannot be replicated by others when taken out of the hands of the original investigators. This "replicability problem" has been extensively reported by Dr. John Ioannidis, chair of the Department of Medicine at Stanford University, and others. In a startling analysis of clinical research published in the *Journal of the American Medical Association* in 2012, Ioannidis showed that only about one-third of proven results can be replicated. These were not just pilot studies, whose test treatments often show a decline effect in subsequent studies; these were failures at replications of established and proven therapies—like the antidepressant I had prescribed to Sarah. Soon, others began to look at research outside of clinical medicine and found that replicability was a general problem in science. Even laboratory and basic research—where we control many more factors than in clinical research—can be replicated only about 30% to 40% of the time. While the decline effect shows that initial findings often shrink or even disappear in the end, the replicability problem shows that even what are thought to be proven effects are usually not replicable. If someone else tries to repeat a study, often the effects of the active agent disappear. What is left are other nonspecific or unknown factors variously attributed to the "placebo effect." As I explain later, I prefer to call these effects—the component that hold the majority of healing—"the meaning effect."

THE DECLINE EFFECT

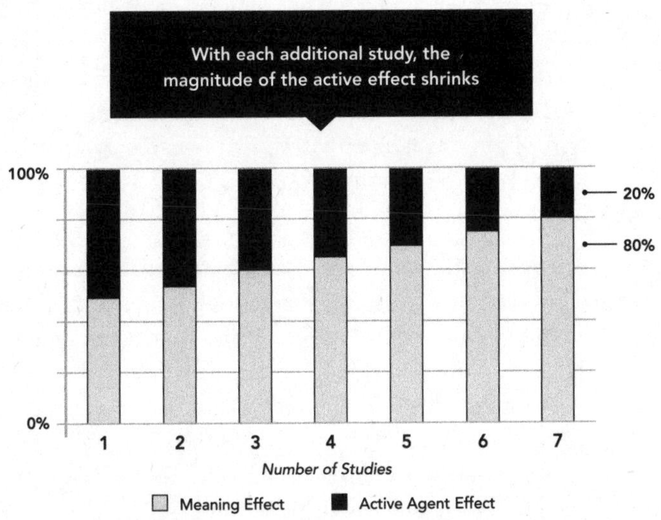

What helped Sarah and her husband was not the fact that the St. John's wort worked for her depression; rather, it was the way I delivered it and the ritual and social events that followed—an ordered house, making a friend, and intimacy—that nudged her out of depression and produced the healing. I couldn't say whether she got a lift in mood from the *Gelsemium*, the St. John's wort, or the sertraline, but I could say that the way she engaged in the treatment allowed her to get out of bed and become her own healing agent. As I had seen with other patients, the treatment context and the meaning response were more important than whether the specific treatment had been proven in rigorous research for her condition.

CERTAINTY FALLS APART

Depression is one of the most common and burdensome conditions in the world. It causes a lot of suffering. And it frequently accompanies other chronic diseases. Sarah had depression after her baby was born. Bill had depression because of his back pain. Sergeant Martin was depressed after his brain injury. Depression frequently accompanies Parkinson's disease. SSRIs have global sales of more than $11 billion a year. St. John's wort, even with all the negative publicity from the NIH studies, still tops $50 million a year in sales. But if more than 80% of improvement in depression from any treatment is from the way it is delivered—the ritual—what are we paying for when we pay for a drug or herb or other treatment? If we are not using the treatment in a way to maximize the meaning response, *we may be* mostly paying for *the side effects*.

Proven treatments that target specific molecular pathways and so create their intended effects, usually also have effects on unintended targets, producing unwanted side effects. Thus, the very treatments that work—those producing the benefit seen in 20% to 30% in randomized studies—also produce unwanted effects. Those unwanted effects frequently impact 50% to 70% of those who take them, including when the treatment did not work. In short: in complex systems like the human body, "specific" treatments have a higher probability of causing harm than good. Judging whether the harms are worth the benefits is the challenge in all of medicine.

STATIN SIDE EFFECTS

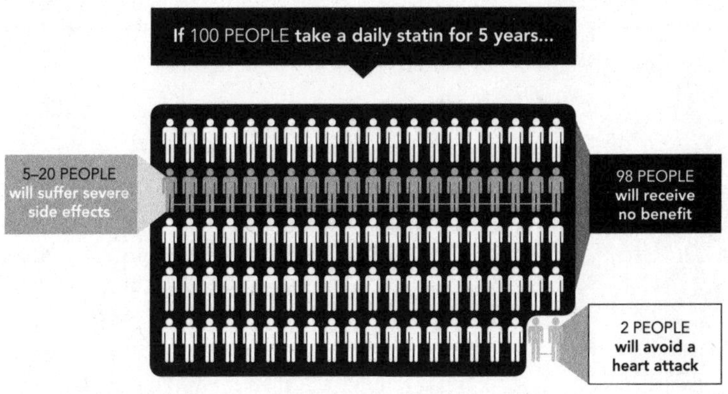
If 100 PEOPLE take a daily statin for 5 years...
5–20 PEOPLE will suffer severe side effects
98 PEOPLE will receive no benefit
2 PEOPLE will avoid a heart attack

The figure illustrates this for one of the most common and beneficial treatments we have for preventing the number-one killer in developed countries: heart disease. That treatment is statin drugs for reducing cholesterol. For every one hundred people who take a statin, two will have their potential death from a heart attack prevented, and ninety-eight will derive no benefit. Most of those same one hundred people will experience some type of side effect, and between five and twenty of those will experience a serious side effect, like major muscle pain or the development of type 2 diabetes.

Not only was my confidence in what I had been taught under threat, but the very scientific basis on which it rested was starting to look shaky. In his 2015 book, *The Laws of Medicine*, Pulitzer Prize–winning author Siddhartha Mukherjee says the laws of medicine "are really the laws of uncertainty, imprecision, and incompleteness. They apply equally to all disciplines of knowledge where these forces come into play. They are the laws of imperfection." He goes on to describe how attempts to apply rigorous science often fall short of giving us a good basis for decisions in health care. Even rigorously done experiments give us only probabilities or shifts in likelihood of benefit. And despite applying strict rules of research and critical thinking to science, decisions are still full of bias—statistical, clinical, linguistic, perceptual, regulatory, and financial bias—which can undermine our efforts at objectivity and certainty. What is more, only about one-third of what is published and "proven" using rigorous, experimental research can be replicated, leaving a two-thirds uncertainty for the gold standard—the best of the best of evidence.

Finally, the negative effects of those treatments for the whole person—with all of his or her complex reactions—are frequent, varied, and often poorly recognized. Layer upon layer of uncertainty began to pile on top of what I had based my whole medical career on, what I had taught to students, what I had used to treat patients. If only a small proportion of healing was from the treatments I dished out, and if most patients were getting side effects from those treatments, then was I throwing out most of the healing—and perhaps producing harm—by always looking for the small and particular effects? To make matters worse, this type of science is also being reinforced with money—lots of money—from companies seeking to get their products approved even when they might be doing more harm than good. Drugs get FDA-approved when they show their benefits go beyond placebo, even by a small amount. This requires very large and expensive studies. Proof now has to be purchased. A "real" treatment must separate itself from the daily processes of healing. It was patients like Aadi and Sergeant Martin who went beyond these rules of evidence and pointed me to the underlying rules of healing, prompting me to think there has to be a better way to heal.

CHAPTER 4

A Science for Healing

The science of the large and the whole.

Before science, we had only superstition or intuition to guide us to truth. Both were flawed when it came to healing. With science, we have approaches for testing our ideas in small ways and making incremental advancements in our understanding. Occasionally, these incremental advances result in a major impact—such as with the discovery of penicillin or vaccines. Before science, an epidemic was considered an act of God. After science, it became a containment challenge. We could now do more than pray. While science is a major improvement over superstition, it does not solve the uncertainty in healing. We sometimes lose sight of this. We think that by precisely defining and classifying disease, by rigorously measuring and instituting robust controls, we can determine the best treatments that will give us the most consistent results. And for many conditions this type of science does just that. When biomedical science works, it can work dramatically—especially when what ails us has a simple or a single cause—an infectious agent, a trauma, or a sudden anatomical manifestation of a chronic process, like during a heart attack. This is when the application of science in health care shines. We find miracle cures and produce magic bullets. We save millions through the application of these discoveries in public health, and we keep individuals alive when they would have died on the battlefield or on the highway or at the end of their life.

We love those discoveries, and we get lured into using this type of science for everything, looking for the cure in an attempt to eliminate the disease we have named. We train our scientists and practitioners to look for those cures. We structure our health care system to look for those cures and treat all diseases and illnesses as if we have found the cures. We pay for these treatments, even when the benefit of the treatment is small, the risks large, and the harms poorly understood. We love this type of science—the science of the small and particular. We love it so much that we use it when we should not. Left to our own intuitive devices, we will pick an attempt to cure over healing or prevention almost all the time. Like the fox who sees a rabbit only when it moves and not the hundred others hiding in the grass, we too tend not to see what happens in our life until something changes. Most of life remains hidden in the background, unless we initially bring those elements into our vision.

Thus the science that successfully stops infections, treats trauma, and saves our lives from acute diseases doesn't work very well for chronic diseases. Not only does it not work well, but it can also mislead us and harm us—by giving us partial treatments for diseases and producing side effects that need to be managed. And by causing us to ignore simpler approaches that produce larger and more whole-person effects. This is why when we do apply a new discovery to chronic illness, we usually get only modest effects—on average about 20% to 30%. Yet there are health care systems and patients who get much better results than that. They have tapped into the other 70% to 80% of what is possible. There is nothing wrong with incremental science, but there is something wrong with the way we apply that science to healing.

WHOLE SYSTEMS SCIENCE

Imagine for a moment that all the chemical, energetic, psychological, and social exchanges of a person could be visualized as a web-like ball composed of millions of interactions occurring every second. When in optimal health, the ball is perfectly round and the interactions are occurring rapidly through a network of nodes or intersections in this web of interconnected links or pathways.

The primary goal of these interactions is to maintain the web-ball's shape—the smooth flow of interactions—even in the face of traumas from the outside and breakdowns in pathways on the inside. When

WHOLE SYSTEMS SCIENCE

Whole Systems Science looks at the web of connections within our bodies.

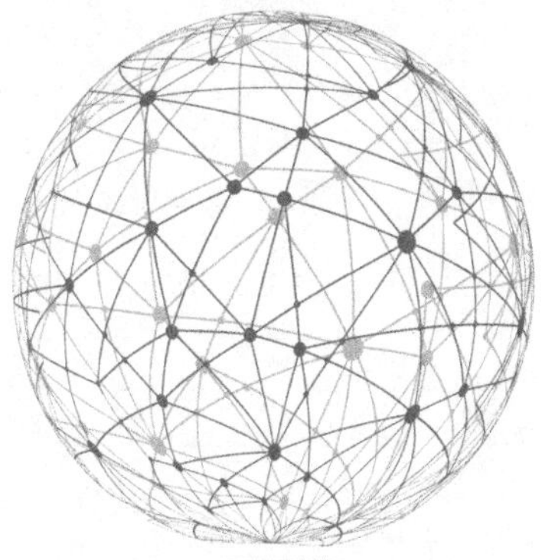

the ball is resilient, whenever a stress or trauma is put on it, the ball rebounds to its established shape and function and so maintains its health and wholeness. This epitomizes resilience. The network of the web also has multiple redundant pathways internally with which to maintain the chemical, energetic, psychological, and social flows when any of the individual links slow or break. Strong pathways can compensate for the weakest links.

Each node and link in the web involves hundreds of thousands of interdependent interactions that create complex chemical and energetic exchanges—billions and billions of simultaneous interactions—all designed to keep us surviving, functioning, and flourishing within a narrow range. If flow and shape are maintained, we experience health. If they break down or are disturbed, we experience disease or illness. We experience these interactions in our life as physical sensations and responses, symptoms and dysfunctions, emotions and feelings, thoughts and perceptions, social interactions with others—and sometimes as connections to unknowable forces beyond ourselves, which give rise to spiritual feelings and insights.

When we are healthy and resilient, this web of interactions exists in dynamic balance and vibrancy. Think of a young child reaching out and playing with his environment; a growing preteen curious and learning about himself and the world; an athlete or an artist at the top of her game and in the zone. We have all seen it. We have all felt it. We have all been there. When we are a person experiencing love, appreciation, peace, joy, and awe and are fully connected in body, mind, social interactions, and spiritual purpose, we then have a taste of full health and well-being. We are in the state that our body and mind is constantly trying to maintain. That is health.

We are not just a sack of chemicals, however. If we open the ball and look inside, we see at least four dimensions that make up a whole person. Manu drew a version of a whole person with three dimensions on his whiteboard when he was explaining to me how Ayurveda approached Aadi and his Parkinson's treatment to me. Modern science has discovered similar (and additional) dimensions that we use for healing. If we were to cut into this web-ball-person, we would see that their network consists of a physical domain on the outside (I call that the body), a set of behaviors under that, a network of social and emotional interactions and then an "inner domain"—involving our thoughts, expectations, intentions, and personal experiences—what we call the mind or spirit.

If we deal with only one aspect of a person—say, the body or the mind parts—we get only partial results, and we produce reverberations (often unwanted) throughout the rest of the person. To fully heal and be well, we need to enhance connections across all four dimensions of a human—body, behavior, social, and spiritual. Healing works by making those connections stronger and inducing us to become more whole and responsive in the world.

Every person has an inherent, automatic set of processes that continually seeks to maintain balance and vibrancy across all these dimensions and maintain the integrity of the entire network. The goal of a

THE WHOLE PERSON FROM THE PERSPECTIVE OF SYSTEMS SCIENCE

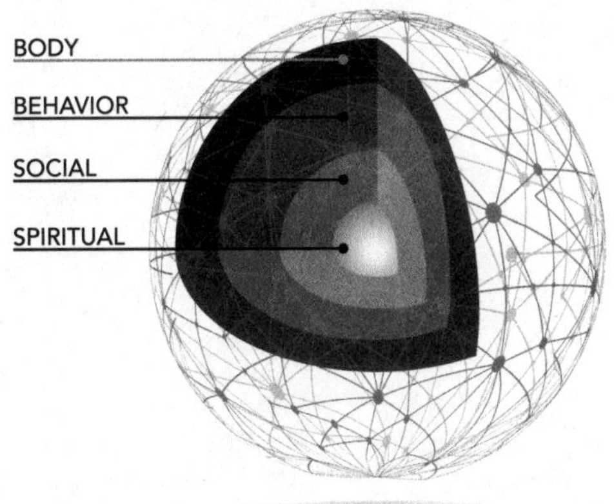

whole systems approach is to keep this in balance when we are well (in medical terms this is called prevention); to return balance when we are thrown off (this is called recovery); and to grow, interact, and flourish even if we have a chronic disease. This latter state is often referred to as well-being and can happen even when we have an incurable disease or are at the end of life. We have all experienced this sense of wholeness, vibrancy, and balance, even if only for a moment. This is health and well-being. Healing is the process that constantly strives to keep us in this state if we are healthy, and seeks to restore us to it when we are hit by trauma, stress, or illness. In medicine this view is called the "biopsychosocial" or "whole person" model of health care, and the science used to study it is called "whole systems science." Whole systems science is the science of the large and the whole. It is the foundation for the future of health care. But you can use it now.

So what happens when things are not working properly and we cannot return to homeostasis? Chronic illness happens when something goes wrong with a person, such that their web of health and healing is distorted.

From the whole systems science perspective, disease is a distortion in the shape or in the web of pathways. When an outside disturbance like a stress or trauma occurs, symptoms are produced as the person attempts to rebound, repair itself, and restore order and harmony again. If the disturbance is from a single cause or event, such as an acute trauma or infection, removing that cause will allow the person

DISEASE DISTORTS THE WEB OF HEALTH, BREAKS DOWN CONNECTIONS & INFLAMES NODES

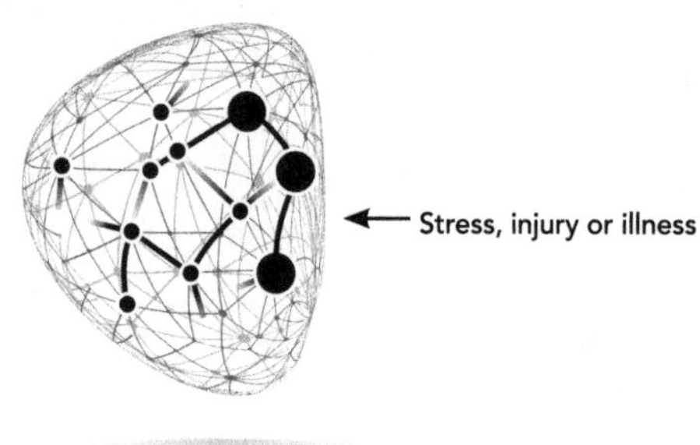

DISEASE-FOCUSED APPROACH

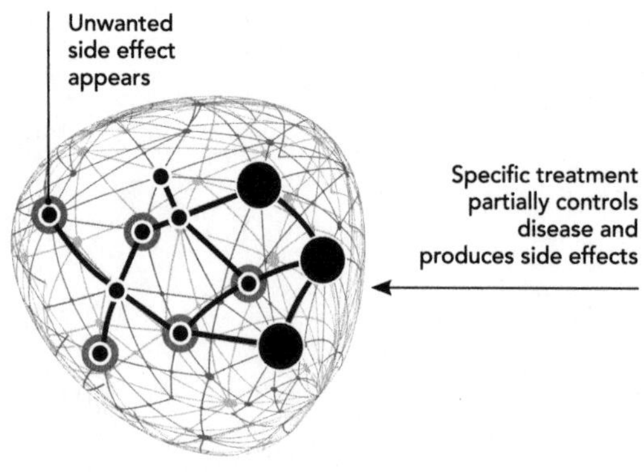

to come back to harmony rapidly. As we saw in the last chapter, if the causes are multiple, as is usual in chronic illness, attempts to control or remove the main distortions may partially control the disease but usually produce only a small or modest response.

A specific treatment is used to control the main disease manifestation. It may do that, but it also produces unwanted side effects in other areas of the body and mind. This is what happens when we apply only specific treatments—treatments derived from the science of the small and particular. It is also why so many of us end up on multiple drugs—each one designed to produce a specific effect. This is how we usually apply science when seeking cures.

THE MEANING RESPONSE

Whole systems science and the biopsychosocial model offer a different approach to healing. It's an approach that taps into this inherent capacity of a whole system to return to balance and maintain its integrity—and to produce the other 70% to 80% of healing. This approach stimulates and supports the person as a whole—connecting all four dimensions and nudging them to recover, rebalance, and restore the harmony that existed prior to the illness.

HEALING-FOCUSED APPROACH

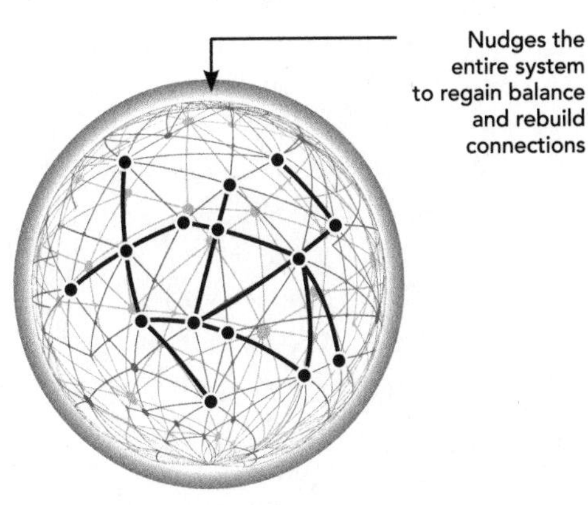

I call how this type of healing happens the "meaning response." Why? The definition of "meaning" is "the intended significance of something: the gist, drift, trend, or purpose." But this word is a bit too cerebral for what actually happens during healing. The word "response" means a reaction to a stimulus, whether that stimulus is a physical environment, a change in behavior, a social interaction, a medical or spiritual ritual, or a word. By combining the word "meaning" with the word "response," we get closer to the dynamic nature of what my patients experienced and what well-delivered health care systems can produce. When the meaning response occurs, the whole person—not just one specific part of the person—is stimulated and supported to return to balance, health and well-being.

This is what my patients had discovered and taught me—though it went against my established knowledge and opinions at the time. Healing works through the meaning response by improving the connections across all the dimensions of a person—by stimulating their response in a meaningful way.

Given our complex, redundant web of pathways, each person's journey to induce their meaning response can follow a different path and may use different tools and modalities. Some enter their healing journey using pills and potions, like Norma did. Some may completely change the setting in which they live, like Aadi. Some may find their journey starts with a change in attitude, like Bill. Whatever human activity is used as the entry point—through the body/external, behavior/lifestyle, social/emotional, or spiritual/mental—the pathway and processes for releasing our inherent healing capacity are similar for everyone. First, a deeply meaningful experience is found—often by engaging in a ritual of care. This helps us find the unique, best, and most enduring path for each of us. Second, all the core dimensions of a person are acknowledged—body/external, behavior/lifestyle, social/emotional, and spiritual/mental. This supports complex healing processes to the full extent and helps us use as many redundant pathways as possible. Finally, we engage in some stimulus for healing—usually a stress or challenge—followed by removal of the stimulus, then rest, so that we can rebound and recover. Periodic repetition of this stimulus keeps our body and mind resilient and responsive and on a continuous healing path.

To help organize this when I work with patients, and to help you organize this in your own life, I define four dimensions of healing for a person—body/external, behavior/lifestyle, social/emotional, and spiritual/mental—within which there are many available approaches, tools, and agents. I then use three processes to activate those dimensions for healing: meaning, support, and stimulus. When a person is well and wants to keep well, or when a person is ill and wants to recover their health, or when a person is dying and wants to find wellbeing, their healing journey involves exploring these four dimensions and engaging in these three processes. When that happens, healing emerges spontaneously and order is restored—like a healthy child recovering from a cold or an athlete rebounding from an injury or an elder dying in peace.

Healing approaches using whole systems science are just beginning to be developed in health care. As with any emerging discipline, it currently goes by many names, including the biopsychosocial model, complexity science, systems biology, systems medicine, personalized medicine, and most recently precision medicine and precision health. The NIH has recently embraced whole systems science with its Precision Medicine Initiative (PMI). PMI performs ongoing data collection on more than a million people in most of the dimensions of human functioning—from genetics to epigenetics—including behavior, medical treatment, and social interactions. Once collected, this database will become a rich source of information for better application of whole systems science and the meaning response in health care.

In the meantime, there are already examples of the power of whole systems science being applied in health care. These also go by various names, such as person-centered care, systems wellness, scientific wellness, precision wellness, functional medicine, and integrative health care. (In the second section of this book, I describe some of these systems and how you can find and use them.)

The late Professor David D. Price, a prominent research psychologist at the NIH, and world-renowned Italian neuroscientist Professor Fabrizio Benedetti analyzed all the research on how meaning and context impact chronic diseases: diseases with pain, like Norma and Bill's; Parkinson's disease, like Aadi's; or depression, like Sarah's. They and others have shown that our brains can produce large amounts of painkillers, anti-Parkinson's neurotransmitters, anti-depression chemicals, and immune modulators—an internal pharmacy used by the meaning response to heal. These chemicals are induced in the brain through rituals and behaviors that not only influence our beliefs and expectations but also stimulate and condition our bodies to respond to those rituals and behaviors in physical ways. Often these rituals involve the use of therapeutic agents such as pills or potions, drugs or herbs, needles or knives; or sophisticated technologies such as implanted electrodes or cell transplants; or softer methods such as massages or physical therapy. From the whole systems perspective, when we set out to heal chronic diseases, the specific agent used is less important than how the treatment is administered; that is, how the ritual of healing is constructed and the meaning response is induced. Armed with an understanding from whole systems science and the power of the meaning response, I could now understand how the remarkable recoveries I had seen provided me and others with the tools and processes for making the same thing happen in others' lives. The mystery of healing—why it happens or does not—was revealed.

BACK TO NORMA

When Norma had gotten better so dramatically from her arthritis and depression as she started taking the pills in the clinical study, I first thought she was on the active treatment, meaning I had discovered a cure for arthritis. When I found out she was on the placebo pill, I then assumed that she had gotten better because I was a good healer and she was suggestible. Her recovery and well-being must have been because I was a good communicator, I thought: I had induced in her a belief that she could get well, reinforced that belief with the treatment, and persuaded her that she could get better. Surely I was a master of biopsychosocial healing.

One of the most influential books in medicine during the last fifty years is a book called *Persuasion and Healing*, by psychiatrist Jerome Frank. I had read the book in medical school, and it influenced me greatly. Dr. Frank demonstrated that any type of psychotherapy has some basic features that account for its effectiveness: an emotionally charged relationship (I was Norma's favorite doctor), a healing setting (the clinic and hospital I saw her in), and a rationale or myth explaining the symptoms and process for resolving them (my hypothesis was that the vitamin could cure arthritis).

Most doctors like to think when a patient gets better, it is because of their treatment and care. This is what keeps us going. It is self-satisfying to think that. But I soon found that the main explanation for Norma's improvement was not the vitamin I had given her nor my miraculous persuasion powers. Norma's recovery was a lot more mundane and less magical than that. When I revealed to Norma that she had been on the placebo, she was with her daughter. Her daughter told me that getting back to her volunteer job in the hospital was one of the most important things her mom wanted in her current stage of life. Before the study, she did not feel like going to the hospital and sat at home, remaining sedentary for long periods. This made her feel worse. Soon after starting the placebo, Norma began to tell herself she felt better and forced herself to start back at her volunteer job. Even before the treatment was supposed to kick in, her activity level increased. After she started taking the pills she began to go into the hospital regularly—at first once a week, then three times a week, then every day.

Now, we know that one of the most effective ways to prevent deterioration and even improve arthritis is to keep active. Exercise reduces pain, improves mood, and slows or reverses the decline from almost any illness—including arthritis and depression. It is one of those general healing nudges. Norma had an important purpose (her job at the hospital), and joining the study had linked that purpose to a behavior that stressed her body with exercise in a way that improved her pain and function and allowed her to nourish her soul with social contact. Her remarkable recovery had little to do with the vitamin or my powers of persuasion. It occurred because she used a compelling life purpose—meaning—to take her outside her physical comfort zone and stimulate her natural recovery capacity through exercise.

I also discovered that something else had helped induce an improvement. She was taking a pill four times a day.

Medical treatments in many systems involve taking pills and potions, whether they are drugs, herbs, vitamins, or over-the-counter liquids or tinctures. Taking a substance, especially if it is accompanied with a sense of feeling better, induces a "conditioned response" in which the act of doing something—especially something requiring a physical act or a substance with a unique smell or flavor—trains the body to respond in a way that reinforces the improvement. Like Pavlov's dogs, which were conditioned to salivate upon the ringing of a bell, we learn to heal upon the swallowing of a pill—including a placebo pill. Our conditioned stimulus (the event that triggers the response) can be almost anything: a pill or a shot, a taste or smell, a needle, a knife or a touch; even an energy stimulus like a light, a sound, or heat or cold. The conditioned stimulus is how our belief and meaning—the reason we seek healing—gets linked to a physical response in our body in a repeated and continuous way. Dr. Kaufmann, who wrote the book on the use of niacinamide—the vitamin I was testing for arthritis—told me that it was very important that patients take frequent doses—a minimum of four times a day rather than using a more slowly absorbed version fewer times a day. His rationale was that the fluctuation of the vitamin in the blood was needed to reduce inflammation in the joints. This, as later studies showed, was not true. Still, he had tried time-released versions of the vitamin that were taken less often, and they didn't work as well, he said. But what he had likely stumbled upon was a universal principle of healing—frequent dosing improves healing through conditioning. In fact, for some conditions, if an effective treatment has the number of pills reduced from four pills a day to two pills a day, a physician has to treat as many as twelve additional patients with the less frequent dosing in order for one patient to benefit. Statisticians call this the "number needed to treat" (NNT). This happens in other diseases also. The effect is seen not just in "soft" outcomes like pain or depression; it even results in different death rates. Several studies have shown that patients with heart disease who take all their medication have a lower death rate than those who do not take all their medications—even when that "medication" is a placebo. Like Norma, they do better if they do it more often. Norma not only took four pills a day during the study, but she was also one of my most eager and compliant patients. At least, I thought, I could take some solace that by interacting with me she had pushed through her pain and gotten on a healing path. What actually happened is that Norma had activated her healing in each dimension of her being. She began to move more (body), she started taking more pills that both she and I believed in (behavior), she engaged with others in her volunteer work (social), and she re-established her purpose in life, which was to help others (spirit). Her healing was not from the agent she took; it was from her own agency she found.

NORMA'S PATH TO HEALING

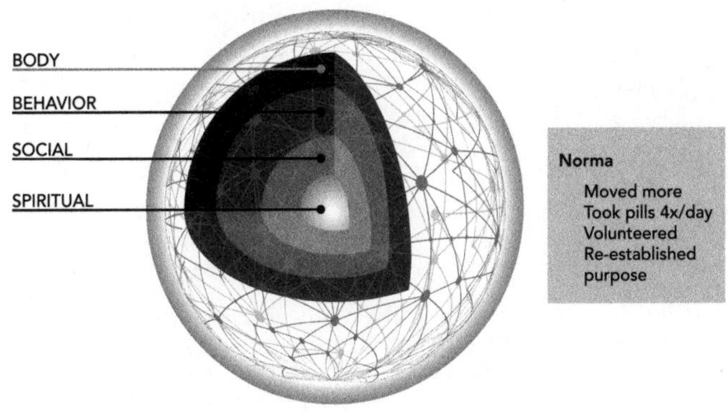

Sergeant Martin found healing through a different path, but by using the same process of finding meaning, whole person support, and using a stimulus to heal.

BACK TO SERGEANT MARTIN

Sergeant Martin hated me. It had not always been that way. For over a year, he and I had worked together seeking the best treatment for his traumatic brain injury and PTSD by juggling various medications, counselors, and social workers. We even tried meditation and "exposure therapy"—the proven standard of care for PTSD in which a patient is gradually exposed to the very things that induce fear and nightmares in them until they learn not to react. He stopped after two sessions. "It was terrible," he confessed to me. "Why would I want to relive that memory again?" I was sorry to see him stop, because the science said that it worked. That is when I referred him to music therapy, and he learned about Beethoven's Ninth Symphony. The music therapist said there was something about that symphony that changed him. Perhaps he identified with the struggle the deaf Beethoven had in writing and performing it. Sergeant Martin listened to it repeatedly.

Soon after that, he and his father came in and insisted I refer him to hyperbaric oxygen treatments. It was my turn to draw the line. The science was clear—hyperbaric oxygen did not work. I wasn't going to recommend a "quack" therapy. Both Sergeant Martin and his father left my office angry. I think their last word to me was an expletive. I was pretty sure my powers of persuasion and empathy were not working with them. It was not my finest hour as a healer.

Almost a year later, when I bumped into Sergeant Martin in the hospital hallway, he was markedly better and off medications, but hesitant to talk with me. But I was truly curious as to how he had gotten so much better, and that convinced him to talk. I wondered: had Sergeant Martin also created the fundamentals of healing—meaning, support, and stimulus—with an ineffective therapy and against my recommendations?

"To tell you the truth, Doc," he finally confessed, "when I left your office with my father that day, I was at my wits' end and ready to give up. I mean, I was ready to give up on everything, including my life. I wanted to commit suicide. But my dad convinced me to go to the hyperbaric clinic and said he would pay for it. I felt bad about how he cursed at you, but what could I do? You had your shot with me for over a year."

I knew he was right. We had tried everything I knew to help him.

"When I got to the hyperbaric clinic," Sergeant Martin continued, "I felt I had come home. There were guys there just like me claiming that they were getting better with the oxygen treatment and putting their lives back together. It was the first time I felt hopeful—that I might be able to heal, to have a seminormal life."

What I immediately thought but did not dare voice to Sergeant Martin was that he had found something he believed in and a group to reinforce that belief. I listened instead. Sergeant Martin went on, "After my first oxygen session, I felt better. There was this rush in my ears and fresh air flowing into my lungs. When I left, my mind was clearer; I had more energy. I even mustered a small smile. And the improvements just kept on coming. Soon, I found that I was the one giving hope to other battle buddies coming in. Guys with brain injury and PTSD who came in hopeless. I told them to hang in there. Instead of me always telling my story, I found that I was listening to others tell theirs, and I could really listen now. I could help them."

Sergeant Martin went on to explain how the hyperbaric oxygen worked—an explanation that has been disproven. He explained to me that there were areas of his brain from the injury that could not effectively use oxygen, and when it was forced into his system under pressure, those brain areas "woke up" and began to function again. I say this has been disproven because good studies have shown that breathing even room air—without high oxygen—and at a low pressure also can also improve function. No more oxygen than usual was getting to the brain in those cases, but people got better anyway. In fact, other studies showed that small doses of ischemia—*low* oxygen—can also induce healing responses in the brain. It was the small physiological stress that stimulated healing. Professor Benedetti, whose research on placebo, pain, and performance I described previously, has demonstrated that many of the physiological and functional effects of 100% oxygen can be produced by room air in people working at high altitude when they collectively believe they are getting 100% oxygen and that they will benefit from it.

While Sergeant Martin believed in his own explanation—that more oxygen was penetrating his brain—what he was actually experiencing was a mild stressful stimulus to his body in a positive environment that, as happened to Norma, that conditioned him to improve. But unlike Norma, whose stimulus involved working through the pain of exercise because of an inert pill, Sergeant Martin got an abnormal physiological jolt of a mild toxin—high oxygen—that his body responded to by rallying a repair reaction. Getting high oxygen may seem counterintuitive. After all, isn't oxygen good for you? Sergeant Martin believed (and his practitioners said) that his brain was getting the oxygen it needed. However, the normal concentration of oxygen in the air and the amount the body is used to is about 20%. Oxygen at 100% delivered under high pressure (as Sergeant Martin received) is actually slightly toxic to the body. This induces the body to protect itself by increasing antioxidant production and other repair processes and accelerates healing. The same healing reaction can be induced with no increase in oxygen or even with low oxygen—or other stressors.

I will describe the ritual he did in more detail in a later chapter, but at this point I had learned that Sergeant Martin found, like Norma, a meaningful way to heal himself by helping other service members with brain injury and PTSD. While his condition and treatments were completely different from Norma's, the healing processes he used were the same. He had lined up a meaningful therapy he believed in, done it in a supportive environment, and used high oxygen as a physical stimulus to condition a recovery response that working with me had not.

BACK TO BILL

This world we live in is a relentless place. Often it seems that traumas and stresses come at us continuously, wearing us down, only to hit us with even more difficult ones. Sometimes, they seem to come all at once—a death of a loved one, loss of a job, a car accident, a serious disease. Other times, it is more like water torture—drip, drip, dripping small and continuous stresses that will not let up and have no end in sight. Regardless of which way life brings us traumas, no amount of treatment or therapy will wipe away suffering unless we also build our resilience and recovery capacity. There is no magic cure for suffering, but there is an ability to recover and be happy—if we are willing to walk the labyrinth of healing and use the tools at our disposal to help. Whole systems science and the meaning response teach us that we have a smorgasbord of healing options—proven and unproven—if we adhere to a few basic principles.

Bill showed me, more than any other patient, how to walk that labyrinth. Unlike Norma, Bill was not a believer in any treatment. Nor was I his favorite physician. Unlike Sergeant Martin, he was not antagonistic toward me. Nor was he looking for any particular type of therapy—alternative or conventional. Of course, he wanted the scientifically best treatments for his back pain, if possible, but even more than that, he just wanted to get better. He had tried so many milder treatments that he wanted something "stronger," as he put it. One might think that having a family member with strong beliefs—like his wife, with her belief in acupuncture, might strengthen one's personal beliefs and help with healing. But this is not always the case. Family members, like physicians, are often trying to "fix" a person with chronic illness—getting them to see the doctor, try new treatments, and change behaviors. This pressure can sometimes backfire, however, making the person resistant to those suggestions, or worse, when the treatments fail, reinforcing their despair that recovery from their illness is hopeless. Over the years, Bill had been to the best pain centers in the world—Walter Reed, Johns Hopkins, and veterans' hospitals. He had told his back pain history hundreds of times, and each time someone had tried to help him with one or more treatments.

Gradually, as Bill told me when he came in for his pre-op evaluation, he needed something stronger because over the years, he had "become" his back pain. It dominated his life. Others helped reinforce that with all their treatments. He had finally stopped seeing doctors until his wife recommended acupuncture. But, like the other treatments, it had only a mild effect. Surgery was his best hope. He wanted to "cut out the pain," he said.

And it worked for a while. Bill got rapid relief from the surgery. It lasted nine months. Then it came back.

Why did it work? Why did it come back? Bill believed in surgery. So did his doctors. Modern cultures generally believe in surgery. It helped him to do what was most important and meaningful to him—to be with his grandkids. But back surgery of the type Bill had is actually not effective when tested in rigorous research—sham surgery works just as well. Still, surgery can be an excellent stimulus for self-healing. Like other treatments, it can work well when the components of healing—meaning, support, and stimulus—are aligned. However, unlike the four pills a day and regular exercise Norma did or the repeated oxygen and social reinforcement of Sergeant Martin, Bill could not repeat the stimulus. Surgery is usually done only once or twice.

It was after his relapse that Bill came back to see me, this time not to find another "fix," but to do the hard work of navigating the labyrinth of healing processes until he found the combination that helped him sustain self-healing. The journey was not quick, and, for Bill, it involved facing some deep traumas from his childhood that he unveiled during one of our visits after he started to keep a journal. As the meaning of who he was and why he was here began to help him connect his body to the emotional parts of himself, a deeper healing began. Once Bill understood the connection between his childhood traumas and his bodily reactions he found it easier to do the things he needed to do to keep his back pain at bay—such as managing his sleep and alcohol use, doing regular exercise, stretching, and having periodic massage. Gradually he broke free of his addiction to cures and learned how to support and challenge himself to continually heal. True to his word, he documented his path, and spoke with me throughout the process so I could better understand how he found healing. One day during our discussions of his process, he came out with it bluntly. "Once I stopped seeking a single fix," he told me, "I realized that all these good-intentioned people and wonderful treatments were actually making me worse. When I decided to find out what I needed for a better life in general, that is the moment I began to really heal from my pain." Bill had become his own healing agent.

BACK TO AADI

Armed with the growing tools of whole systems science, I went back to India to explore if it could help me understand what was happening to Aadi and his Parkinson's disease. Did they align with the components of healing and the concepts of whole systems science I was discovering? I took a deep dive into the ancient medicine of Ayurveda with this new lens.

Like Bill, Aadi was not a religious or even very introspective man. His approach to everything was businesslike. He wanted to know what needed to be done and how to do it. Like Bill, problems were to be fixed when they arose so he could move on to the next one. The bottom line of life was the measurable advance in prosperity for him and his family. When Parkinson's disease struck, he approached it in a similar way. Here was something to be fixed too, and the doctors were ready to help him to do just that.

But when visits and treatments from the top doctors in the world did not allow him to get back to work, he grew despondent. That is when his wife visited the Ayurveda hospital and asked for an astrology reading for him. She felt that they needed to seek a deeper understanding for his illness and why the treatments were not working. Aadi thought it was ridiculous. He had no time for "pseudoscience," like astrology or prayer to the Hindu gods, in whom he had no belief. Like Bill, he agreed to go to the clinic to get his wife off his back. Anyway, he thought, it might give him some rest. That, he admitted, he needed.

Like me, Aadi was a bit startled to meet Dr. Manu for the first time, with his impeccable Oxford English and his knowledge of Western science.

Dr. Manu said that there was no requirement for Aadi to believe in any of the treatments. "Ayurveda has been honed over thousands of years to produce a fundamental change in your mind and body," he said. "All that is required is that you go through the treatments for at least thirty days. Parkinson's is a serious and difficult problem, so each treatment is essential in restoring balance and recovery." Aadi agreed. He also liked the idea of having my team explore the possible biology of what he was doing.

But the evidence using the science of the small and particular was bleak. First, there was no evidence that the treatments and lifestyle changes Aadi undertook could help Parkinson's specifically. Although he did get some sleep, the process was not a picnic. Each morning he got up early and went to a prayer ceremony in which a Hindu priest went through a long series of chants and rituals. While Aadi did not believe in any of the gods to which they prayed, the rhythmic tone and repetitive motions produced a calming effect to start the day. Since no alcohol was allowed, he soon found his mind much clearer than at home. By the second week, he looked forward to this start of the day. In two weeks, the mental worries around his work and family began to fade. His sleep improved; he began spontaneously waking up early with a clear mind and more energy. Dr. Manu said that Ayurveda had a name for this mental state—*sattvic mind*. This mental state, he said, is one of the core goals of all Ayurvedic treatment and a foundation for healing. In the West, the closest term we have for this state is the *relaxation response*, coined by Dr. Herbert Benson at Harvard Medical School in the 1970s. Dr. Benson was one of the first scientists to study monks in India who meditated for many hours a day. In the 1960s, he measured the profound changes in their brains and bodies that resulted. Since then, he and others have shown mind-body practices that induce what he calls the relaxation response improves physiology, biochemistry, and genetics for a number of conditions. Eight weeks of mindfulness practice (a method to induce the relaxation response), for example, has been shown to grow areas of the brain that often shrink in Parkinson's disease.

Beyond that, however, the morning ceremony and other sattvic mind practices allowed Aadi to explore more deeply why he was so driven to succeed in business. He was the second of five children; his father had always praised his older brother for excelling in school and entrepreneurship, and he'd given him money to develop a small business. Aadi, who was four years younger, could never meet his father's expectations. So he had tried harder. Although he'd become a highly successful businessman, his father had died before seeing his success. Still, the pattern was set from a young age—keep your head down, work hard, compete, and grow wealth. Aadi realized by the end of his thirty days at the Ayurvedic hospital that he had internalized that drive, which often made him callous to others and even caused him to ignore the pain of many whom he loved—and any pain he felt himself. He began to think more about his family and what his life and legacy were about.

Had this been all the mental work Aadi did, it would have been little more than a type of psychotherapy. However, other practices were used to reinforce this relaxation and induce a physical response to the soul he was discovering. The goal was to deepen the meaning he found and embed it into his bodily response. The chief method for this was yoga and diet. One hour of yoga each day not only reinforced the relaxation response and improved circulation to all areas of Aadi's body but also strengthened his muscles and reduced his tremor and unsteadiness. It was not easy; in fact, it was at first downright stressful.

"I didn't like yoga," Aadi admitted. "I was never one to exercise, and this was hard. My muscles were sore the day after the sessions for the first fifteen days." What yoga was doing for Aadi was like what Norma's activity did for her—it introduced a mild traumatic stimulus that produced healing. Over thirty days, Aadi's mobility, strength, balance, and flexibility improved, and parts of the activity—primarily the ending—started to grow on him.

"I loved the ending of the yoga sessions," he said. "It is a posture called 'the corpse' in which you just lie still on your back with arms facing up. It was then that a flood of love would come to me. I would imagine my wife and children and all the affection I had for them and them for me. It was wonderful. I saw and felt what was really important to me."

Finally, his sattvic mind was linked to his body through an oil massage once a week. But the oil massage of Ayurveda is not like the spa treatments given in the West. Two masseurs, one on each side of the body, would rub his body with warm sesame oil in a coordinated and rhythmic pattern, infusing his body with oil and heating it. This was followed by running a small stream of warm oil over his forehead (a procedure called *shirodhara*) with the goal of inducing a sense of relaxation and mental clarity. I asked Manu about this seemingly strange practice.

"Both yoga and shirodhara are done for the same purpose," he said. "To cleanse the body and mind and to help link the understanding Aadi is getting from prayer and meditation to his body, so that both his spiritual and physical life are balanced and function as one."

I did not buy that explanation. When we looked at these and other practices Aadi received, we found the primary molecular changes they produced had nothing to do with cleansing. Instead, they all seemed geared toward inducing nonspecific changes in Aadi's psychological and physical healing responses through repeated mild stress and trauma, followed by deep relaxation during which repair occurred. This happened also with the diet and herbal treatments he underwent. The prayer was followed by a light breakfast, the yoga, a midday meal, and sometimes cathartics and enemas all geared toward "cleansing" as Manu explained. But the food served during his stay was very different than his normal fare. It was all vegetarian and high in curcumin, garlic, and other Indian spices. Fasting was also introduced. Once a week, he fasted for a full twenty-four hours, taking in only vegetable broth and water. Basically, Aadi was undergoing a controlled form of starvation. I was shocked. How could mild starvation help heal Parkinson's?

THE STIMULUS TO HEAL

While periodic starvation may sound harsh and not healing, studies show the exact opposite—when carefully done. Extensive research on large populations, as well as in controlled studies with animals and humans, shows that periodic low-calorie intake, whether through eating foods with lower caloric density (vegetables and fruits), fasting, or simply removing protein from the diet for short periods of time, rapidly stimulates a number of healing responses. Would short episodes of fasting and low protein intake, like those Aadi had been experiencing, increase biochemical mechanisms that preserve and repair damage produced by eating?

To find out, I asked Dr. Mark Mattson, a senior scientist at the National Institute of Aging, part of the NIH. He has been studying effects of diet and fasting on healing and aging for over thirty years. Dr. Mattson is one of the most cited scientists in the world. I asked him, "Could periodic fasting and low-calorie or low-protein intake, like Aadi went through, produce benefit?"

Dr. Mattson had a long and detailed answer, but the short version was a definite yes. Eating both nourishes and causes damage in the body. It supports and feeds the body with nutrients, and it stimulates oxidative and inflammatory processes that, over a lifetime, accelerate aging and damage organs. Refraining from food, or certain types of food, both helps heal some diseases and reduces the risk of chronic disease. Managing the dance between eating and not eating is key to healing and longevity. Periodic fasting (not prolonged starvation), according to Dr. Mattson and other brain researchers, enhances a whole soup of gene and biochemical factors associated with better health, lower disease, and longer life. It also improves mental function and lowers the risk for several diseases of aging, including diabetes, heart disease, brain decline, and cancer. Like exercise, Aadi's lower protein and calorie intake was a periodic stimulus to healing, which conditioned him into a regular pattern.

"The problem," Aadi readily admitted, "is that it was hard to keep up these behaviors once I left the hospital. Outside I relied more on supplements and herbs." But, he concluded, "they were not as powerful as what I got at the hospital. That is why I come back every year or so for a booster." Then he asked me, "So what did you find out about these treatments? Is there any science to them, or are they all just magic?"

They were not magic, but they were also not proven with the science of the small and particular. Were the potions and pills he was given specific treatments for Parkinson's disease? Not likely, I said, given what I had seen about both drug and herbal research for Parkinson's. But from a whole systems science perspective, the rationale of these treatments made a lot of sense. Most of the herbs Aadi was given had anti-inflammatory effects, as did the spices in his food. One, a powder from a tropical legume, *Mucuna pruriens*, had been studied for its effect on the level of L-dopamine in the brain, but the amount was too little to produce the magnitude of improvement he had experienced.

As I pieced together the various approaches Aadi underwent during his stay at the Ayurveda hospital, it became clear that the most likely explanation for his recovery involved the same factors that had healed Norma, Sergeant Martin, and Bill—just differently organized and in a different context. These had helped Aadi find meaning in his life, even though he did not believe in astrology or Hindu gods. The space and time to reflect, think, and talk; his improved sleep; and no alcohol all helped him gain insight and grow new brain cells. This helped him discover meaning and guide him toward recovery. He exercised more, and his nutrition improved with the plant-based diet and spices. More omega-3 and omega-6 fatty acids from the oil massage reduced the inflammation in his brain and nourished his neurons. The herbs and supplements increased his dopamine level—although mostly through the placebo effect from simply taking them. Finally, numerous methods for regularly stimulating a healing response with low-dose stressors were administered. Yoga, fasting, cathartics, massage, heat, and enemas were given rhythmically to keep up a steady response. From a whole systems perspective, these small challenges induce stress proteins and genes that our bodies use to repair and defend itself. These were the nudges to his whole system that induced healing.

The problem with the traditional systems is that the practitioners do not know if what they are doing is, in fact, properly dosed or delivered. While I discovered several healing approaches with factors that could enhance healing, the effects of these treatments were not measured or tracked, except for the patients' subjective reports. No modern science had been applied to them. Of course, that does not mean this science can't be done. Recently, a growing number of studies has looked at the intersection of whole systems science and traditional medical systems. An example of this growing intersection is a course taught at Harvard and the Massachusetts Institute of Technology by Dr. V. A. Shiva Ayyadurai, CEO of a systems science company called CytoSolve. The course examines the relationship of whole systems science and Ayurveda. Clinical verification of these concepts is also beginning. A 2016 study by researchers at the University of California, San Diego, examined more than fifty metabolic pathways altered by a six-day course of treatment using ayurveda approaches like those Aadi had received.

THE PRINCIPLES OF HEALING

In condition after condition, system after system, and person after person, I found three common factors that induced healing: (1) the rituals that helped a person have a meaningful experience, (2) the support of the whole person, and (3) the regular stimulation of a biological response. The specific treatments and agents used varied by person, culture, theory, and place, but the processes were the same. Whole systems science showed us that a person is an ecosystem—*more like a garden to be cultivated than a car to be fixed.* In systems science, the safest and greatest effects occur when the whole person is nudged toward a meaning response, using the universal need to maintain dynamic stability as the healing force. By taking advantage of this force, health and resilience emerge. Instead of manipulating our network nodes and attempting to produce specific effects (and side effects), we strengthen our network links and stimulate our own healing capacity in nonspecific ways to achieve a deeper and more lasting healing.

Healing emerges when we support and strengthen the connections within us—body, behavior, social, and spirit—making us more whole. Using the science of the large and the whole, we now understand that both healing and wholeness involve the same processes and that inducing a meaning response enables both.

Whole systems science, the biopsychosocial model, and the meaning response also allow us to personalize healing in precise ways using almost any agent or behavior. This understanding opens new worlds of opportunity. Treatments usually dismissed—because they do not fit the science of the small and particular—now become available for effective use in a new way. We know that both before and after a diagnosis, and between states of health and disease, there are health-promoting conditions and actions that can prevent, slow, or reverse chronic disease, strengthen overall health, improve function and quality of life, and enhance overall resilience and well-being. We can reduce suffering, regardless of a person's illness or stage of life, provided our behaviors are meaningful, they support and nourish us, and we challenge ourselves to respond.

This is how healing works.

section 2

THE DIMENSIONS OF HEALING

CHAPTER 5

Coming Home

The place where you live can heal.

Our external physical environment affects our mind and body in ways that heal or hurt us. And that happens mostly outside our awareness. Sometimes, if we simply immerse ourselves in a healing environment, our body responds and we get better. Sometimes the environment is what is making us sick. Cultures around the world have systems to design a space and environment to impact the mind, body, spirit, and well-being. The Japanese tea garden is a well-known example of this. Other approaches include sacred geometry, healing design, feng shui, anthroposophical systems, and Ayurvedic systems. Until recently, modern health care has largely ignored the effect of space on health and well-being. Yet everyone can describe a place they have been where they feel whole and well. And some of us have spent time in "sick buildings."

The key to using the external environment to stay or get well is connecting the physical aspects of your life—the aspects you can see, smell, hear, and touch—with the inner aspects of you—the ones that give your life deep meaning and value. This involves paying attention to how your body and mind already respond to the space you are in, and then organizing the elements of your own healing environment to maintain and restore health. Create your own stage, so to speak, for the drama of healing to happen.

As I sat down to write this part of the book, my wife, Susan, and I were given the challenge of navigating this healing path again. She has given me permission to tell our story.

SUSAN

Our three-month-old grandchild discovered Susan's breast cancer. Well, the baby did not actually discover it, but it was because of him that Susan, who was helping take care of him, found the cancer. Cradled in her arms, the baby's head pressed against the area in her left breast where the cancer was, triggering her to notice the growth. For years, we had been looking forward to having a grandchild, and we were overjoyed when he came. However, his mother had complications after the birth and required some extra care, so my wife enthusiastically volunteered to help care for the baby as our daughter-in-law recovered. Susan loved the job, exhausting as it was, and would hold and carry the baby during the day and even part of the night.

"I think he must have bruised my breast," she told me one evening. "I have a small sore spot where his head presses. But it is not going away."

We both immediately suspected something more ominous. You see, Susan had had breast cancer before—twenty-five years before, and in the same location. She also had a personal and family history full of cancer. Her father had died at fifty-seven of lung cancer. Her paternal aunt and cousin had died at a young age from breast cancer.

This was also her fifth time with some type of cancer—breast, melanoma, basal cell, and squamous cell. Susan's first breast cancer had appeared when she was thirty-five. We had three young children. We cried for days that first time. Her father had suffered a lot as his lung cancer progressed, and we were only a few years out from that experience and his passing.

We had built a treatment and healing ritual that helped her to recover and be cancer-free for twenty-five years. Now, when the MRI and biopsy confirmed another cancer—a different type of breast cancer this time, likely induced by her treatments for the first one—we had a good idea of what we were up against.

The treatments—three types of chemotherapy, a bilateral mastectomy followed by antiestrogen drugs—were going to require that Susan tap deeply into her own capacity to heal, not so much from the disease as from the therapies. As is too often the case in health care today, healing is needed as much to recover from the treatments as to deal with the disease. We are in an age of heroic medicine where there is a thin line between the benefits and harms caused by treatment. This is especially true for cancer treatments. Dealing with the disease *and* the therapy requires resilience and the ability to recover. We needed to tap deeply into her healing capacity.

BABIES AND GRANDBABIES

You would think that the first thing someone would think about after being diagnosed with cancer is survival. And for most this is true. Almost all of medicine and biomedical science is thrown at that issue. Finding a cure for cancer is a constant mantra in medicine; it is what drives some of our most extreme treatments. Alleviating suffering tends to take a backseat. You can see it in the response people have when they hear the diagnosis, and you can hear it in the words our culture uses to fight it—the war on cancer, cut it out, burn it out, poison it, eliminate it, get rid of it, cancer is the enemy, victory over cancer. Oncologists focus on cure data, mostly by doing large studies to calculate the five- and ten-year survival rates under various treatments. You get cured only when the disease is gone—and gone for a long time. When a patient learns she has cancer, she seeks out anything that looks like a magic bullet—something proven to eliminate the disease. Many treatments have permanent effects that people must cope with for the rest of their lives. We usually accept those treatments even if the benefits are small and the side effects large (even when eliminating the tumor is not the most important thing for us). For Susan, the first thing on her mind was not a cure—it was the grandbaby.

It was not that Susan did not want to live long enough to enjoy the child and the family and have more life for other things. It was just that she realized life was more than a quantity; it was also a quality. Because she'd experienced cancer and its treatments before, she knew firsthand the lifelong impact of chemotherapy, radiation, and surgery. And her reasons for long-term survival are different now because all our children are grown and doing well. And she knows from experience the rather modest improvement that treatments make to survival rates. Twenty-five years ago, they did not know if chemotherapy for her type and stage of breast cancer was of any benefit. Now they can tell more precisely what it would add to her chances of living over the years. Whatever the reason for her perspective, the quality of the *now* became as important as the probability of a *later* for her.

None of the physicians asked what her main goals from treatment were. They assumed she would follow their recommendations to increase survival, even by a small margin, at almost any cost. They did not ask what was most important for Susan at this stage in her life. They did not ask if she wanted to weigh the harms of treatment against the potential gains. They did not know about the grandchild. Yet it was our grandchild who dominated many of Susan's decisions for what treatments she would undergo and when, and how she would organize her healing rituals. Without a word, our grandchild not only helped find the cancer but also was influencing its management. The dominating question for her became, how could she undergo the intensive treatments needed and also spend time caring for her grandchild? The path to this was not obvious.

TO CURE OR TO HEAL?

Susan and I have always been very different in our responses to her cancers. I, like most physicians, am a doer—always looking for something to add or manipulate in a person with the idea it will cure them. Susan is more of a be-er—weighing the value of these recommendations with her own values and desires. When faced with a challenge, my instinct is to do it all and look everywhere. If there's a hint of evidence for benefit, I like to try it out, provided the risks are not too great. My wife, on the other hand, is a minimalist; her attitude is "Tell me what I absolutely have to do and I'll do it grudgingly, folding up inside my shell and sleeping until it's over." Healing requires both responses, but not too much of either one. Most important, the response must be created by and meaningful for the person in need of the healing. The methods, whether trying out multiple treatments or holing up in bed, are all simply techniques for navigating the maze of responses when our health and life are threatened.

During her first breast cancer twenty-five years ago, the first thing she did instinctively was to reach out to friends and family and find support for her children as she underwent treatment. Fortunately, our children attended a school that was extremely nurturing to everyone in the family and took special attention to care for them during the process. Second, Susan had an older friend who became a surrogate grandmother and "adopted" us. A joyful and caring woman, she not only helped Susan through chemotherapy, surgery, and radiation, she nurtured the children as well. This support network (and Susan's age) allowed her to undergo intensive chemotherapy and recover rather rapidly, but not without some long-term residual problems including increased weight, early onset of menopause, some cognitive impact (called "chemo brain" in the medical literature), lymphedema, and mild damage to her nerves—peripheral neuropathy, which causes numbness and tingling in the fingers and toes.

Meanwhile, I was out looking for cures. At that time, I fully drank the biomedical Kool-Aid. I was convinced that science- and evidence-based treatments were out there for cancer. I read about and collected articles and books about cancer treatments. I talked to my colleagues to get their thoughts and recommendations. I urged Susan to do many of these treatments. Often, they were not available locally. She complied for a while as we traveled around and tried many of them—me looking for a magic bullet; she rather reluctantly. Most of those treatments turned out to be useless, and some even diminished the quality of her life—and mine. At the time, I did not understand about the decline effect whereby treatments initially look beneficial but further research demonstrates their limited impact. I was only beginning to understand the role of the meaning response in healing.

When Susan was diagnosed with breast cancer the second time, the first thing I explored was the possible benefit of her getting other types of therapies besides the conventional chemo and surgery. I considered supplements to prevent neuropathy and chemo brain, immune therapies to prevent recurrence, and lifestyle changes—exercise and diet—for overall health and recovery. But the evidence for most of these approaches was modest or nonexistent. In addition, the local oncologists had no expertise in these approaches; you had to travel to find them. Susan had promised and wanted to help our son and daughter-in-law take care of the baby. So running off to another part of the world to try other treatments and tests was simply out of the question. Even seeking out those treatments would remove from her one of the most meaningful activities she had in her life.

"We need to find something else," she told me, "close to home and just as good." We then found out that advances in breast cancer management would make that challenging in a different way.

In the last twenty-five years, there have been major advances in the management of breast cancer. These new approaches are guided by genetic testing. The nice thing about genetic tests is they can help tell what the survival benefit from chemotherapy will be for many patients—so they provide that therapy for only those it will help and avoid harming all the others. Susan had those tests and hoped she would not need chemotherapy. Unfortunately, her tests demonstrated that Susan was highly susceptible to a recurrence of the tumor. New chemotherapies like paclitaxel that hadn't existed twenty-five years before might be helpful to reduce that risk. The additional benefits of chemotherapy were modest, improving her ten-year survival chances by 7%—from 88% to 95%. Also, new and sophisticated imaging tests showed that she had atypical cells in her other breast that might become cancer in several years. *Might* was the operative word in this case. We had no idea whether that would happen. Between 30% and 50% of breast cancers detected by these new imaging methods will likely not advance to become problematic. We just don't know which patients those will be, so we treat them all as if they are at high risk. Genetic testing is helping us find out which patients may benefit from treatment and which patients the treatment may harm, but there is uncertainty for many. Still, none of this was known twenty-five years ago. For Susan, however, it soon became clear what she wanted to do. Chemotherapy would reduce her chances of recurrence by 7%. The genetic tests, the abnormal findings in her other breast, and her own personal and family history of previous cancers moved her to decide that the best approach for improving long-term survival involved several rather harsh treatments. She was at high risk for recurrence, so she decided to "hit it with all barrels"—twenty weeks of three types of chemotherapy followed by a double mastectomy followed by ten years of an antiestrogen drug. She would need to tap into her 80% healing capacity just to withstand the cure. The healing would be hard.

So would taking care of the baby. How was she going to undergo all these treatments, attempt the supplements and lifestyle changes I suggested, and be with the baby? These three seemingly incompatible forces converged on her. Navigating between her most meaningful activity—being with our grandchild—and the steamroller of medical treatments that might compromise both her short- and long-term function would be daunting. How could she find the right path toward healing?

Susan was now faced with a dilemma that many of those with chronic illness often confront: the clash of two systems with very different goals. Our cure-focused medical systems are by far the dominant force, populated with well-trained experts and bolstered by the best (but always uncertain) evidence that modern medical research money can buy. Rarely does this system spend the time or money to investigate or provide care for what the whole person needs for healing—their social and emotional situation; the strength of their physical, nutritional, and mental fitness; the lifestyle and behavioral resources available to help them heal; and the value and goals they have for a meaningful life. We have no integrative health system for the delivery of both curing and healing in cancer, for bringing together evidence-based medicine and person-centered care.

Susan and I discussed this dilemma as we sat in the preoperative suite waiting to have a vascular port inserted into her chest through which she would receive her weekly chemotherapy. She lay in bed dressed only in an operating gown, with the nurses, technicians, and physicians moving in and out. They checked the marks where they would open her neck to bury the tube running into the veins. The port would be used every week to draw blood and check her white blood cell count and to deliver the three chemotherapies. How, we wondered, could she be empowered to find a meaningful path forward under these circumstances? It was not obvious. Instead of deciding what to do, she paused in the now, meditated, and listened to her innermost self. She wanted to understand how her current disease and treatment might link to her soul. As they rolled her into the operating room, she heard a song over the intercom. It happened to be a song she had listened to the summer before while walking the Camino de Santiago (The Way to St. James) in France and Spain with our daughter. The song was "All of Me" by John Legend. Suddenly, the memory of that wonderful, spiritual walk came back to her and she felt deeply loved, not just by those around her, but by her own God—even in the midst of this difficult life challenge. She relaxed and released her worries about how to solve the dilemma she now faced. As she drifted off under anesthesia, she had a flash of insight. To embed meaning into her healing and integrate it with her cancer treatment, she would need a healing space in our home. We needed to redo our bedroom.

HEALING SPACES

It may seem strange that what emerges out of a sudden, almost spiritual insight as you are rolled into an operating room is that your bedroom needs to be changed. But this type of sudden and certain insight, which my wife had come to trust, turns out to be one of the best ways to discern a meaningful healing journey. I often work with patients to find ways to increase these insights—using practices like journaling, mindfulness, or dialogue—to help align evidence with intuition and curing with healing. While joy and intuition are important parts of a person—connecting to the emotional and spiritual dimensions—a full healing response must also connect to the external dimension of a person, the physical spaces that impact the body. The physical space is often a good place to start a healing journey. Physical spaces are easy to see and change. Almost everyone knows the calming effect of a beautiful vista, a sunny day, or the sound of flowing water. We have good scientific evidence that physical spaces influences healing for many chronic conditions. And there is a growing understanding of the mechanisms in our brain that do that.

Neuroscientist and immunologist Dr. Esther Sternberg spent thirty years at the NIH investigating the links between stress, stress management, our external environment, and our mental and physical health. She discovered that the physical environment directly impacts our ability to heal, independently of what goes on in that space. While Dr. Price and Professors Kaptchuk and Benedetti have been showing us how the rituals of health care affect our brain's ability to deal with pain, depression, Parkinson's, immune diseases, and other disorders, Dr. Sternberg is showing us how the space itself does the same thing. In her book, *Healing Spaces: The Science of Space and Well-Being*, she summarizes much of that research, demonstrating how the physical environment can trigger our "brain's internal pharmacies," making us sick or healing our ills. She and others have demonstrated that the brain is built to respond to the place we are in—directly, continuously, and unconsciously. The brain structure at the center of our response to space is the hippocampus—a part of the brain that is key to building memories. It also determines whether the physical location we are in is safe, telling us if we need to act to get safe or can relax where we are. It integrates signals from our sensory input—what we see, hear, and smell—to create a sense of place. It also sits near and continually communicates with another brain structure, the amygdala, which controls emotional arousal and response—often called the fight, flight, or freeze response. Thus the hippocampus creates a sensory impression of where we are and connects it to any emotionally laden memory that determines if we should respond or relax. Think of it as the GPS of the brain, which locates us not only in physical space but also in emotional space and puts the two together. This continual arousal or relaxation response produced by where we are signals other organs—including the heart, gut, and immune system—to be on alert or to engage in rest and repair. This happens mostly outside our conscious awareness. The hippocampus reacts to where we are and influences our mind-body response by comparing our space to memories that induce either fear or safety. Through this mechanism our physical space continuously puts our body on alert or into recovery mode, emitting a steady stream of chemicals that can hurt or heal. The place we are in is a powerful pathway to inner healing.

Until the science of this process was understood, the influence of the hospital environment on our internal healing capacity was largely ignored. Hospitals were built for physicians to deliver treatments. The hospital I did my training in was a typical example. Six floors of stacked rooms—usually two to four patients to a room—adjacent to a noisy road with no parking. Doctors had their own entrance in the back, and the emergency room entrance dominated the front of the building. Sirens blasted on and off day and night. Two wings of this concrete block formed the center of the hospital; it was built with little attention to light, noise, color, air flow, or nature. When the hospital needed to expand, other wings were added—usually through long corridors extending from the main lobby. After a few of these were added on, the place became a confusing web of hallways, often without clear markings for directing patients where to go. The larger the hospital became, the more confusing it became—and it had the ambiance of a warehouse rather than a healing environment. This was the typical hospital during most of the twentieth century. Then in 1984, environmental psychologist Roger Ulrich did a pioneering study called "The View from a Window." In that experiment, patients recovering from surgery were randomly assigned to either a room with a window view of a brick wall or a room with a window view of a grove of trees. To everyone's surprise, patients who had a tree view did better in all ways. They had less pain and used less pain medications, needed less nursing care, made fewer complaints about their care, and recovered more rapidly—leaving the hospital a whole day earlier than those looking at the brick wall.

Ulrich launched a research field exploring the effect of space on healing outcomes. So far this growing field has shown that:

- Single-bed rooms in hospitals can reduce infections; reduce falls; improve patient sleep; improve patient, family, and staff communication; and improve satisfaction with care.
- Natural light can reduce medical errors and length of stay; improve sleep, depression, and pain; help premature babies gain weight faster; and improve patient and family satisfaction.
- Exposure to nature can reduce pain, the stress of hospitalization, and the length of the patient's stay, and improve satisfaction.

Other space and environmental characteristics also impact health, including noise, ventilation, artwork, furniture arrangement, and the availability of family and private spaces. Recent research shows that the health care environment can save money, reduce employee turnover, and attract patients—all good for the bottom line. This research is now known as evidence-based design and optimal healing environments (OHE)—an area in which I have focused much of my own work (more on this shortly).

Most changes to create an OHE have been done in acute care. But when used for chronic illness, as done in many cultures over centuries, the impact of an OHE can bring about significant and sustained healing. Clara, a patient of a colleague of mine, used the external dimension to heal herself, when even the best of medicine could not.

CLARA

Clara had been a vibrant and loved teacher at a school for foster children in Baltimore. With three grown children of her own, and a supportive husband, she had retired from teaching to devote her time to community work in the city. All was going well in her life when she was struck by a mysterious illness. It started with fatigue and gradually progressed to muscle weakness and then muscle wasting. She lost an alarming amount of weight and became depressed. Her work in the community was important, but the disease progressed and forced her to give up the work and spend more and more time in bed. Even going to the kitchen to fix breakfast exhausted her. "What is happening to me?" she lamented.

With the help of her husband she began to look for a cure. She had access to and saw specialists throughout the country—at Johns Hopkins, Columbia, Harvard, Wisconsin, Stanford, and UCLA. Multiple hypotheses were entertained. She received multiple diagnoses and tried multiple treatments, some with reasonable evidence, some experimental. What was it? Chronic fatigue syndrome or myalgic encephalomyelitis? Autoimmune myositis? A prion disease? Multiple chemical sensitivity syndrome? Mitochondrial deficiency? Major depression? Psychosomatic disorder? Clara needed a name for her illness, but no one could give her one.

Her hair began to fall out. Soon she needed to hire someone to help her with basic activities of daily living—dressing, cleaning the house, and getting around. She then went to nutritional and alternative medicine doctors. They suggested other causes. Food allergy? Nutritional deficiency? Adrenal fatigue? Yeast overgrowth? Dysbiosis? Chi imbalance? Dosha imbalance? Soul loss? She got a lot of names—but no relief.

It was all the more puzzling because Clara seemed to already have all the elements of health and healing in her life—a supportive family and friends, a good diet, a nice home, and access to the best medical care, both conventional and complementary. Still, she could barely function. One day a friend was visiting and the conversation went from updates on events in the community to Clara's future. Instead of considering what else she could do, her friend asked Clara if there was a place she loved the most and felt happy and well. Clara immediately knew. "Well, yes," she said. "It is in the mountains. My husband and I have a small cabin up in New England. I love being there. It is deep in the woods on a small lake. The animals visit. The light and sounds change by the moment. The silence is wonderful. I can see the mountains from our back porch. The place restores my soul every time I go. But I have not been able to go for a long time because of my illness." There was a pause in the conversation as her friend just waited for her to continue.

In that moment, Clara knew what she was going to do. She had to go to the mountains. It would be difficult, as she could barely take care of herself. But her caregiver would go with her, and between her caregiver, her family, and her friends, she just might be able to stay for a while.

"But what about your doctors and therapy visits?" her friend asked. "What will happen to you if you give those up?"

Clara thought a moment. "I don't know." She took a deep breath. "All the diagnoses and treatments I have done so far have not helped. I think I need to take things into my own hands now." So, with assistance from friends and family, she traveled to her mountain cabin, determined to stay until she either recovered or died.

Her recovery began almost immediately. At first, all she wanted to do was sleep, day and night. "It was," she said later, "as if I was dead most of the time. Except that when I woke up, it was to the peace and silence, the clean water and the cold fresh air. It made me sleep deeper than I had in months. And when I was awake—oh, the beauty. I felt as if I was living in a Mary Oliver poem. I could open my windows and see the glowing green mountains, hear the nearby brook, feel the soft light of the moon at night. Everything changed by the minute. Animals, small and large, crossed my view. Rain and sun moved over me—alternating fire and water. The wind rippled through the trees. They seemed to be in constant prayer." Friends and an assistant helped her eat, bathe, dress, and go outside. For two weeks, other than beholding beauty, her physical condition did not change. And then it did.

It was not a sudden, miraculous improvement. It was slow and incremental, like the waxing and waning of the moon. A little different each day. A bit more energy. A bit less pain. After two more weeks, she was able to go out on the back porch herself. In four weeks, she could walk for thirty yards to the stream behind her house. In six weeks, she ventured into the local town—with help. In eight weeks, she went there on her own. Also on her own, she gradually reduced her medications. Her pain pills, her antidepressants, her steroids. She hoped she would not relapse when she did this—and she did not. After three months in the mountains, Clara woke up one morning, got out of bed, and fixed a cup of coffee before she realized that she had not yet thought of her illness. That is when she knew she was solidly on the path to recovery.

Other things in her life also came together during those three months: the realization that she truly loved her family and wanted to spend more time with them; a clear view of the toll that her sacrifice for others—first teaching and then community service—had taken on her; a deep appreciation for being able to physically move and exercise, which was something she had never liked before. She had a deeper love for her body, as flawed and dysfunctional as it often was. When she returned home, she found that taking care of herself emotionally, physically, and spiritually was no longer an annoying chore, but a privilege—no, a necessity—for her life.

Several years later, Clara confessed to me, "I don't know why I got sick. I had no more understanding of my illness than the doctors had. But I do know that I recovered by doing what I loved most. And in the process, I became more myself—more whole—than I had ever been before." It was a profound and meaningful change in place and space that started Clara on the path to that wholeness—and to healing.

OPTIMAL HEALING ENVIRONMENTS

"Since the beginning of humankind," writes architect Marc Schweitzer, who analyzed data on the effects of environmental design on health, "it is likely that people have been seeking safe shelter in which to heal." Making simple changes in space can improve healing, function, and well-being inside and outside health care—in homes, worksites, and schools. Patients assigned to a room with a view recovered a full day faster after an operation, and two and a half days faster if hospitalized for mental health problems. Premature babies exposed to full-spectrum light that cycles like daylight gain weight faster than those exposed to continuous light—even though they have literally never seen the light of day. Students in classrooms with windows that open progressed 7% to 8% faster on standardized tests in one year than students in rooms with windows that could not be opened. Children allowed outside to play during school hours have fewer behavioral problems and do better in school, including on tests. Richard Louv, in his book *Last Child in the Woods*, summarizes the remarkable impact that exposure to nature (or lack of such exposure) has on children's health, functioning, and happiness. (The book is a must-read for parents and teachers.)

An increasing number of hospitals around the country are now becoming the OHEs I introduced earlier. Samueli Institute, the organization I directed for fifteen years, created a model to measure whether a health care setting was impacting healing, not just curing. We showed that specific architectural elements—including lighting and interior design—can reduce stress and anxiety, increase patient satisfaction, improve morale and performance of health care workers, and promote the health and healing of patients. OHEs don't just enhance well-being and improve clinical outcomes—they also save money.

Our definition of an OHE is a system and place designed to stimulate and support the inherent healing and wellness capacities of its inhabitants. In short, an OHE delivers healing-oriented practices and environments (HOPE) in a way that integrates them with medical disease treatments. I will show you how I use HOPE later, but for now, simply know that an OHE is a holistic organizing framework applicable to all health care organizations and health care systems. Consistent with its preventive and palliative role, it is also applicable in schools, worksites, and community locations. It is a way of connecting many models of care that share similar goals and philosophies—models such as relationship-centered care, patient-centered care, family-centered care, holistic care, integrative medicine, and the medical home, as well as worksite wellness and optimal learning environments. I briefly describe the OHE in the following section. More detail can be found on my website, DrWayneJonas.com.

THE FOUR DOMAINS OF AN OPTIMAL HEALING ENVIRONMENT

Note that these domains of an OHE parallel the dimensions of a whole person that Dr. Manu drew on his whiteboard in India (see page 46) and also those that whole systems science identified as elemental for how people remain healthy and recover when ill—body, behavior, social, and spiritual. There are four OHE domains as well—internal, interpersonal, behavioral, and external.

Internal Domain

Healing intention: This is a conscious determination to improve the health of another person or oneself. It incorporates the expectation of an improvement in well-being, the hope that a desired health goal can be achieved, the understanding of the personal meaning that is attached to illness and suffering, and the belief that healing and well-being will occur.

Personal wholeness: This is the experience of well-being that occurs when the body, mind, and spirit are congruent and harmonious. Personal wholeness can be developed and fostered with mind-body practices that reinforce wellness and recovery.

Interpersonal Domain

Healing relationships: These are the social and professional interactions that foster a sense of belonging, well-being, and coherence. Nurturing healing relationships is one of the most powerful ways to stimulate, support, and maintain wellness and recovery.

Healing organizations: An organization's structure and culture is important for implementing and maintaining an optimal healing environment. The vision and mission of an organization contributes to the development of a healing culture. A successful OHE organization also has a strategic plan for meeting goals, as well as leadership support, stable funding, and a flexible, resilient evaluative culture.

Behavioral Domain

Healthy lifestyles: Healthy behaviors can enhance well-being and can prevent, treat, or even cure many diseases. Making appropriate dietary choices, engaging in physical exercise and relaxation activities, and managing addiction are important to lifelong health and wellness.

Collaborative medicine: This is team-based care that is both person focused and family centered. It also includes thoughtfully blending the best of complementary therapies with conventional medicine.

External Domain

Healing spaces: These are built environments designed to optimize and improve the quality of care, outcomes, and experiences of patients and staff. Design components that foster wellness and recovery include evidence-based architectural design, color choices, and access to nature, music, art, and light.

When working with hospitals to use the OHE model, I often find it easiest to start with the external domain and then link it to the other domains. Many hospitals are now putting healing design into action. Next time you seek out a hospital or clinic or ask your insurance plan about coverage, ask if they provide or are becoming an OHE.

HOW TO BRING HEALING HOME

When I assist patients in discovering their own healing capacities, I always ask questions about where they live, work, learn, and play. Exploring these elements with patients helps them find and create the proper physical healing space—the space that their body dimension occupies.

While each of the elements in this bodily external dimension has evidence for its value, the purpose of exploring these is to find just a few—or even one—that is the most meaningful for them. We are seeking how to connect the external space they are in to the patient's inner space of mental, emotional, and spiritual response. Susan would change her bedroom to simplify and sooth her sleep and ease care for

ELEMENTS OF THE BODY AND EXTERNAL DIMENSION

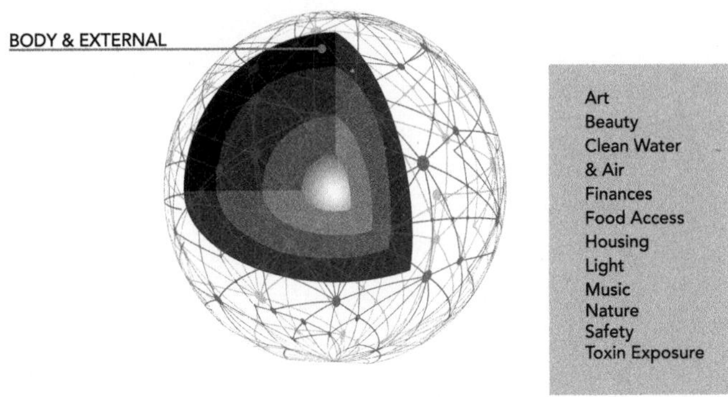

her grandchild. Clara changed her location to soak herself in nature. Both used the external environment as an entry point to induce a meaning response for them and pave their path to healing.

Many healing traditions pay attention to space. In my research group's global studies, we found traditions such as feng shui were used at the Great Wall Hospital for Xiao, and *sthapatya ved*, the ancient healing architecture of India, used at the ayurvedic hospital where Aadi was treated. In some Native American belief systems, "sacred geometry" assigns specific healing properties and meanings to each of the compass directions. Greek temples surrounded patients with nature, music, and art to restore harmony and promote healing. Florence Nightingale attributed differences in the survival rates of patients to differences in crowding, light, and ventilation. And unbeknownst to Clara, she was engaging in an ancient Japanese practice called *shinrin-yoku,* or "forest bathing." Research has shown that immersing oneself in nature influences the body through more ways than simply the beauty and calm, as important as those are. Trees also emit chemicals called phytoncides that stimulate the immune system, something Clara likely needed. Being in nature also lowers cortisol and reduces heart rate and blood pressure. It increases our brains' natural painkillers. Phytoncides allowed Clara to rest more deeply and experience less pain.

Most people are so familiar with the places they live that they no longer take note of the details of the space or its impact on their lives. However, when I ask them to tell me the ideal environment that evokes a positive memory of joy, awe, or beauty—their ideal place—they can almost always tell me. Is there a window from which to gaze out at nature? What are the colors of the walls and furniture that they love the most? Is there clutter to step over or move aside to get past? What attracts them to a place? Are there elements of a place that allow them to look beyond a chaotic, disorganized space to an image that brings peace and a smile? Most people know their own healing space when they see or imagine it. It is easy to tell when someone realizes his or her healing space—the face lightens, the breath deepens, the muscles release. The signs of a healing response become evident in the person's posture and demeanor. My neuroscience mind sees my patient's hippocampus integrating sensory cues of the place the patient is in with the emotional cues that produce relaxing and joyful memories. The patient reacts as if she were settling into her mother's arms, like she has found a home. I then know she has connected her external environment to the inner dimensions of her life—social, emotional, mental, and spiritual—in a meaningful way. If she can make that a permanent space in her life, she more easily taps into the 80% of healing capacity that routine health care leaves largely untouched.

THE BEDROOM

When Susan came out of the operating room after her port placement, she knew how to solve her dilemma. She'd had an insight that she could use our bedroom as a healing sanctuary to recover from the chemotherapy and surgery and also to have a place where our grandson could be with her and play—with help, of course—during the most difficult times. She had never felt our bedroom had been a comfortable place to sleep—it was too cluttered inside and too open to the outside elements through a large French door and palladium window on one wall. And the colors were not right—too dark in some places and too bright in others. It did not feel like a calming, safe place to rest and bring a baby into. So of all the elements in her external dimension, it was the bedroom that Susan found most meaningful for her as she faced cancer and its treatment again.

The bedroom Susan created for herself was a simple, soothing place with natural light bathing the room in a soft, heavenly glow. A new and more comfortable bed was placed against our too exposing (for her) French doors. This allowed the light to penetrate the room indirectly from the top of the room. White opaque curtains were hung from ceiling to floor. The walls were painted a light blue-gray and kept bare except for a solitary painting placed on one wall—an abstract that almost blended into the wall. It looked like angels off in the distance emitting light—harmonizing with the feel of the room. It was painted by a good friend of hers, which further personalized its meaning. A small mobile of folded paper cranes (a Japanese symbol of healing she had come to love) hung from the ceiling. This too was personal—handmade by friends from the school her children had attended and where she had been chairman of the board after her first cancer.

The closet was expanded to eliminate clutter in the bedroom. Every piece of clothing, every shoe, every dress and sock now had a place. If it didn't have a place, she gave it away. A soft gray-and-white stool stood in the middle of the closet.

When the transformation was complete, I thought the room looked as if it was already part of heaven—glowing, ethereal, simple, uncluttered, peaceful—a picture of the world to come. "Just in case I don't end up in heaven if I die," she humored me one day, "I want to feel a little bit of it on earth now."

In the corner, Susan set up a small play area for the baby and some chairs where others could sit when her grandchild was in the room. As she began to take on the weekly onslaught of chemotherapy and then after that the surgery and other medications, she spent a lot of time in that room often feeling deathly ill, but now continuously healing by sleeping, reading, listening to music, visualizing herself in a better place, and being with the baby in a way that was safe for both of them. “Just being there felt close to God,” she said, “and those I most loved, whether I was awake or asleep.” She had created her own healing space.

More difficult, however, for Susan (and for most people) was the next dimension of healing—changing behavior and lifestyle.

CHAPTER 6

Acting Right

How behavior heals.

Seventy percent of chronic disease can be prevented or treated with a healthy lifestyle—by not smoking, consuming minimal alcohol, maintaining an improved diet, exercising, and minimizing stress. But which diet works best? A low-fat diet or low carbohydrates? Paleolithic or Mediterranean? Ornish or Atkins? With some alcohol or none? We were told for many years that we should not eat eggs or butter, but now they are okay. Coffee was bad; now it is good. Low fat was good, now it has caused the obesity epidemic. Exercise is good, but increases injuries. Stress is bad, but some stress builds resilience. It can all get rather confusing. Although there is general agreement on some harmful behaviors—smoking is definitely not good for your health, for example—science seems to flip-flop on the specifics of what is good for us. More important, even when we know what healthy behavior is, most people cannot embed those behaviors into their lives. Less than 5% of people engage in these top-five healthy behaviors. It may be good for you, but if you can't or won't do it, it won't do you any good.

What is the secret to the tapping into the 80% of our healing capacity through lifestyle? A patient named Maria taught me even as she learned it herself. The secret to healthy behavior is not willpower; it is something else.

MARIA

"I think we need to start you on insulin," I said to Maria about seven seconds into our visit. "The medicines we are using now are not controlling your diabetes."

I was not prepared for her reaction. "No," she said flatly, "I can't do that."

There was a fire in her voice I had never heard before. Maria had always been a pleasant and cooperative patient, accepting and using all of my recommendations.

"My father started insulin and then soon lost his legs! He went downhill from there and died. I can't do it! I won't do it. I am sorry, doctor." She burst into tears.

"But Maria"—I tried logic, even though it was clear that was not her operating mode at that moment—"it was the diabetes that caused your father's legs to be amputated, not the insulin."

She was not persuaded. "I am sorry, doctor. You are a good doctor. Can't you find me another way besides insulin? I will do anything. What about a special diet? I can go off sugar," she implored. "I can lose weight."

I was skeptical. Maria was from a large Mexican family—the first child of eight. Her mother and grandmother had been her role models for domestic care and order. Maria had married an American and moved away from Mexico, but she'd brought a lot of it with her. She had six children and had created a home of her own, of which she was proud. To say that food was a major part of her home was an understatement. She loved cooking. And her family loved her cooking. She prepared it with love and from scratch, every day, three times a day, seven days a week. Often the family would invite friends to the feasts and enjoy her marvelous meals. She did it because she grew up that way, she knew how, and it made her and others happy. Maria loved food and cooking. Unfortunately, the food did not love her back—it had given her diabetes.

Maria had been overweight most of her life; she had had diabetes for seven years and was gradually getting worse. I had referred her to the dietitian—twice—with little effect. Would she really be able to stick to a diet? The Diabetes Prevention Study, just completed, demonstrated that lifestyle modification could prevent the progression of prediabetes to diabetes better than medication. But Maria had full-blown diabetes already, and in my opinion she needed insulin. I had her on the maximum doses of an antidiabetic drug called metformin. At the time, none of the newer antidiabetic medications, such as SGLT2 and DPP-4 inhibitors were available. Insulin was the recommended next step.

"Well," I said, unable to conceal my hesitancy, "there are some major dietary and lifestyle changes that might control your diabetes. But you don't have lot of time to show improvement. We could give it a month—two at the most."

Maria looked eager to hear more. So, with little hope and even less thought, I wrote down the names of two books that had reported rapid improvement in diabetes patients who use them. Both involved very low fat, no sugar, and an organic vegan diet. No meat, no processed or packaged foods, no added anything.

"See what you think of these," I said, "and come see me in about two weeks and we will see if these make sense for you."

Despite my lack of enthusiasm, Maria was overjoyed. "Thank you, doctor. I will cure my diabetes. You will see." She left with vigor in her step. *False hope*, I thought.

She didn't return for six weeks. I had just asked my nurse to give her a call and ask her to come back in when I saw her name on my schedule.

She looked much different. "I did it!" were the first words out of her mouth. "I cured my diabetes with your diet."

Maria had lost fifteen pounds, and a check of her short-term blood sugar was normal. I was still skeptical, but pleased. "That is great, Maria," I said. "Let's check your long-term sugar."

That too showed improvement. It was still abnormal, but better. I was impressed and a bit more hopeful.

"How are you feeling?" I asked.

"Just fine, doctor. Can I avoid insulin now?"

I agreed to have her continue and check back with me monthly. Each month we checked her weight and the long-term blood sugar marker called HbA1c. Over the next five months, her weight largely stayed the same, but her blood sugar remained stable and continued to improve. But something else was happening to her that I couldn't quite put my finger on. Her moods had changed. Instead of the cheerful, agreeable Maria I had known, she seemed sad. I wondered if something stressful was going on at home. Had someone died? Were she and her husband not getting along? It took a few more visits for her to finally tell me.

"Doctor," she said flatly, tears now running down her cheeks, "I didn't want to admit this, but I cannot do the diet anymore. At first it was okay—new and different. But over the last several months I have become very sad. My family hates the food I prepare now, so I cook two meals, one for me and one for them. But, frankly, I hate the food, too. We no longer have friends over for dinner. When my family visits from Mexico, they want someone else to cook. I have lost energy for the kitchen. I cannot care for them like this. I can't care for myself like this. I have failed. Put me on insulin. I will lose my legs and life rather than my family."

Now I had tears running down my cheeks. Maria sounded despondent. She had been so afraid of insulin and so determined to cure herself with the new diet that she had gutted her primary identity as a cook and homemaker. She was afraid to talk with me about it because she thought I would confirm that she had failed and put her on insulin—a death sentence in her mind. In the process, she had also likely reduced her fat intake so drastically that it was affecting her neurotransmitters and contributing to her mood problems. But the main problem was that she had tried to make a lifestyle change that she was not ready for, a change that removed joy from her family and her life. Like many who try to make a radical behavior change without linking it to the central purpose and meaning in their life, it could not be sustained.

"Maria," I said gently, "you have not failed. You have succeeded. Your blood sugars are much better, and you don't need insulin. But for this to last, you will need to find a way to balance this diet change with your love for food and meals that you and your family have always had. Let's work together to figure out a way to do that." She agreed.

We also agreed to take up the conversation in full at another visit. But I actually hadn't the foggiest idea of how to help Maria. In the meantime, she would make herself and her family a wonderful Mexican meal to celebrate her success—and not worry about what was in it.

The next time I saw her, the old sparkle had returned in her eyes. Her blood sugar had also risen a bit. We would work out a plan with her that was better than the last one, I promised. I suspected it would require we bring in not just another dietician, but a chef to help her take her favorite recipes and make them healthier, and a health coach to help her move her goals forward in a more incremental and meaningful manner. I knew that part of Maria's improvement had to do with the lower sugar content in her diet. But part of the improvement was also the partial starvation she induced in herself by such a radical shift in protein and calories. Like Aadi, she had induced her body to begin healing through a physical stress response. But the process could not be maintained if it removed something so important in her life.

LIFESTYLE MEDICINE

Every year, nearly a million people in the United States die prematurely because of unhealthy behaviors. And chronic lifestyle-related diseases are rapidly becoming the major causes of death worldwide—and soon will surpass infectious disease and malnutrition. Behavior is the primary contributor to the six leading causes of death—heart disease, cancer, stroke, respiratory diseases, accidents, and diabetes. These collectively account for almost 75% of all deaths. And they are all largely preventable. Lifestyle also contributes to diseases of the brain, such as depression and Alzheimer's. Even more disturbing is a new trend: the recent increase in adult-onset (type 2) diabetes in children and teens, which is caused by obesity, lack of exercise, and environmental toxicity. The behaviors that can prevent these premature deaths and diseases are fairly simple—no tobacco and minimal alcohol and drug use; maintenance of proper weight; consumption of nutritious, unprocessed food; clean air and water; physical activity; social support; and good stress management. Most people know this. Shelves of popular books are written about this. Multiple national scientific bodies make recommendations on this. Governments try to regulate behavior for this. Yet despite these efforts, less than 5% of people engage in all of these basic behaviors. And, in an ironic alignment of numbers, less than 5% of medical funding is spent on primary prevention—supporting efforts to help people make these behavior changes. We get what we pay for. Willpower is not the solution to this dilemma. Maria had great willpower yet ran into common social and personal obstacles to using behavior as a path to healing. When left to our own devices, often we can't do what's necessary—or we do it wrong.

Behavioral change is difficult for us, not because we are "weak," but because we are unaware of how our environments and experiences—the health care system, our culture, our past personal history, and the media—are influencing us. When we have this awareness, we can create personal environments where healing behavior easily occurs. We do not have to struggle. We can create a new reality, as one of my other patients showed me.

JEFF

Jeff's dad had died short of age sixty-five of a massive heart attack. Jeff, also a smoker, worried this would happen to him, and he hated the coughing and the smell and the cost of his smoking, but he just could not stop. He had tried nicotine patches, smoking cessation classes, vaping, hypnosis, and acupuncture, but nothing worked for more than a few weeks. He was chemically and psychologically addicted. Then he asked me for help. We did a healing-oriented evaluation (a HOPE assessment, which I will describe later), during which I asked him questions about the dimensions of healing in his life—his external environment, his behavior, his relationships, and his inner life. Surprisingly, what emerged from our discussion was the idea of running. He enjoyed running for short distances; it made him feel better, and he loved both being outdoors and the rhythmic, almost meditative movement; he even liked the soreness he felt after a workout. He had played basketball in high school but hadn't been to the gym since he graduated. Despite liking running, he had never run more than one mile at a time. "I don't think I could do more than that," he noted. "Especially since I started smoking."

If Maria had been a ten on the "I can do it" scale, Jeff fell closer to a one or a two.

I heard about a program that offered marathon training for people who had never run before. I suggested that he stop worrying about trying to quit smoking and sign up for this program instead.

"I can't do a marathon, doctor," he scoffed. "I can barely run a mile." But he agreed to check out the program anyway. Neither of us expected what followed.

At the first meeting of the group, the leader asked people to take off their watches and pedometers and just follow him on a short, easy run. They could stop any time during the run and walk instead, if they wanted. They set off at a moderate pace and ran a flat or downhill route.

Jeff had no problem with the run. In fact, he loved it, especially running with others, which he had not done before. When they stopped, he was shocked to learn that he had just run four miles, something he thought he was incapable of doing. He had broken through a mental barrier.

Over the next few weeks, he started making friends with his fellow runners, enjoying both the social contact, being outdoors, and the discipline of the training. He also noticed that he was smoking less and less, even though he had not made any conscious decision to quit. He was simply not craving cigarettes so much anymore. He was craving running instead.

There are biological explanations for Jeff's response. When you smoke, your body is stimulated to produce neurotransmitters such as dopamine, serotonin, and norepinephrine. These transmit messages to receptors in your brain that make you feel good—just as a nicotine high does. This is the reward that smokers are addicted to. When the nicotine is removed, they feel bad. But other behaviors, such as vigorous exercise, switch on some of the same brain receptors stimulated by nicotine. Many runners, myself included, experience this feeling as a runner's high. By stimulating his brain's reward system with running, Jeff was simply substituting running for cigarettes to satisfy his brain's craving and to get the reward. By the time he ran his first half marathon a year later, he had not smoked a cigarette in three months. Rather than futile battles to overcome a negative addiction—smoking—Jeff had a new ritual that became a positive addiction—a healthy one. This method of change can work for many behaviors and negative addictions, including overeating, alcohol, and drugs, by developing a healthy behavior in a manner that feels equally rewarding. A year later, he was still running—and not smoking.

Jeff did that successfully. Maria did not. She and I still needed to figure out how changes in her food behavior could become more rewarding. We had to connect her behavior change more deeply to what she valued in life.

THE PLACEBO LIFESTYLE

Even healthy behaviors can produce both benefits and harms, depending on how we view them and use them. Maria's healthy diet improved her diabetes but harmed her mental well-being and family life. Current biomedical science attempts to tease out what produces the benefit of specific behavior changes by using the science of the small and particular. This type of science approaches behavior, such as eating, as it does drugs, herbs, and other treatments. We examine the content of certain diets and try and separate out the effects of their content—low or high fat, low or high carbohydrate, low or high protein, and so on. We dissect different types of exercise, such as running, walking, swimming, weight lifting, yoga, tai chi, or gardening. When we investigate methods for stress management, we scrutinize various approaches, such as meditation, visualization, music, mindfulness, biofeedback, and intentional breathing. This is all well and good, except that the more rigorously we do these studies—with better controls, larger sample sizes, more accurate measurement methods—the smaller the effect from the specific behavior is—just like with drugs and herbs.

However, there is a different path to such knowledge, especially when we want to put that knowledge into action in a whole person. Whole systems science helps us understand how to use behavior to maximally stimulate our internal healing capacity and minimize the harms. We saw in chapter 4 (see page 87) how the work of Dr. Mark Mattson of the NIH and others showed that fasting and episodic calorie reduction produced a general reparative and healing response—leading to improved function and longer life. Aadi, Xiao, and Maria were all using dietary manipulations similar to fasting to stimulate healing. Other behaviors can be used in a similar fashion. Exercise, for example, stresses the body—especially the heart, lungs, and muscles. It produces inflammation and generates oxidative damage. In addition, it causes small micro traumas in our muscles, which our body repairs during rest. Provided it is not overdone (yes, you can get too much exercise), these stresses and physical microtraumas become small stimulants to healing that induce our whole system to repair itself and keep us in good health. This is largely how exercise maintains health and increases healing. This is the same mechanism that stimulated Norma to function better with less pain from her arthritis, helped Aadi to improve his brain function, and allowed Bill to finally ease his back pain. Dr. Jordan D. Metzl, author of *The Exercise Cure*, has summarized much of the research on physical movement and health and provides a step-by-step approach to improving the time you spend moving, even if you have never purposely exercised. Research shows that even small and incremental steps toward greater movement are beneficial for most people. Only at the extreme athlete level do negative effects begin to appear. The type of exercise matters very little.

This happens with mental exercise also. Differences in the effects of various stress management approaches are minor compared to the general goal of inducing a relaxation response. For more than fifty years, Harvard's Professor Herbert Benson, author of *The Relaxation Response*, demonstrated that almost any type of relaxation inducer—prayer, meditation, rhythmic breathing, visualization, or biofeedback—can rapidly reverse the more than five hundred genes that are turned on by stress. In addition, those who regularly practice a relaxation method have better long-term health, recover faster from health challenges, and use fewer medical services.

Was the specific content of the food Maria switched to in order to lose weight and control her diabetes the most important part of her improvement? While the emerging evidence currently points to a Mediterranean-type diet as good for overall health, it appears that simply changing our eating patterns to almost any whole-food approach provides the most benefit. In a large network meta-analysis published in 2014 in the journal *JAMA Internal Medicine*, researchers compared all the major diets being used for weight loss—Ornish, Atkins, paleo, Mediterranean, Weight Watchers, high carbohydrate, high fat, and others. While the high-fat diets worked better for weight loss in the short term, in the long run (after a year) all diets were equally effective. How much of the benefit that we get from healthy behaviors comes from the specific behavior we adopt? Is much of it actually—like the benefit from taking a drug, herb, or other treatment—more like a placebo effect, derived from the context and meaning of a behavior?

As you can imagine, it is a bit challenging to create a placebo behavior. Bill and Aadi knew they were doing yoga, and Maria knew she had changed her diet—those are hard to fake. However, researchers have developed ways to improve the rigor of studies on behavior by producing "placebo lifestyle" approaches and modifying the expectation of benefit from a behavior. These studies have found that much of the improvement from behavior change is produced by what people *think* about the behavior they adopt. Professor Alia Crum of Stanford University has been studying this idea of mind-set as a determining factor.

One ingenious study was set up to evaluate the role of mind-set on the benefits of exercise for health. Everyone believes that exercise is good for health—and it is. But is the benefit from the exercise itself or from the belief and meaning we give to it? That was Professor Crum's question, and she devised this study. Hotel workers who clean rooms all day get a lot of exercise—making beds, cleaning bathrooms, as well as vacuuming and hauling stuff—a workout every day. It should be good for them. The researchers divided a group of these hotel workers into two groups. One group was instructed about the health benefits of activity from the work they did. They were given specific information on how their work activity helped their health. The other half was not instructed in any health benefits associated with their work activity. After one month, the researchers asked the groups about their perceived workload and the management about their actual workload. The researchers also did health measures such as weight, blood pressure, and body mass index. On average both groups did about the same amount of daily work activity—each worker cleaning fifteen rooms. However, the group who knew details about the health benefits from their activities and thought they were getting good exercise showed significantly more health improvement than the group who did not have that knowledge. This included improvements in objective measures, such as decreases in weight, blood pressure, body fat, waist-to-hip ratio, and body mass index. It seems that, as with drug effects, what we know and believe about exercise contributes significantly to its health benefits, well beyond the actual exercise itself! A significant part of the "exercise cure," then, is the meaning response.

Does this happen with food, too? We know that how a drug or herb treatment is labeled has a major influence on its psychological and physiological effect. Pairing a smell or taste with substances that produce biological effects enhances those effects through a process called "conditioning"—remember the impact of Norma taking her placebo pills four times a day compared to two times a day? The very act of doing something with the intention of benefit produced an effect. We know that the social environment and learning from others further enhances this process—remember Sergeant Martin and his hyperbaric oxygen group all getting the oxygen together and reinforcing its positive effects with each other? Eating combines all these factors. Think about how you have eaten all your life. Every meal is infused with your belief in its relative health value (or lack thereof); you get daily conditioning of that belief from its smell and taste; and, most of the time you get social reinforcement of that belief from what and how you prepare and eat together with family and friends. Are the health benefits of eating, something you do several times a day, also influenced by the meaning response? Professor Crum also investigated this question by examining the impact of food labeling on our hormone responses. In an experiment called "Mind over Milkshakes," she examined whether the nutritional label and information about food produced biological effects. One milkshake was called Sensishake; the label said it had no fat, no sugar, and only 140 calories, and was "guilt-free." It seemed very sensible from a health point of view. A second shake was called Indulgence; the label said it contained 640 calories of combined fat and sugar—and delivered the "decadence you deserve." In truth, both shakes had 300 calories and the same nutritional content. Before and after people drank one shake or the other, they had their level of a hormone called ghrelin measured. The ghrelin level rises when you are hungry and drops when you are satiated and don't feel like eating any more. It also slows metabolism, so more calories are stored as fat rather than burned. The study found that ghrelin levels dropped three times more when people drank the "indulgent" shake compared to the "sensible" shake. When people thought they had eaten a heavy, calorie-laden food, their bodies responded as if they had. As in drug studies, most of the effect was due to the belief combined with the ritual around the food—not what was in the food itself. Almost all nutritional science tells us what is healthy or not—based on examining the content of what we eat rather that the process of eating itself. This dilemma contributes to the confusing claims.

Does this mean the content of our diet does not matter? Of course not. Lots of research shows it does. However, how much it matters and the health response generated by food content are markedly influenced by the meaning we attach—individually and culturally—to what we eat. Professor José Ordovás, a senior scientist and director of the Nutrition and Genomic Laboratory at Tufts University in Boston, has studied the effects of the Mediterranean diet on genetic factors related to health. He studies what cultures are eating and measures how those food patterns trigger gene changes related to health and disease. While your doctor may measure your cholesterol and blood sugar and recommend diet changes based on these, Professor Ordovás studies how those factors are influenced by the food-gene interactions that are precursors for them and explain much of what your doctor measures—using the very tools of whole systems science. During his Mediterranean diet research, he noticed there are practically no situations in which the food—healthy or otherwise—is ingested in isolation. Most of the people in countries where the Mediterranean diet is consumed prepare and partake of that food in family and community groups—usually in an atmosphere of friendship, fellowship, and love—like Maria did with her family and friends. When Ordovás measured the gene expression (in the urine) attributed to the Mediterranean diet during the meal preparation, he found that many of the gene expression changes attributed to the health benefits of the food were turned on before a single bite was taken. Eating does not just involve taking in a bunch of chemicals—it is a meaningful social and personal behavior solidified around the "agent" of food. The meaning infused into that behavior influences our bodies—from genes to hormones to cholesterol to our weight. So to help Maria, we had to link her healthier behavior around food to its association with her family and the joy it produced in her life. We needed to use food to induce a meaning response.

HEALTHY BEHAVIOR

While there is scientific evidence for the value of each of the elements I explore with patients to help them find and create healthy behavior, I discuss them with patients not in order to tell them what to do, but for them to find just a few—even one or two—that are the most meaningful for them. Jeff used exercise to stop smoking because he loved to run and be outdoors. He used this love to create a positive addiction to replace smoking. Maria used food to facilitate the cure of her diabetes, but in a way that did not bring her joy. Jeff linked his behavior to meaning, which allowed it to penetrate deeper into this life. Maria simply tried to comply with a dietary change that helped her body but created side effects. Both used the behavioral dimension as an entry point on their path to health and healing. Both did the behavior; however, only Jeff induced a meaning response. Maria did not, even though she seemed to have more willpower.

In most major health systems around the world—both ancient and modern—lifestyle is a cornerstone of disease treatment as well as disease prevention. In ancient China, for example, the head of each family paid the doctor only if everyone in the family remained healthy. When someone became ill, the doctor received no money until the patient recovered. (Think how that would go over in today's managed care!) The system used lifestyle (diet, exercise, exposure to nature, and energy "chi" balance) for both prevention and treatment. It applied the same practices and principles at different intensities depending on whether they were meant to maintain health or restore it.

ELEMENTS OF THE BEHAVIOR AND LIFESTYLE DIMENSION

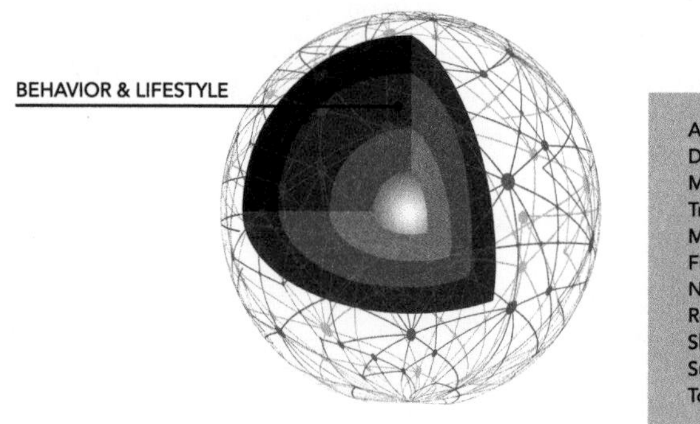

Alcohol
Drugs
Medical Treatment
Movement & Fitness
Nutrition
Relaxation
Sleep
Supplements
Tobacco

In the equally ancient Ayurvedic system of India, we saw how Aadi's Parkinson's disease was treated with a personalized regimen of diet, yoga, prayer, meditation, and oil-based massage customized to his body type and emotional makeup. These same approaches were used outside the hospital to prevent the disease's return. Both these medical systems are at least five thousand years old. In another part of the world, in the fourth century BCE, Hippocrates, the pathfinder and inspiration for modern Western medicine, declared that food is the best medicine. The ancient Greek health center of Epidaurus provided gardening for teaching nutrition, sport and exercise to regain physical fitness, theater to work out social and mental health issues, and hot and cold baths to cleanse and stimulate the body to promote healing. Prevention and treatment used the same tools and processes. It was one system. But modern biomedicine has split these goals—prevention and treatment—and developed very different ways to accomplish them.

MINDING THE GAP

In health care today, we have two very different health systems and a gap between them. One system focuses on acute problems such as injury, heart attack, stroke, and infection; the other emphasizes prevention and health promotion through activities like vaccinations, sanitation, and lifestyle changes—like smoking cessation, improved nutrition, exercise, and stress management. The two systems operate in virtual isolation from each other, as if they were in separate buildings—and in most communities, they usually are. What happens, for example, when you have a heart attack? You are rushed by ambulance to a hospital, where elaborate and expensive medical resources are mobilized to help you: a fully equipped emergency room, surgeons, anesthesiologists, nurses, imaging technicians with their machines, and an operating room filled with a dazzling array of medical technology, just to begin. Then, when you have been stabilized with angioplasty, a stent to open up a clogged blood vessel, or surgical removal of a blood clot, you are moved to a hospital room, where nurses, orderlies, technicians and health aides, support staff, and the billing office tend to your needs. All this happens under the supervision of an attending physician, and if you are in a teaching hospital, residents, interns, and medical students join in as well.

After treatment, you need a calm, peaceful environment in which your body can recover from the medical assault. Instead, machines, staff conversations, and loud announcements over the paging system surround you. You are awaked in the middle of the night, stuck with needles to draw blood, and have devices attached to measure your vital signs. If you're in the intensive care unit, these machines are a constant presence, with blinking and beeping readouts on display—blood pressure cuff, finger clip to monitor oxygen levels, electrodes, and maybe a catheter. You are given meals high in sodium, animal fat, and refined carbohydrates like white bread or white rice. And when you are out of acute danger, depleted by the ordeal, you are sent home, usually as soon as possible, with minimal home care planning and often without anyone talking to you about the lifestyle that caused your heart attack in the first place. Once you have been labeled with a disease and have crossed the diagnostic threshold to enter the world of acute care, an entire industry awaits you. Everything in this "building" of the medical system is based on the acute care model of health: namely, that there is a single cause for disease. If an artery is blocked, open it up. If cholesterol or blood pressure is too high, lower it with medication. If you have mild to moderate depression, prescribe mood-elevating drugs. The detailed manipulation of the body by this system is impressive—and expensive.

By contrast, the other "building" in the modern health care focuses on prevention of disease. Here, health care practitioners and public health specialists try to educate you about ways to modify your lifestyle through diet, exercise, stress management, and smoking cessation to address the underlying causes of disease and prevent problems from developing. They supplement your milk and bread with vitamins; your water with chlorine and fluoride; and, repeatedly urge you to eat better, stop smoking, exercise, and, oh, see your doctor for checkups. With a few exceptions, there is still a huge gap between the systems that prevent disease and the systems that treat disease, because they operate from completely different health models.

So, the first step in creating a personal environment that promotes healing behavior is awareness of this gap and exploring ways to fill it in your life. If you find yourself crossing the diagnostic threshold into the acute care system, you can ask your doctor to help you bridge the gap between prevention and treatment by giving you information on and assistance in finding a health behavior change meaningful for you. Armed with this information, you can then find lifestyle changes that will prevent future problems. At the end of this book, I give you specific tools to help you in that conversation with your doctor.

You must be persistent in finding this help within the medical system, however. Although primary care, like family practice, is supposed to help fill the gap, payment for primary care is still based mostly on the episodic visit in an acute care system, with minimal coverage for prevention, lifestyle, and healing. So even those tasked with bridging the gap usually cannot. Remember, only 5% of the measured expenditures in our health care systems target lifestyle treatments, health promotion, and prevention. And 95% is spent on treatment of acute disease with nonlifestyle approaches, so don't expect the medical industry to do this very well for you. When it comes to bridging this gap between prevention and healing, the situation is changing, but it is nonmedical organizations such as companies and even the military that are leading the way. An example of that is Total Force Fitness in the U.S. military.

TOTAL FORCE FITNESS

One of my assignments in the U.S. Army was to develop ways to close the gap between prevention and health promotion and treatment. The military realized that very often behavior could both prevent and treat disease, and they wanted to help close this gap for service members and their families. In 1991, the Army Surgeon General launched a massive health promotion and prevention program on all Army posts. I was its medical advisor. Every soldier was to get a

Health Risk Appraisal Assessment (HRAA). The HRAA screened all soldiers for their lifestyle habits and risk factors, such as smoking, high-fat diet, alcohol use, exercise, and stress. It measured physical health factors such as cholesterol, blood pressure, blood sugar, weight, and percent of body fat. It explored each person's stress management and mental health issues. The HRAA eventually replaced the annual physical, which had been around for over a century and was shown to be largely useless.

Armed with this new information, each post commander was instructed to work with the hospital commander to take care of any problems that were found. And a lot of problems were found. Although generally healthier than the average population, soldiers were found with previously undetected high blood pressure, cholesterol elevation, smoking and excess alcohol use, weight problems, and depression. What were commanders to do? Most sent these soldiers to the medical treatment clinics, where they received "quick fix" solutions from the acute care system: medications and instructions to change their habits. These clinics and hospitals were all set up on the acute care model of health care that I described earlier. Their environments were neither preventive nor particularly healing. In general, clinic doctors, when confronted with a patient with high cholesterol or high blood pressure, would prescribe medications, rather than taking the time to look at the underlying lifestyle causes of the disorder or manage the more complicated process of behavior change. To be fair, even if they took the time to do this, the acute care system was not organized, nor did it have people with the right knowledge and skills, to deliver effective health promotion. So physicians' hands were largely tied. When commanders realized that a medical solution was not the answer; they created health promotion programs in military units and the community. There was a great need to set up bridges between these two worlds, which was my job. So various "bridging" programs were set up throughout the military and eventually reached the top leadership in all four branches of the military.

In 2007, working with Admiral Mike Mullen, then Chairman of the Joint Chiefs of Staff, my team helped develop an approach called Total

Force Fitness. This whole systems science model sought to link healthy behavior not only to health care but also to service members' deeper psychological and spiritual needs. It was a whole person approach designed to address the body and mind and also the person's social and spiritual dimensions. (The whole person healing–oriented approach of Total Force Fitness was subsequently implemented military-wide in a variety of programs and is now being expanded to whole communities such as the Healthy Base Initiative, Operation Live Well, and a seven-state Building Healthy Military Communities program.) Samueli Institute worked closely with the military to explore ways of bridging specific health behaviors and meaningful daily life. This was done on the military bases, but also in civilian communities, where most service members and their families come from, live, and return to every day. We also assisted programs to address the specific dimensions of healing behavior such as stress management and healthy eating programs. These included programs such as Healthy Kitchens, Healthy Lives, which taught healthy shopping and cooking skills; the Metabolically Optimized Brain, which connected community food access to resilience and enhanced mental health; and the Family Empowerment program, which set standards for implementing science-based, mind-body stress management programs in schools and worksites, teaching people how to improve the relaxation response and build mental fitness. It was from these programs that I learned the key to unleashing the healing power of behavior and lifestyle: connecting behavior change to a personally meaningful life. I didn't see this clearly, however, until another patient, Ensign Rogers, gave it to me straight from his hospital bed. He also gave Maria and me the answer we were looking for.

ENSIGN ROGERS

Ensign Rogers had just had a major heart attack. A retired cook and food service supplier with thirty-four years in the Navy, he had become overweight and developed high blood pressure. After he retired, he developed diabetes. Now he was in the hospital, recovering from the heart attack. I visited him there and we discussed what had happened.

Ensign Rogers' heart attack was, as he put it, "the big one." His recovery was prolonged. It gave him time to think about his life. Rogers, as they called him when he was on active duty, had provided food for sailors throughout his career, first on ships, starting as a server on the line. Then he became a cook and gradually rose in the ranks to become the main supply person for delivering food to ships—from small patrol boats with fewer than twenty passengers to large aircraft carriers with more than six thousand personnel on board. His duties had gone from peeling potatoes, to overseeing food delivery during training, to supplying food to boats during wartime. Later he was responsible for food for entire Navy communities, including families on bases. He knew a thing or two about food. After he retired from the Navy, he became a consultant for food services for the military. Now he advised all four services on how to provide more fresh fruits and vegetables at low cost. "Health food," he said, with some irony, "from scratch. Just like in the old days."

"You know, Doc," he mused, his heart monitor beeping in the background, "unlike medical care, which you only get when you need it, food has to be there all the time—three times a day and 24/7 for all sailors." He had never failed in that job. When he first started, they used to peel the potatoes and cut the vegetables themselves. He learned how to cook then, "from scratch" as he put it. He wasn't a bad cook; not a gourmet chef, but he could put a meal together—usually several hundred at a time, anyway, most from fresh ingredients.

He remembered exactly when cooking from scratch started to change. At first, it was expensive to get the packaged and processed food. But people wanted it. It was quick and easy and scientifically based. "Who wanted to peel all those potatoes every day, anyway?" he reminisced. If you added up the number of people it took to prepare food from scratch, the packaged food became cheaper and easier just to buy—preprocessed food in bulk. "We called it 'industrial food' because it came from the food industry, not our kitchens." he said. Food budgets got thinner and the war mission started to accelerate. "The sailors didn't have as much time to sit around and talk or eat. They needed food quickly and lots of it. They needed high-calorie food, and that's when the cans and packages came in," he reflected.

Instead of ordering pounds of potatoes and carrots, beans, and steak that he had to cut up himself, he received complete meals in packages. Packages of tasty high-fat, high-salt, high-calorie foods—just what the young sailors wanted. "The main drivers of this were the food companies that were selling packaged food at very low prices. And the military could negotiate even lower costs, so things got shifted into those packages," he recalled. Efficiency increased by not having to make food from scratch; now it mostly required only opening and heating. Industrial food had arrived.

Meanwhile, what was labeled "industrial food" inside the military was called "fast food" outside the military. American families were getting conditioned to fast food—a trend that spread and is still spreading around the world. In 1970, only 27.9% of daily meals were eaten outside the home. By 2012, it was over 43%. Ads for high-sugar, high-fat foods began to flood television, further reinforcing fast food as both fun and cool for the modern life. Women, increasingly working outside the home, wanted more rapid ways to feed hungry children. After a full day at work, a drive-through food run became just the ticket.

"The new sailors wanted this food, which they were getting used to as children before they came to the military," Ensign Rogers recalled. "It wasn't too long before the sailors started asking for that kind of food. So, while the industry pushed it as more convenient and cheaper, soon it was the sailors themselves who were the pushers. If we didn't supply it, they would go off base to get it. If they didn't eat in the dining halls, then our budgets were cut further. We couldn't have gone back to fresh foods if we wanted to." He paused for a long time. "I guess now the military leaders want fresh food back again." An even longer pause followed. Finally, he said with a sigh, "I wish them luck."

As the United States entered WWII in 1941, they found so many young men underweight that the military feared they would not be strong enough to endure a grueling war. So the government started feeding programs in schools, including free school lunches, to try and bulk up young men before they entered the military. That, and the need for large amounts of nonperishable, shippable food during the war, had spurred the development of industrial food. What was originally supposed to be a special type of feeding needed for large numbers preparing for battle, soon became the basis for feeding the entire population all the time.

After the war, the military type of fast food was converted into the fast-food industry the succeeding generations now wanted. During this same period, the rate of obesity began rising. Soon being overweight, rather than underweight, became one of the top reasons potential military recruits were turned down. By 2008, over 27% of all recruits and 40% of women wanting to come into the military were too fat to fight. That meant that they were disqualified for entry because they didn't meet the minimum standards for height/weight or fitness that the military considered essential to even start training.

"That is why they hired me as a consultant now, I guess," Rogers said, "to help them reverse this trend. I had seen it happen."

As Ensign Rogers looked up from his hospital bed, we discussed the health consequences of those shifts. He realized that in his career he'd done more than simply find cheaper food to fill the bellies of sailors in less expensive and more rapid ways. He had unwittingly become the architect of his own illness and converted many others into candidates for the costly, high-tech medical care he now received. He was grateful for the procedures, medications, hospital care, and stents that saved his life. He was grateful for the medications that controlled his diabetes and hypertension. He had developed hypertension in his mid-forties and had been put on several medications. He had already been on cholesterol medications. The diabetes medications came a bit later. Toward the end of his career, he didn't meet even the Navy's maximum weight standards, which are generous, and he was afraid he was going to get kicked out early. He starved himself before the biannual weigh-ins. After he retired, his weight ballooned, and that's when the diabetes and hypertension got worse and hard to control. During his thirty years in the Navy, the obesity rates had increased to almost 25% of all service members. He realized now that when he got together with his buddies in the NCO Club, he wasn't the only one with high blood pressure, diabetes, and heart problems. They were all talking about their doctor visits, and almost all were on cholesterol, hypertension, or diabetes medications. He just took it as a normal part of good medical care. After all, they had good medical care even after retirement.

But now, as an advisor to the military, when he recommended that a few million dollars be spent to try to prevent these diseases from happening to others, he heard that either the money was not available or they had to show that buying fresh food would reduce costs. In addition, most of the nutritionists worked at the hospital and didn't have time to help redesign the purchasing and preparation of healthier food. However, he did see a nutritionist when he went in for his diabetes checks, and a great new cooking class had been added to the cardiac rehab program for those with a history of a heart attack. The nutritionists were hired by one part of our health care system—the acute treatment part—but they did not have time to bridge the gap to the other part of our systems—the health promotion and prevention part. The payment system also did not bridge the gap. Military leaders were including only costs for the supply, preparation, and delivery of the food—24/7, three meals a day, without fail. Food was fuel for these young service personnel; they had a mission to accomplish, and that mission came first. They didn't count the cost from the medical consequences that would pop up years later. Nor did they count the personal costs Ensign Rogers now faced.

Like many military members, however, Ensign Rogers had always dedicated his life to service. So even as he talked from his hospital bed, he began to wonder if he could help the admirals and other ensigns with their situation. How could he help them see the long view—a view that had taken him nearly forty years to see himself?

After his discharge from the hospital, he started to attend cardiac rehab. While most of that focused on exercise, he also took a new twelve-week "healthy eating" class for heart patients that the base

Community Wellness Center offered—an offshoot of the Total Force Fitness program. In that class, nutritionists and chefs joined forces to teach heart patients how to cook—from scratch, he noticed—in ways that were both healthy and delicious. In addition, the group culture of the class helped people help each other make the behavior changes permanent. If you had a challenge—be it with blanching vegetables or balancing your budget or getting your family on board—usually someone had a similar problem and could help you solve it.

"But," Ensign Rogers told me in a follow-up visit about six months after his heart attack, "for most of these heart patients, the horse had already left the barn. That was not the time to start to prevent their disease. They already had it. I needed it thirty years ago. It can't be just for people who have already had a heart attack."

I agreed.

One year later, Ensign Rogers partnered with a chef and started such a course for everyone at the base Wellness Center. He volunteered his time. "Eat for Life," he called it. Anyone with a risk factor for heart disease—overweight, diabetes, high blood pressure, high cholesterol, smoking, or a family history of early heart problems—could come. Family members could come, too. Meeting once a week for twelve weeks, participants learned how to select, buy, and prepare healthy food; how to make it taste great; and how to involve family and friends in the process.

Brilliant, I thought to myself. It was exactly what I was looking for to help Maria—to see if she could put meaning back into her medium of healthy food. I introduced her to the program as soon as I heard about it. She loved the idea and signed up for the next class.

After taking the class, Ensign Rogers and Maria decided to develop a version focused on Hispanic food—something Maria knew well and Ensign Rogers wanted to learn. With some help from a master chef, and a bit of guidance from a nutritionist, they began a community cooking class for prevention of the country's leading disease killers. Maria found an outlet for her passion, Ensign Rogers for his experience—and both found a new purpose in life. The "side effects" were many. Their diabetes remained under control, their energy improved, and their life expectancy lengthened. And they were helping others do the same. They had tapped into their own healing agency using the "agents" of food and behavior change.

MAKING BEHAVIOR MEANINGFUL

People are creatures of habit. Whole systems science shows that self-regulating systems—like people—constantly work to return to the same form and behavior after they have been stressed or traumatized. That automatic rebound response—the same response that fuels healing and recovery—also makes behavioral changes uncomfortable and hard to implement for many people. Behavioral change can be much more difficult for some than for others. Difficulties implementing long-term behavioral change often occur because of experiences and patterns set in childhood. Maria found a process to merge her healthy eating needs with the contribution she made to family and friends through cooking—something she had learned to do and was rewarded for as a child. Once she linked that meaningful activity to healthy food, the change came naturally and easily.

My wife, Susan, found changing her behavior much more challenging, even when she had reason to do so. Healthy behavior not only prevents disease and reverses many chronic conditions, but it can also blunt the side effects of curative treatments like chemotherapy and surgery. Cancer patients who exercise, eat healthy food, and engage in stress management, tolerate and complete therapy better, recover faster, and suffer fewer consequences of treatment long term. Susan had firsthand experience with the long-term consequences of cancer and its treatment. After her first cancer, she suffered the long-term effects of chemotherapy, including weight gain, nerve damage, and fatigue. Had she been able to engage in extensive behavior change—intensive exercise, careful dietary control, and major stress management—some of the consequences from her disease and treatment could have been mitigated. But Susan was not able to engage in that kind of intensive behavior change for several reasons. For one thing, our two health care systems—one for disease treatment and cure and one for healing and prevention—rarely bridge the gap and integrate, even in the crisis of cancer. During Susan's first breast cancer, oncologists had made no recommendations on healthy lifestyle during or after her treatment, and some even minimized it. There were few places to find assistance in learning and engaging in these changes. There are no profits to be made from building systems to help people make behavior change, so those systems are minimal. We went on with our lives as before.

During her second breast cancer, twenty-five years later, things were somewhat better. There are now lectures on nutrition, yoga classes, and support groups for cancer patients. There is a Society for Integrative Oncology (SIO), where mainstream oncologists explore the integration of healing practices with the cure-focused treatments in cancer. The role of behavior is now at least acknowledged as important in cancer survivorship—although physicians are not trained in how to use behavior. Advances in the science of healthy behavior are still not integrated into the delivery of cancer care. Our oncologist, one of the best in the region, did not know about SIO. There were no health coaches or coverage for behavior change available to Susan.

The second reason behavior change is hard for Susan is because of her childhood. As Maria discovered, the ability to make behavior change was linked to her childhood experiences, but in a different way. In three major areas of healthy behavior, Susan's childhood was stacked against her. First, while growing up, Susan frequently felt like she did not have enough food. Her family struggled financially, and food was carefully purchased and allocated to feed a family of six. As the "smart and most responsible one" and the oldest girl of four children, she was also expected to help take care of the family. By the time the food for dinner had been passed around, she often did not get enough. Her brother was a competitive swimmer and was constantly hungry, so she intentionally took smaller portions so he could have more. She said nothing about this, but later as an adult the idea of limiting food intake—especially food she could not get as a child—was very challenging to her. She experiences any change in possible food intake as a threat to her well-being, especially when things are stressful. Second, she was not encouraged to participate in sports and exercise. As was true for many girls of her generation, sports was something you watched boys do. She developed no skills or experience in keeping physically fit. Exercise was more difficult for her than for me; I had been involved in many sports. Finally, stress levels were high in her house. Her father had a volatile and unpredictable temper, often flying off the handle, yelling and screaming. She became the peacekeeper of the family, constantly on the alert to anything that might upset him and taking the emotional consequences of his abuse. Susan's stress management tactic for this was to anticipate possible emotional discord and compromise her own needs and desires in order to keep things calm. The only time she was relaxed was when there was social and emotional peace in the family, which was rare. Even today, she still habitually (and automatically) scans the social environment for any developing discord. That makes it hard for her to breathe deeply and induce the relaxation response when awake. Sleep is her only escape, especially when faced with a major assault like chemotherapy and surgery.

These types of adverse childhood experiences (ACE) have been shown to produce lifelong challenges to health and healing for many people. Not only do those with high ACEs have more mental and physical health problems, such experiences establish behavioral, neurological, and physiological patterns that are difficult for people to change. They are a double whammy—producing poor health and inhibiting behavior change to improve that health. If physical or sexual abuse is also involved, these problems are literally beaten into the brain and body of a person, making the induction of healing through behavior especially difficult. Until a person learns to reprogram those automatic emotional and physiological responses, repeated attempts at behavior change often fail, further reinforcing the difficulty. Such reprogramming can be done, but to pull it off requires extra assistance with environmental and social support. This assistance focuses on developing a readiness to change. Once the readiness has been properly prepared, actual behavior change becomes easier.

BRINGING HEALING INTO HEALTH CARE

Just as there is no magic bullet for chronic illness with specific medical treatments—no drug or herb or needle or knife that by itself will make you well—there is also no magic diet or other behavior change that will do this. After my patients and research taught me that most healing was not coming from the treatments I was prescribing, I discovered that the same thing applied to lifestyle. Add to that the paucity of science being applied to understanding lifestyle as therapy, and you can see why we have a plethora of self-care books running the gamut of recommendations. As important as healthy behavior is, if you want to access its healing capacity beyond what you can expect from simply making a change, you must connect that behavior to your life in a unique and meaningful way.

Healing can happen by applying medical treatments like Norma, Aadi, Sergeant Martin, and Xiao did in earlier chapters. It can happen by changing the external environment as Susan and Clara did in chapter 5. It can also happen with behavior changes like those that Jeff, Maria, and Ensign Rogers made. In each case, they found the right combination of approaches for their lives. To do this, however, we needed to focus less on finding a cure—the magic bullet or latest self-improvement fad—and more on how to connect healthy behaviors to our deeper personal dimensions.

One fundamental sign that a medical treatment, physical environment, or lifestyle will tap into the 80% of your healing capacity is the return of joy—a joy that comes from the experience of meaning and purpose. Another sign is an intuitive sense of certainty—a gut feeling that goes beyond belief and superficial desires for things to be a certain way. This gut feeling alone, however, is not sufficient to ensure it's the right healing choice for you. Any treatment or other healing approach should be verified with scientific evidence. What you decide to do should make sense to you and your doctor rationally, feel right to you emotionally, make sense socially, and be doable logistically. It is a committed embrace of the decision and follow-through that comes from your whole being. Many cultures describe this feeling in spiritual terms, but it is rarely seen that way in modern biomedicine. Modern medicine calls this approach by many names, such as person-centered care, precision health, or integrative medicine. The methods used to obtain this may involve personalized care planning, shared decision making, and health coaching. But optimal healing goes beyond the limited concepts of those terms. It involves the whole person and is produced by the meaning response. An emerging field that captures this most completely is called "integrative health."

Whole system sciences is providing powerful tools to more efficiently track when and how healing happens—providing objective ways to check your gut feelings. For example, as part of the million-person NIH Precision Medicine Initiative I described previously, researchers at Stanford University tracked nearly two billion measurements (250,000 a day) on sixty people to see how their day-to-day patterns of behavior correlated with health or illness markers. By analyzing patterns of change in this data over several months, the researchers could predict risk and illness as well as what produced improvements and healing in those people. Currently, this tracking is cumbersome and expensive for a clinic or person to do—but soon it will be relatively easy and some of it is being offered now. Technology is advancing our ability to measure, analyze, and monitor the whole person in ever more rapid and refined ways. Dr. Eric Topol, director of the Scripps Translational Science Institute and editor-in-chief of Medscape, describes this brave new world in his book *The Patient Will See You Now*. Technology is increasingly able to continuously monitor the core components of chronic disease and its risk factors and directly guide patients on how to monitor their own behavioral changes to prevent such disease. Integrative health will take this same technology and flip this monitoring on its head. That is, you will be able to get a continuous "healthy aging" readout and adjust what you do, think, and take to keep in your optimal health and well-being zone. The goal of whole systems science is to see the impact of this whole-person healing approach—be it from conventional or complementary medical treatments, lifestyle medicine or behavior change, social relationships, thoughts and feelings, or maybe even what happens in our soul.

That information will be at anyone's fingertips. As this happens, we are creating a true science of whole person healing, and our ability to use it will improve. We will increasingly have precise ways to find the drugs to help each person, provide guidance on the environment to support optimal health, monitor the effect of daily behavior, and interpret a person's intuition.

You don't have to wait for this future, however. Much of this is available to you now—if you seek it and ask for it. There are already clinics and self-care tools delivering integrative health. These clinics and tools coordinate behavioral therapy, nutrition and lifestyle medicine, health coaching, and spirituality along with regular medical treatment. You can find them both inside and outside of medical centers. Those that are part of medical clinics are now delivering healing approaches and merging them with the approaches that seek to cure. I describe them and how you can access or create them at the end of this book.

The gap between our two health systems—between treatment and prevention—is being closed. But the area of behavior and lifestyle is not the widest gap between curing and healing. To understand what is, we must delve even deeper into how healing works—into the dimensions closest to the core of what it means to be human.

CHAPTER 7

Loving Deeply

How love and fear affect healing.

What are these other fundamental dimensions of being human needed for healing? Simply put, they are the emotions of love and fear—or more precisely, how we experience and manage them. How and what we love is intimately tied to our ability to find deep meaning and stimulate healing. The flip side of love is not hate; it is fear. Fear is the primary emotion alerting us to danger and drives our bodies to react—by fighting, fleeing, or freezing. Our entire brain (and body), with all its complexity, is constantly screening the environment for threats to our survival, asking what we should worry about and act on and what we can let go and relax around. When it thinks it has found a threat, it alerts us with fear and all the psychological and physiological reactions that accompany it.

If there is a single secret to how healing works, it can be found in how we handle our loves and fears. Love and fear are not intangibles—they have a physical effect and are, as we'll explore in this chapter, a matter of life and death. Love opens. Fear contracts. Both of them are needed for healing.

One of the myths about love and fear is that we have no control over them—that they just happen to us. We "fall" in love. We are "seized" by fear. Being subjected to the slings and arrows of emotion is indeed how many people experience their life. But whole systems science has now shown that not only can we learn to manage these emotions, but our health and healing depend on having just the right balance of them in our lives—both to get healthy and to stay healthy. Modern medicine's failure to take advantage of the social and emotional dimensions that help us manage love and fear leaves much of our healing potential untapped. When health systems have made these social and emotional dimensions central to their operations, those systems universally produce better outcomes and reduce costs.

The importance of managing love and fear has actually been shown in the laboratory—using rats and rabbits. Let's start with that.

THE RABBIT EXPERIMENTS

The rabbits were not dying, and that was a problem. How could the scientists find the cure to heart disease if they could not produce it? To study the effects of diet on heart disease, researchers fed different diets to two groups of rabbits and then compared the effects. One group ate a diet very high in fat and cholesterol; a control group ate a normal rabbit diet. Most of the rabbits who ate the high-fat, high-cholesterol diet developed high levels of cholesterol in their blood and blocked arteries in their hearts, putting them at increased risk of heart attack and stroke. It was a standard research test model that reinforced the cholesterol hypothesis of heart disease, a model demonstrated in laboratories all over the world and previously verified in the researchers' own laboratory multiple times.

But this time the results for one group of the fat-eating rabbits were different. Although they developed high levels of blood cholesterol, the rabbits in cages on the lower laboratory shelves had fewer blockages in their arteries and were not dying. The researchers checked and rechecked both the type and the amount of food that the rabbits ate and made sure that these rabbits were identical to the other rabbits used in the experiment. However, they could come up with no explanation for the lower-shelf rabbits' apparent immunity to the unhealthy diets. The researchers were confused. And then they talked to the lab technician.

The lab technician, a short woman, was taking the rabbits in the lower cages out of their cages every day and playing with them. She held them on her lap and petted them. She talked to them. Soothed them. Basically, she loved them. Then she would clean the cages and put them back in. Since she could not reach the higher cages, another technician was taking care of those animals. Those rabbits were not being petted—and they were dying at the normal rates.

The researchers were skeptical that simply soothing and petting an animal could negate the effects of a proven disease-producing diet. To have this effect, the loving touch these rabbits were getting only once a day would have to produce powerful chemicals that reduced the inflammation in the endothelium (lining) and the deposition of cholesterol in their coronary (heart) arteries and reduce blockages.

Most scientists would have not been distracted by the idea of love and simply told the technician to stop petting the rabbits. After all, their grant was funding them to test the diet-heart disease hypothesis, not the love-your-rabbit hypothesis. But the lead investigator was curious. Was love really overcoming diet? To rigorously test that hypothesis, the researchers designed an experiment that randomly divided a new set of rabbits into separate groups. They instructed the technicians to take the rabbits in certain groups out of their cages every day, play with them, stroke them, and love them for different amounts of time. They were to leave the other groups alone, except for routine feeding and care, without taking them out of their cages or touching them, except to transfer them quickly. They then studied the effect of this caring on cholesterol, endothelial function, artery narrowing, and heart disease.

What happened? Despite eating large amounts of fat and cholesterol, and even having elevated blood cholesterol levels, the cuddled rabbits had 60% less plaque in their arteries than the ignored rabbits, even though they were comparable in every other way—genetically, diet, weight, serum cholesterol, and heart rate. The factor that made the difference was love. The researchers were stunned. If only a few minutes of petting each day could reduce heart disease by 60% in a laboratory animal, imagine what power a lifetime of love (or its loss) could have on humans!

One patient in particular showed me clearly the power of love to heal the heart.

MABEL

Mabel was the "grand dame" of a large extended family. At eighty-four, she was the matriarch; for fifty years she had fretted, cared, and cooked for, disciplined, raised, and loved several generations. She was a sister, mother, grandmother, and great-grandmother to a family of nearly sixty—most of them relatives, others having showed up at her door and been "adopted" into the family. This included seven children of her own, nineteen grandchildren, and twenty great and great-great-grandchildren. Every week for three decades, the family had gathered at her house after church on Sundays for food, fellowship, and fun—and some of Mabel's continuously dispensed wisdom. Usually, her advice started with the phrases "Lead with love" or "Love first" or "The Lord loves everyone." If a child misbehaved, she might look at him sternly and say "Child . . ." Then she would advise the person to manage his anger or guilt or attitude better. "The Lord loves all people," she would say—"you and them. It's your job to catch up to the Lord." Not everyone took Mabel's advice, but everyone loved Mabel back.

Mabel's emotional heart may have been healthier than most, but now her physical heart was failing. I had admitted her to the hospital with shortness of breath and a very low cardiac output, a sign that her congestive heart failure—a condition she'd had for more than a decade—had progressed to the end stages. Congestive heart failure (CHF) is one of the leading reasons for hospitalization and has a very high mortality rate—killing more than five million people a year in the United States alone. The death rate from CHF has increased by 35% since the 1990s as the population has aged and our ability to keep people from dying of a sudden heart attack has improved—leaving them to live with damaged hearts that are more likely to fail later. CHF is also one of the most expensive conditions to treat, with more than one million people a year hospitalized—30% to 60% of them more than once. Annual costs of treating CHF in the United States are estimated at $40 billion a year. Mabel had not been hospitalized for more than a year as we had kept her heart functioning, and her overall care improved at home. But that increased home care had a consequence.

Three months before this hospitalization, I had recommended that a home caregiver come in to help her function better in her house. She didn't want that, but the family agreed with me so they found a home health care nurse. In addition, her family began to rotate coming over to be with her and help care for her each day. She didn't like that either. She had always been the one to care for them—not the other way around. Mabel couldn't love others in the way she had done before.

After admitting her to the hospital this time I found her numbers were off—her weight was up, largely from accumulation of water as her heart did not pump effectively. Her ejection fraction—a measure of how weak her heart was—had dropped. Her blood oxygen levels had also dropped—a sign that her lungs were filling up with fluid and not getting sufficient oxygen into the blood. I adjusted her medications and oxygen and diet to help these, and in a few days the numbers were better—but she was not.

One morning when I came in to check on her, she said, "Doc J, I appreciate all you doing for me. Just seems like too much bother, though." She was clearly discouraged.

"No bother, Mabel," I replied as I listened to her lungs and checked her weight. "That's my job—to get you better."

The next day she still complained of shortness of breath and weakness, and her blood oxygen was not quite as good. I prescribed physical therapy, upped her oxygen, and readjusted her medications a bit more. Her numbers improved again. But two days later, she was worse, as were her numbers. I checked a few more things—were her kidneys failing, too? Was her family slipping her salty snacks? Was she on the wrong medications? Was her heart just at the end of its life? Nothing seemed amiss. But this pattern repeated itself. This time I did not adjust any therapy. The numbers improved, then worsened, then improved. Her heart failure was going up and down almost independent of my treatments. I was not sure what was going on.

"Doctor Jonas," the head nurse said to me one morning, "I think you might want to talk to Mabel's family—especially Jason, her grandson. He and the pastor think she wants to die."

Jason, as it turned out, had gone to college and earned a degree in psychology. "My love child," Mabel had once told me about him. "He just sits and listen to me and gives me no grief. Always was that way."

I scheduled a meeting with Jason and the pastor. Indeed, they confirmed that ever since I had prescribed the home nurse and the family came in to care for her, she had complained about being a "burden" and "useless" to her family. "I'm better for you-all dead," she would sometimes blurt out. The family members tried to counter that attitude, imploring her not to say that and insisting that she was still loved. That seemed to make things worse. Jason told me that ever since this hospitalization, she had confessed to him that she was trying to decide whether she should go back home or die right then and there. As family members came and went, she would feel better for a while, but then fall back into her "I'm a burden" attitude. Back and forth this went. I suggested she was depressed, and I prescribed a mood-elevating drug, but it would not become effective for several weeks. Besides, that would not address the core issue that she was struggling with now—the meaning of her life with advanced CHF.

Then the pastor made a suggestion. If we could get the family to agree not to try and "take care of" Mabel on their visits, but to seek out learnings and wisdom from her—let *her* take care of *them*—maybe that would help Mabel feel useful again. Jason agreed. Although he had suggested to individual family members that they not counter Mabel's comments, they had never discussed a coordinated plan for how to receive her love and wisdom. If the doctor and the pastor recommended and helped organize such a plan, he was sure that most of the family would go along.

So, working with the family, we set up a plan to let Mabel love again. Jason and the pastor gathered most of the family together, and they agreed when visiting Mabel to ask her questions related to struggles they were having in life and to seek her wisdom. The basic question they would seek from her was—"What has love got to do with it?"—a question they knew she could answer. The gathering was arranged. I had to transfer the other patient in her room out just to fit in all the family and friends who came—more than thirty in all. The pastor said a prayer, and then the family asked her if she would do this.

"Well," she said between labored breaths, tears in her eyes, "I guess I can try that for a while." The pastor, to my surprise, suggested they sing the old African American spiritual "Ain't Got Time to Die." They all knew the words.

Within three days, Mabel's numbers stabilized—basically back to where they were on the medical regimen I had put her on when she was first admitted to the hospital. She went home with oxygen and hospice. She lived six more months, and she died with her family around her at home. She never entered the hospital again. She had found her healing power through to the end.

THE SCIENCE OF LOVE AND LOSS

From the time we are born to the time we die, life is punctuated by loves—people, places, pets, and passions—that we get deeply attached to. Life is also punctuated by the loss of those same people and passions. Our mind and body are constantly alert to find such loves and on guard against their losses. We instinctively seek the former and avoid the latter. Survival may sometimes depend on it. Yet the world is both ugly and beautiful, inflicting on us trauma and cruelty, and also inducing in us healing and compassion—sometimes all at the same time. How do we find peace in the face of pain and grief? How can we feel whole when we are broken and battered? Why do we try so hard to avoid pain, suffering, and death, even at the risk of not fully living?

It is not an easy task to face suffering, and almost impossible if we are alone. When illness and injury come, when our life is threatened by disease, and our body and soul buried in pain or sadness, it is the presence of a caring person that can often carry us through that suffering into healing. Facing loss is especially difficult if our early experiences with others were not caring, if our first ventures into love were met with rejection or loss or, worse, with anger or violence. If experiences in our childhood involved too much pain or trauma, we may be too afraid to open to the love of others, even when it is offered. Yet it is by sharing our suffering with others—and by its presence as we explore our fears—that healing and wholeness come, because some of the most meaningful experiences humans can have is when we are cared for and care for others. We are social beings; we are not whole without love.

Sociologist Dr. Ian Coulter, chair of integrative health research at the RAND Corporation and a professor at UCLA, described the scientific aspect of this to me in detail. Sociologists define a person as an individual embedded into a social network of mental, physical, and personal interactions. That network not only defines us as a person but also influences what happens to us on all levels of our being—including in our body.

Harvard physician and social scientist Professor Nicholas Christakis and his colleague James Fowler summarized many of these influences in their book *Connected: The Surprising Power of Our Social Networks and How They Shape our Lives*. They say, "As we studied social networks more deeply, we began to think of them as a kind of human superorganism. They grow and evolve. All sorts of things flow and move within them. . . . Seeing ourselves as part of a superorganism allows us to understand our actions, choices, and experiences in a new light." I agree. Who you are connected to—not only your family, but even your "friends' friends' friends"—impacts large swaths of your health and happiness, whether you know it or not. Everything from obesity to smoking to infection to alcohol use and depression are mitigated and influenced by your social network—often in ways you cannot see. Not only does this help us understand and explain how we change along with others, but it also applies to individual healing. If we look at a person as if he has a literal social and emotional body—and treat any injury to this body with the same importance as we treat a cancer or heart attack—we can unleash that aspect of our healing potential. When we do that, this social and emotional dimension of healing provides us with powerful tools for resilience, recovery, and repair.

Extensive evidence shows that social support protects us from disease and death and enhances recovery from illness. In studies with subjects who had similar conditions, strong ties to family and friends reduced the risk of dying by 50% compared to those who were alone. Isolation and loneliness are strong contributors to chronic diseases—both mental and physical—and work primarily through the body's stress and fear responses, inducing inflammation in the walls of blood vessels and in the brain and impairing the immune response. Dr. John Cacioppo, professor of cardiology at the University of Chicago, summarizes much of this research in his book *Loneliness: Human Nature and the Need for Social Connection.* Lonely people have a 45% increased risk of dying from all causes and a 64% increased chance of dementia in later life. The magnitude of increased health risks for people who are socially and emotionally disconnected from others and the comparative protection for people who are well connected are comparable to well-established risk factors such as smoking, obesity, injury, substance abuse, and environmental quality. Here's a specific example: Two studies compared men who had experienced heart attacks. The men who reported being in loving relationships had lower death rates than the men who were not in such relationships. The increased odds of dying after that for those not in loving relationships was as great as if they smoked a pack of cigarettes a day. Research has also shown a significant relationship between a patient's recovery after a heart attack and the extent of the spouse's social support, family stress, marital satisfaction, and sexual comfort. Other studies have found that patients are statistically less likely to die after a serious illness if a nurse simply calls them weekly to check on how they are doing. Several researchers have tested the mental, physical, clinical, and economic impact of making even short but deep emotional connections. Like the rabbits in the study mentioned earlier, connecting to someone who cares for you—even a little—reduces the odds of illness and premature death and helps you heal.

Loneliness is not the same as simply being alone, which for many can be a welcome and enjoyable state. Loneliness refers to the quality and depth of relationships—or lack thereof. It is not about the number of connections, either; rather, it is about how deep those connections are and how happy they make us. When people feel love and safety with others, their stress reactions in the brain and body are diminished and reparative functions improve. Professor Cacioppo points out that in the absence of social safety, stress hormones surge, triggering the release of cardiovascular and inflammatory chemicals and activating genes that lead to damage to mind and body. Socially disconnected people are more prone to arterial stiffening, leading to increased blood pressure—a risk factor for heart disease and stroke. Their bodies are also less efficient at repair and maintenance functions: their wounds heal more slowly, and their sleep—a vital restorative function—is less effective. Connections associated with love and safety increase heart rate variability—a moment-to-moment marker of relaxation and health risk. Increased heart rate variability—that is, a rate that quickens and slows with the cycles of inhalation and exhalation—correlates with resilience, good health, and increased lifespan. Heart rate variability can be tracked minute by minute, making it a good marker of the quality of one's relaxation state, emotional connection, and physical health. Mabel's heart rate variability decreased as her CHF progressed. When she felt love, however, it improved. I smiled as I thought of the science behind social and emotional connection. I could just imagine Mabel saying, "What did I tell you? Love heals with every heartbeat!" It does.

A HEALING PRESENCE

The first time my wife, Susan, went through chemotherapy, she did it largely alone. I was so busy with my job in the military that I often could not be present for her. Like many doctors, I hated feeling helpless, so I was compelled to take action, even when there was no good evidence that any action would help. I didn't know how to feel comfortable just *being* with Susan. It felt like I lost my power and control. So I worked. She found a supportive network to help her through, seeking strength in her spiritual life and the need to care for our young children. She did well.

When she started chemotherapy for cancer the second time around, I told her that this time I would be there—that we were in this together. She believed me and appreciated it, but realized how difficult it would be for me. She also knew that my periodic presence was not enough support for what she was about to go through. After all, she pointed out, I was running a large research organization, had to continue doing my job for our income, and had many demands on my time. Because of that, Susan reached out and gathered helpers around her: our daughters, our son and daughter-in-law, my sister, her sister, her mother, her sisters-in-law, other family members, and friends. Her goal was to take care of herself and help take care of our new grandchild. I didn't realize that she needed more than psychological support from me; she needed my physical presence—with my emotional body.

I should have known this. I had done research showing that the physical presence of a loving person does more than provide psychological support. The physical presence of another person has a direct impact on a person's body and mind. For example, the electromagnetic waves from the beating heart of one person can be detected in the brain of a person standing next to them. The beat of your heart is picked up and produces a sort of reflection in another person's brain. This might partly explain why when you are near a very calm person, you also start to feel calmer. That calming feeling also increases heart rate variability and the activity of the parasympathetic (relaxation response) part of the nervous system and stimulates the vagus nerve. Increased activity in the vagus nerve creates a biochemical and physiological cascade of effects that reduce inflammation and increase resilience to stress at the organ, cellular, and genetic level. Thus a person's physical presence—without her doing anything at all—can influence another person's brain and their other organs, immune system, cells, and genes, as well as bring a feeling of peace. This is probably the underlying reason that some people are said to have a "healing presence." People are probably picking up on the physical emanations from the person's relaxed and calm heart.

There are additional ways in which physical presence influences healing. We know, for example, that electromagnetic waves in the form of heat and infrared radiation emanate from the body, especially the hands. Through meditation, biofeedback, and breathing techniques, people can increase or decrease the amount of this heat and infrared radiation. Infrared radiation, especially in the frequencies of 400 to 800 nanometers, is absorbed by a chemical in our cells called cytochrome c. Stimulation of cytochrome c increases the amount of adenosine triphosphate (ATP)—the energy-producing molecule found in all cells. In dozens of experiments done at Walter Reed Army Institute of Research, investigators found that individuals who put their hands around test tubes containing immune cells while meditating increased the amount of infrared radiation emanating from their hands, which stimulated the immune cells to produce more ATP and energy. After this exposure those cells were more resilient—that is, they survived better when hit with stresses such as heat and chemical shocks. Remarkably, the kind of meditation and visualization that was the most effective for increasing the amount of ATP and resilience of these cells looked like love. Cultivating a feeling of love—such as gratitude, affection, and appreciation—produced the greatest effect. Mental activity such as counting backward or thinking about the weather did not increase ATP or improve cellular resilience.

I knew all this research—had even done some of it—but for some reason I didn't think it was relevant for helping Susan heal. Scientists (including me) are generally skeptical of any research purporting to objectively measure and explain emotional and social interaction or the energy it creates. The area is considered too intangible and subjective to be reliable, so it is dismissed without looking at whether the research is rigorous or relevant. My skeptical doctor side had also dismissed it as an interesting laboratory findings but not relevant for patient care. I wanted something more doable—a medication, supplement, or behavior. I wasn't going to simply wave my hands over her head or take naps with her. What good would that do, I thought? So even as Susan began to lose energy and feel poorly from the chemo infusions, week after week, I didn't think my presence could really make a difference in how she did.

Then one week, I went away on a boating trip through the Grand Canyon with our daughter. We were off the grid for a while, and I was not with Susan for more than a week. When we got back within cell phone range, I received a call from her. While I was away, her white counts had dropped precipitously and she had developed a fever. The oncologist had given her a shot to boost her white blood counts and put her on antibiotics. If it persisted, she would be hospitalized and isolated.

I came home, fearful that this drop in white blood count was likely to recur the following week, because the effects of chemotherapy tend to be cumulative. But something about just being together started to make her feel better. Then I remembered the research at Walter Reed. Still skeptical, I decided to try a little of this laying on of hands—this healing presence process—myself. I recalled from the research that the technique that affected the immune cells most powerfully involved breathing, imagining a soft white light filled with love being transmitted through the top of my head, down through my arms and hands, and out into her body. After a few minutes of trying this, I could feel warmth coming into my hands from increased blood flow and heat. Susan also said that she could feel something—and then she fell asleep. The session lasted about fifteen minutes.

The next day, her energy was much improved—she was up early and out pulling weeds in the garden, something she had not done for months. Was it from more ATP, I wondered? At her next chemotherapy session two days later, her white blood count had recovered practically back to normal—so she did not need the immune-boosting shot. Were her white blood cells more resistant to the chemo? She was clearly less fatigued, slept less, and was more active during the day. I was stunned. Had the simple physical presence of another loving person produced this response? I decided not to go on any more trips for a while. From then on, my job was to just make sure my body—in all its physical, social, and emotional dimensions—was around.

OPENING UP

Although little research has been done on the therapeutic effect of the physical presence of another person, there is extensive research on the impact of making emotional connections. When our encounter with another person results in connecting to our emotional self—especially to a part we have avoided dealing with because of fear or grief—the healing can be profound. In his book *Opening Up*, social psychologist Dr. James Pennebaker summarizes much of this research. A single sharing of a deep trauma or loss with another can improve health. Some of the most remarkable studies in this area are with Holocaust survivors. Even decades after the war, most Holocaust survivors have never discussed their experiences in concentration camps or the trauma, fear, and losses they endured. In the research, these survivors were asked to write or speak about those experiences to another person who simply listened in a safe and confidential environment. The investigators then measured the impact of this sharing on the survivors' biology (inflammatory response or blood pressure, for example) and health. Compared to those who wrote or spoke about something superficial—the weather or what they had to eat that day—this single deep sharing resulted in significant health improvements. The improvements were wide ranging and lasting—better immune function, less pain, improved mood, and less need for medical care, even a year later.

Other studies have shown that such sharing of deep feelings about trauma and loss can also help heal specific diseases. Patients with rheumatoid arthritis report significant pain reduction after a single episode of such sharing. Patients with asthma have improved lung function—measured objectively with a spirometer—a month after a similar single sharing.

More prolonged or repeated social and emotional exchange has profound and often permanent healing effects, especially if done in an emotionally safe environment and framed and guided in a positive direction with others to witness. An emotionally safe place is a social environment where a person can trust others to stay with them through difficult emotions, to care for and respect them, and to honor their deepest experiences as real and of value. My experience in the military, treating service members and veterans with PTSD and chronic pain, demonstrates this. For example, typical treatments for PTSD with drugs and psychotherapy have a positive but limited effect—usually helping only 20% to 30% of veterans. Exposure therapy—in which the veteran is gradually exposed to his fear triggers—can be a bit better, but it is complicated, and many veterans—especially those who have experienced sexual trauma—will not go through it. But two other approaches that tap into the meaning response have shown larger and often permanent healing.

One approach is a therapeutic retreat, during which veterans are guided to open up to their fears, anger, anguish, and grief in the presence of other veterans who understand, accept, and love them. Dr. Joseph Bobrow describes the profound and prolonged benefit from these retreats in his book *Waking Up from War*. In follow-up assessments of veterans who attend such retreats, a majority experience long-term improvement and restoration in their lives. A second approach is inducing these deep meaningful experiences with hallucinogenic substances. Recent research reports that when even a single dose of such substances is administered, a majority of deeply depressed patients suffering from advanced cancer had major improvement in their mental and emotional state.

It is important to note that the success of this approach depends on the patients being professionally selected, cared for, and guided to experience deep meaning from the episodes. Simply taking the drug by itself does not produce the healing—and in fact can cause significant harm. The drug isn't key; the meaning is. Healing does not necessarily require a drug—hallucinogenic or not—provided the meaning response occurs. A meaningful experience often occurs spontaneously through what are called exceptional emotional experiences. These occur most often when people are suffering and open up to their emotions. Loss of a loved one—through death, divorce, or another type of separation—increases the risk for disease and death several fold. Between 30% and 50% of people who have experienced a major loss

ELEMENTS OF THE SOCIAL AND EMOTIONAL DIMENSION

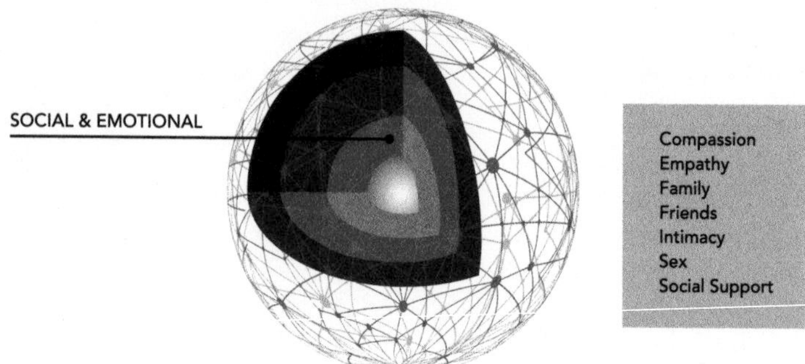

will subsequently have an exceptional experience, often described as spiritual—such as seeing or feeling a deceased person returning or seeming like a ghost, or experiencing a profound sense of the unity of all things. If those experiences are treated respectfully by others and the person is guided toward understanding and acceptance, this can be profoundly healing. If they are dismissed or treated negatively, the experience can damage a person permanently. Healing comes from how meaning is made from those experiences. It involves the social and emotional body.

THE BEAUTY WAY

To help my patients use their social and emotional dimensions to heal, I ask them about their social relationships during a healing-oriented visit with me.

The purpose in exploring these elements is not to do psychotherapy or tell them how to feel. The goal is to help them learn how to use their feelings to find deeper meaning in their lives. Mabel and her family found meaning in her wisdom, love, and teaching—and arranged a way for her to express that. Susan used her social connections and her grandchild to help increase the level of social support and love in her life during a traumatic time that needed enhanced healing. My veteran patients find meaning through deep encounters with their own losses and the support of others who understand and travel with them through their anger, fear, shame, and grief. Whatever the form or method used to create this opening up to deep emotional experiences—groups, drugs, herbs, psychotherapy, energy practices, spiritual encounters, or simply spontaneous acceptance—healing comes from the way meaning is made of those experiences.

Many cultures, both ancient and modern, use the social and emotional dimension to enhance healing capacity. I mentioned how Epidaurus—where the Hippocrates school of medicine in ancient Greece originated—had a theater at its center. In this theater, physicians helped patients learn how to deal with and heal the traumas of life by acting out the drama of emotional connections and disconnections.

Other cultures acknowledge and use this dimension for healing. Consider, for example, the way in which the traditional Navajo culture handles mental illness. Rather than thinking of mental illness as an individual problem, the Navajo consider it a social problem, shared by the whole community. They make no distinction between individual illness and social illness. In their view, we are all swimming in the same body of social "water." Whether we are aware of it or not, we need the water in order to survive, and a disturbance in one part of our individual world affects the world of all the community who "swim" there. The traditional Navajo treatment for mental illness involves the entire community in special healing ceremonies. One is a social ritual called "the Beauty Way," intended to restore beauty, wholeness, and coherence to the community, tribe, and family. There are different versions of the Beauty Way ceremony, but it often consists of a combination of prayers, offerings, rituals and sweat baths, sand paintings, chants, and singing—sometimes for days. The ill person and the community are thought to have lost *hózhó*, the sense of beauty and integration with the universe. By surrounding the ill person with beauty, this appreciation is restored in the social environment, and the individual recovers his sense of meaning and order.

Could incorporation of the social and emotional dimensions as in the Beauty Way ceremony bring healing back into modern medical care? If so, how would that affect the experience of health care and health outcomes, and how much would it cost? Dr. Don Berwick, founder of the Institute for Healthcare Improvement and former director of the Centers for Medicare and Medicaid Services (CMS), pointed me toward one system that has done just that: the Nuka System of Care, developed and run by the Southcentral Foundation (SCF) in Anchorage, Alaska. What attracted me to this system was not just Dr. Berwick's recommendation but also the major impact that SCF produces on the people it serves. In 1982, when the SCF was first formed, the health care services for Alaskan Native peoples provided by the Indian Health Service (IHS) in Anchorage was abysmal. Their rates of alcoholism, diabetes, obesity, domestic violence, suicide, and life expectancy were some of the worst in the country. Premature births and infant mortality were similar to sub-Saharan Africa. It was not that the IHS-provided medical care was bad. In fact, state-of-the-science medical visits, prescription drugs, and specialty care were all available. IHS poured millions of dollars into providing this medical care with costs rising every year. So why was it failing its patients?

From 1982 to 1989, SCF gradually took over health care delivery from the IHS. The results were astonishing. Twenty years after fully taking over health care delivery and after creating its own care approach, the foundation has markedly improved rates of obesity, diabetes, alcoholism, family abuse, and adverse childhood experiences. The need for costly emergency room and urgent care visits has dropped by 36%, primary care by 28%, and hospital admissions by 36%—all while improving the health of the community. Patient satisfaction rates have soared to more than 90%. Employee morale also improved, as shown by steady improvements in workforce commitment and reduction in annual staff turnover and employee satisfaction to 96%. SCF's overall revenue has gone up and, compared to IHS days and to the rest of health care, costs per person have gone down.

What were they doing differently? Had they found some new treatments that science had missed? How had they improved the outcomes of their delivery system so dramatically? I decided to go see for myself.

RELATIONSHIP-CENTERED CARE

When I visited SCF's Anchorage Native Primary Care Center and some of their more remote clinics in 2015, they were running a training program for other health systems on how to improve care and healing. I took the training; talked with employees, health care providers, and patients; and visited with system leaders. SCF had first asked to take over parts of health care for the Alaska Native people from IHS in 1982. From the very beginning, SCF set up "listening circles," in which the people talked about their needs beyond medical care—needs in the physical, behavioral, social, and spiritual dimensions of their lives. The listening circle approach was an adaptation of an Alaskan Native process for social connection and reconciliation traditionally used by many of the tribes. SCF leaders used these circles to directly address the social and emotional dimension. One leader, an employee named Dr. Kathleen Gottlieb, opened up about the deep wounds and adverse childhood experiences in her family. Others followed, revealing the impact of illness and trauma in their lives. Soon these listening circles became Learning Circles, as participants developed deeper relationships and began to help—and challenge—each other to engage in whole-person healing, not just disease treatment. Gradually, this process was embedded into SCF, and, with Ms. Gottlieb as President/CEO, relationship-centered care became part of its standard delivery processes.

The Learning Circle is a safe place where people can address trauma, fear, and grief and deal with their loves and losses with others' support. In the process, they become more whole—more connected to their own social and emotional "bodies"—and healing sets in. One person I spoke with told me she grew up in a family where physical and sexual abuse, alcoholism, suicide, and obesity had been growing problems for more than four generations. By coming to a Learning Circle, she had could break that cycle and raise children who were largely freed from these adverse experiences. She did it by sharing some of the deepest traumas and losses in her own life. Others walked the healing journey with her as she learned to take these behaviors out of her own family and adopt other, healthier behaviors. For those who engaged in this process, life quality improved, and life expectancy jumped by decades—especially for their children. Over the years, this focus on relationships became a core part of the SCF health care operations. Today at SCF the patients are no longer treated as people whose medical services are delivered by strangers. Patients are now treated as customers and are owners of the company. They have continuous input on their own needs and the needs of the community. The use of the social and emotional dimension for healing was incorporated by bringing "behavioral health" into all the clinics. All employees, including physicians, are required to understand and participate in Learning Circles—through SCF's Relationship-based Core Concepts workshop, which is now offered to other health systems.

But I wondered: were the medical treatments provided by SCF somehow more evidence-based, more scientific or state-of-the-art than they had been before they developed the Nuka System of Care? The answer was no. Access to good, evidence-based medical treatments had been part of the IHS before SCF took over care, and that good medical practice had been continually updated for decades by IHS. Yet outcomes had continually worsened. The types of medical treatments and the agents used—drugs, surgery, counseling, emergency, and preventive care—are all part of the current Nuka System of Care and provided by IHS elsewhere. SCF had no unusual medical interventions, no better science, no more magic bullets than other systems. They still make diagnoses and deal with research and medical guidelines, insurance coding, and reimbursement. The doctors and nurses come from standard medical schools and use standard treatment tools. What has changed is relationships and customer ownership. SCF added the social and emotional dimension of healing to their delivery of health care. This allows them to tap into this previously ignored capacity for human healing.

THE FACE OF LOVE

Most of the medical community ignores this data, just as I had. Most physicians and scientists think these dimensions are too intangible, so they seek more material ways to treat illness—preferring to lower cholesterol rather than increase love; to raise brain serotonin rather than deal with grief. Not that lowering cholesterol or raising serotonin are bad things—but they are only a small part of what humans need to heal. Love may be a many-splendored thing—the stuff of poets and songs and mystics—but that splendor does not pay off like a drug or supplement. So, nothing further was ever done with the rabbit data on petting and heart disease, yet we have a multibillion-dollar drug and supplement industry selling you a way to lower cholesterol. Little has been done with the data showing reduced mortality with reduced loneliness, yet we have a multibillion-dollar drug industry to increase serotonin so you can worry less about your loneliness.

After I flew back from Alaska, where I had seen relationship-centered care in full operation, I could not find a health system in our area that integrated this into the care for my own family. When Susan got cancer again, we needed such a system so we had to figure out how build one on our own. Fortunately, we had the awareness and social networks to do so.

After six months of chemotherapy, Susan now faced another, even more traumatic event—the surgery. A double mastectomy and simultaneous DIEP flap reconstruction (deep inferior epigastric perforators, named for the associated blood vessels) this meant a twelve-hour operation involving three surgeons, two anesthesiologists, and four nurses. She would be cut from neck to pelvis, with the top part removed and the bottom part shifted up to the top—her body reorganized. Thank science for anesthesia and antiseptics! The recovery would be long and painful; the physical loss alone would be large. The surgeon said she would bounce back in no time—two weeks. The nurse indicated that she should not lift the grandbaby or even have him on her lap for eight weeks. The risk of suffering would be great; the possibility of falling into sadness and depression was present every day. While Susan had difficulty with the behavioral dimensions of healing that could prepare her for this onslaught—exercise, improved diet and supplements, meditation and visualization—she was good at relationships. During her first cancer she had sought divine love through prayer and meditation and a spiritual meaning for her illness. This time she looked again for love, but not the divine kind of love that spiritual healers describe. This time she sought a different kind of love—the common love of ordinary humans. It was a love that emerged largely from the females in our family, at least in acts and presence. Those who showed up at the door to sit with Susan when she couldn't move were people like our next-door neighbor, Rose Ellen. Rose Ellen doesn't cook, so she didn't bring any meals; she said she couldn't help with the grandchild because she wasn't good with babies. But she came over anyway and said she would be available for anything Susan needed any time, day or night—just let her know. Rose Ellen isn't a romantic type of person, nor is she particularly spiritual or complicated in how she lives her life—but she offered true caring and presence on an as-needed basis.

Others came, too. Susan's friend from college, who'd had a similar procedure a few months before, showed up and stayed for several days cooking, cleaning, and making conversation. Our two daughters came. One, a chaplain—the "analytical one" of the family, who had worked for over a year as a hospital chaplain ministering to the depths of suffering—knew exactly how to be, from lying down in bed with her mother to setting up an online meal chain system that brought food from friends on an organized schedule. Our younger daughter is a singer and teacher, the "creative one" in the family. She recorded a special set of songs for each phase of recovery and brought humor and laughter into the house—sustenance for the soul. Through both chemotherapy and surgery, one person after another showed up—all people Susan had loved and served in her life. Some we had not known well before. Some we had. Our niece from California flew out for ten days to help with the grandbaby and to cook. My sister followed her and did the same thing. I realized from watching this parade of faces—all bringing their physical bodies and human love to our house—that this was also the way that divine love leaked in. No special spiritual healers or waving of hands needed. The support first, Dr. Geller explained, setting up disease-focused groups emed the right approach. But then he realized that, like Gloria, the ajority of people with chronic illness didn't like going to a group iere everyone seemed sicker or more depressed than they were. In dition, many were also lonely, and that loneliness was preventing em from healing.

ven if they were not lonely," Geller said, "connecting with others was t a bad thing for anyone. It's like social exercise. Nobody can pay for ychotherapy or gym membership anyway. The patients who come this clinic are poor, and life has not been filled with opportunity. any of them don't even have the five-dollar copay we ask for. So I cided to start a bunch of groups based not on my desires or their edical diagnoses, but on their preferences and friendships. If they in a group they like, they stick with it. If, at the same time, they get idance from me, our health coaches, or each other to help change to ealthier behavior, they get better. And best of all," Dr. Geller noted, articipants become empowered to be healthier because they are supported by others and others need them. They feel important again."

nd that is exactly what happened. Groups began to form that did t conform to the usual medical categories the health care sysm was trying to treat—like weight loss, cancer support, pain, or st–heart attack. Instead, groups were formed around friendships. ften these took the form of youth groups, men's or women's groups, groups of mothers and seniors. Some combined these categories ecause the members just got along with each other. Says Dr. Geller, atients who found and attended a group they liked not only made iends, but their health improved faster than in disease-based groups. ow many of the groups are run by other patients—with help from ır staff."

r. Geller and his staff have set up a way to tap into the healing power f the social and emotional dimension for people with few other sources than their ability to find friends and the common human ve that accompanies it. It would have been the perfect solution for loria and many like her.

we got from this network of other human beings allowed me to spend time sitting with Susan, helping her to the bathroom and the shower, sleeping next to her when she slept, bringing our new grandbaby up the steps into her room—and going to work. I took periodic breaks to take care of myself, and so I could, with this help from others, be present for her in the long run. We may not have had a Nuka-like health system to deliver relationship-centered care, but Susan used a network of friends and family to bolster the social and emotional dimension of healing on her own. And it worked. Her white count stayed up, her surgery recovery was like clockwork, and the grandbaby brought us joy and thrived. Eight weeks after the end of chemo and surgery not only could Susan lift the grandbaby, but she also had planned a trip for the extended family to Florida during the holiday season. The medical treatments for her cancer may have added only an 7% chance to her ten-year survival, but the quality added to all our lives by the social and emotional dimension of healing was immeasurable. We had found our own Beauty Way.

GLORIA

Not everyone has the network Susan does to tap the social and emotional dimensions of healing. However, that does not mean this dimension can't be used effectively by everyone. Gloria demonstrated that to me. She had retired three years earlier from her job making omelets and doing kitchen work at a local golf club. The club, an old one with an established staff, had been her home for forty years. She started working there when she was twenty-five. It paid reasonably and provided benefits, so she stayed. With that income and her husband's, they raised three children—two of whom had gone to college—something she was very proud of because she had not finished high school. She had retired at age sixty-five, and soon after that, her fatigue and muscle pains became progressively worse. She was diagnosed with fibromyalgia and chronic musculoskeletal back pain. She was told to exercise and rest, given painkillers to take "as needed," and sent to physical therapy and acupuncture. These helped some, but her pain levels hovered "around four to five out of ten all the time," she told me on our first visit, "especially in the morning."

"It is pretty bad. Sometimes it takes me an hour to loosen up and have enough energy to get out of the bedroom"—a common situation with fibromyalgia.

Gloria was referred to me by her primary care doctor because she wanted to do better and heard that I prescribed fewer drugs than other doctors. As we went through her healing-oriented assessment, I found very little amiss in her life. She had a comfortable clean house and a "nice husband who works a lot"; she tried to eat right and walk outside every morning. She went to Catholic mass each Sunday and prayed daily—"for others," she mentioned nonchalantly. Her ten-year-old grandchild (she had five grandchildren who lived some distance from her) had come to stay for the summer. He was a "nice boy, very active, and in camp most of the day." A year previously she had gone to an acupuncturist that her health system covered, which helped her back pain for a while, but then her insurance stopped paying for it. "It did not seem to help my fibromyalgia or my tiredness," she said.

When we got to questions about her social and emotional life, I noticed a shift in her voice. "Do you have good friends you spend time with?" I asked.

Her voice softened as if she did not want me to hear. "Well, doctor," she said slowly, "to be honest, ever since my retirement I have missed everybody. I was at the club for forty years, rarely missed a day. I miss it now. But they are all so busy. I don't want to bother them."

Gloria, it turned out, was lonely. And she was not alone in that. Each year more than sixty million people in the United States suffer from chronic loneliness. It is common after retirement when routine interactions and friendships at work are suddenly stopped. Although her medical diagnosis was fibromyalgia, her problem was loneliness. Was it a coincidence that her chronic pain and frequent visits to the doctors began soon after her retirement? While I had no objective test that could prove this connection, I did know that reconnecting her to a meaningful social network would help her heal. But how to do that? We needed to find a group that Gloria could join.

She seemed to read my mind. "I went to one of those chr
support groups, but I didn't like it. Everybody was so sick. I
afterward."

Back to the drawing board, I thought.

"Well, Gloria," I said after a pause. "It seems to me that
benefit from finding a place to go each day to work with oth
things that are meaningful for you. Let's think about how t
She agreed.

Gloria ended up volunteering at a church food pantry and
running it. Her pain improved by 80% in about six mon
the day she started, she said she felt better, and gradually
returned. My guess is that she was largely cured. Her reco
have been shortened and even more effective had she acces
like Dr. Jeffery Geller's.

DR. GELLER

Dr. Jeffery Geller is one of the world's experts on heali
illness through social connection. He does this through g
conducted at a community health center in Lawrence, Mass
the poorest county in that state. Some of his groups gather
illnesses—like for weight loss, diabetes, cardiovascular
chronic pain, like Gloria had. Some of his groups are
behavior—like for fitness, cooking, or stress management.
no theme other than improving health and well-being in
Dr. Geller has a different agenda from all of that.

"What I am really treating," says Dr. Geller, when only sligh
"is loneliness. More people get better, and faster, when I fo
ing them with that than if I only treat their disease or tr
their behavior." He went on to tell me how he came to th
was using group visits so I could treat more patients. Th
the clinic is high and our reimbursement is low. Paying fo
instruction in wellness and lifestyle was not possible. M
need help with the same things—diet, exercise, stress,
management—so why not do it as a group?"

THE CAKE

The tools used and exact path in a healing journey are different for everyone. Yet the basic processes are the same. Bill gave up seeking cures, then realized the childhood source of his pain and eventually found a path to self-care that kept him largely pain-free and functioning. Jeff continued to smoke after joining a group to help him quit—but he eventually succeeded by substituting a healthy behavior for an unhealthy one. Maria jumped right into the behavioral change without preparation and planning—and suffered from it. Later she found a way to connect it to something more fulfilling in her life. That is when it became a long-term solution and lifted her out of sadness and struggle—and improved her diabetes. Susan and Clara began their journeys in a different dimension: the space they lived in. Susan also added tools from the social and emotional dimension of healing. Accessing the love and care of others helped her recover during her most difficult time in the curing of her cancer—when she felt she could not go on. And it came in an unexpected way.

About the tenth week of Susan's weekly chemotherapy, a deep fatigue hit her. The word *fatigue* does not really describe it adequately. It's hard to describe using any language. It's like having a hundred-pound millstone around your neck and being thrown into the bottom of a river. You can move around a little bit, but you can't get back to the surface. The amount of oxygen is low, and the effort it takes to move is huge. You know you can't get back to the surface, so you are just watching and waiting as the world goes by. Sharks and other scary animals seem to be swimming nearby in the murky water. I too felt her fatigue, especially toward the end of the day when there was a lack of will to even speak. It was more than the fatigue we expected and she'd had from the start of chemotherapy. It kicked in most drastically in the middle of chemotherapy and stretched out for several weeks and into the summer.

On this particular Fourth of July, we had four generations of family with us, including my mother and the grandbaby. But I was worried that she would not be able to participate in one of her favorite family holidays—the Fourth of July and especially the making of The Cake.

This was not just any old cake—it was The Cake. It was a cake Susan prepared for the family gathering every year for over thirty-five years. Everyone looked forward to it. It was, of course, a depiction of the American flag. Susan had been making this cake since before we were married. She usually served it after the family dinner when all were gathered to celebrate Independence Day—a ritual revealed right before the fireworks. Originally, The Cake was made from a cake mix, with thick cream cheese frosting, and decorated with blue and red food coloring and sprinkles. Not the picture of healthy food. Over the years she had substituted healthier ingredients such as blueberries for the starry field and strawberries for the red stripes. She also began to make a light whipping cream frosting with healthier fat and less sugar. I tried to encourage her to use whole grains in the cake mix, but that never quite worked, and I must admit it didn't have the same result as the good old Betty Crocker cake mix, so we ended up sticking with the latter.

But on this particular July Fourth, Susan had just received her tenth weekly chemo treatment and was very tired and anemic. She had not cooked for weeks. Still, despite how she was feeling, she decided to make it.

My ninety-year-old mother, who has moderate dementia, had come to visit, along with my sister and her daughter. We had the core family and more—it was the first July Fourth also for our new grandchild. Despite her dementia, my mother responded with tremendous joy when she saw her great-grandbaby, a reaction that was infectious to us all. Perhaps it was this joy, and that all of her family was together, that motivated my wife to make The Cake. Others helped. Susan made the cake part with the Betty Crocker mix, and our daughter prepared the whipped cream frosting and decorated The Cake while the others played with the baby.

After dinner, Susan placed The Cake on the table to an enthusiastic reaction from everyone. My mother, who had never seen The Cake before, reacted with more great joy.

"It's beautiful!" she said. "I'll have a big piece."

My sister, who usually goes sugar-, gluten-, and dairy-free, ate three pieces. My son, normally not a cake fan, had two; and I—remembering the rabbits—had one myself. The kitchen was cleaned up. We went outside and shot off fireworks and shared music together. When my mother left a couple of days later, her final words were, "Thank you for having me. It was such a joy to see the baby." Then, after a pause that made us think she was confused, she turned to Susan and said "And oh, thank you for that cake!" There was an understanding in her eyes, rarely seen any more with her advancing dementia.

The next day we saw a clear change in Susan. She began to make travel plans. She wanted to go to a wedding we'd been invited to; previously she had been noncommittal, but now she looked at the calendar to plan the trip. She started talking politics again—something she loved. She mentioned walking the Camino de Santiago again, and planning a visit to see her mother and family in Florida the next winter. She spoke of taking care of her grandchild more fully next spring. She considered resuming her volunteer work teaching English as a second language. The Cake had become a healing agent and helped turn things around. It didn't change the physical side effects—she still had the fatigue, her red blood cell count and hemoglobin were still low, and her hair kept falling out—but after The Cake was made and served, she recovered something she had lost during the treatment. It was something even more fundamental than her hair, her toenails (which she also lost) and her white blood cells. Her soul was returning—and along with it, the joys of her life.

CHAPTER 8

Finding Meaning

How mind and spirit heal.

From birth to death, we humans are constantly trying to understand and make sense of the world. We are meaning-making machines. But unlike machines, we operate in nonrational ways, most of which occurs outside our awareness—even while we sleep. These attempts at sense-making continuously take in information and compare it to both past experience and the current context, determining how to respond. That response is triggered (or not) depending on subtle judgments we make concerning our safety, the social situation, and our very survival. We absorb and integrate that information from many sources at once—our body, sensory perceptions, relationships, memories, beliefs, and hopes—and use that information to create our universe and trigger biological responses.

Meaning is more like a thought field shifting between people and their environments, and it emerges from multiple interacting judgments rather than a single thought. What we believe and expect drives what we see and how our minds and bodies react. Stress, for example, with all its physical, emotional, and mental consequences, often has less to do with an actual threat than with what we believe the threat to be. Meaning is not simply held in the mind; it is constructed in our body by our culture.

The way to access our healing capacity depends on using tools from any of the dimensions of a person to find and construct meaningful responses. We have talked about three of those dimensions—the external environment, our behavior (including lifestyle and medical treatments), and how we use our emotions and social relationships.

But the most powerful way we have for making healing work is our own automatic assumptions about whether healing is possible; that is, the story we, our family and friends, and culture tell us about the way things are and can be. In this chapter, I describe patients who have broken out of limiting assumptions and experienced dramatic healing. As in other chapters, I will show you how systems science documents how this healing works and can be enhanced in daily life. My patient Jake showed me how simple and powerful this process can be if we take control of it.

JAKE

Jake was on the edge of death—now for the third time. No one knew why. He had been a tobacco farmer all his life—as had his father and grandfather before him. They did not own the farm; they only worked it. He did not smoke, did not drink, and worked hard every day except Sunday. At eleven years old, he was pulled out of school to work the farm when his family needed extra hands and money to survive. That lasted the rest of his life, even as he grew up and started his own family. Farming, family, and church were the anchors of his life. Jake was a mild-mannered and deeply faithful man. A man of simple needs and little talk. Content with his life. His only major venture outside the farm was a short trip to Vietnam in the military. He was drafted and shipped over with an infantry division just before the end of the war. His unit left six months later and he was discharged back home. That was years ago. He had been healthy all his life, as far as he knew. But he rarely visited a doctor. Then, for reasons neither he or his doctors could explain, he ended up in the intensive care unit (ICU)—not once, but three times—each time on the verge of death.

Each ICU admission had the same pattern. Jake developed a fever and began to get short of breath. X-rays revealed a sudden, severe pneumonia—in both lungs. "A whiteout," they called it. As the doctors watched in frustration, the pneumonia spread, eventually covering his entire lung fields and dropping his blood oxygen to dangerously low levels. The first two times that happened they needed to intubate him (insert a breathing tube) and put him on a breathing machine. Sputum and blood cultures did not reveal a cause. No bacteria were found, and viral levels were also inconclusive. The infectious disease specialist we called in assumed it was a virus and said Jake must have an immune problem. The immunology specialist we called in suspected the same, but no specific immune problem was found. Each of the first two times this happened the pneumonia lasted about six weeks—with two weeks on the breathing machine—and then it gradually cleared up. It took Jake about four months after that to fully recover and get back to work. Now, for the third time in as many years, it was happening again.

When I visited Jake in the ICU, the specialists were debating when to intubate him again. "Probably tonight," said the internist in charge of his hospital care. His pneumonia was spreading as before, and his oxygen levels were beginning to drop. The oxygen by mask was barely keeping him in the range needed for survival. Jake's breathing became more labored by the hour, and he was tired. But the internist wanted to delay as long as possible. Being intubated is never a very good idea unless you absolutely need it. I sat by Jake's bed to see how he was doing and explore what he was thinking of all this.

He was circumspect. "Well, Doc," he said between labored breaths, "I guess . . . the Lord . . . has some purpose in it. . . . Maybe . . . I done somethin' . . . bad or maybe . . . he just wants . . . to test my faith. . . . We all have . . . our cross to bear."

Did he have others pulling for him? I asked

"Oh sure, Doc . . . my family . . . and church prayin' . . . for me every day. . . . I prayin', too. . . . most all day. . . . nothin' else to do . . . I guess."

I was struck by how calm he was, even with his labored breathing, on the edge of intubation and possible death. Could he go through this illness again, having been weakened from the last two times? Then, mostly out of desperation, I had an idea. I tried to frame my proposal in a way he might find meaningful.

"Jake, would you be interested in trying something that might help all that prayer you are having?" I had decided to explore working with Jake's deep faith rather than provide long explanations we got from this network of other human beings allowed me to spend time sitting with Susan, helping her to the bathroom and the shower, sleeping next to her when she slept, bringing our new grandbaby up the steps into her room—and going to work. I took periodic breaks to take care of myself, and so I could, with this help from others, be present for her in the long run. We may not have had a Nuka-like health system to deliver relationship-centered care, but Susan used a network of friends and family to bolster the social and emotional dimension of healing on her own. And it worked. Her white count stayed up, her surgery recovery was like clockwork, and the grandbaby brought us joy and thrived. Eight weeks after the end of chemo and surgery not only could Susan lift the grandbaby, but she also had planned a trip for the extended family to Florida during the holiday season. The medical treatments for her cancer may have added only an 7% chance to her ten-year survival, but the quality added to all our lives by the social and emotional dimension of healing was immeasurable. We had found our own Beauty Way.

GLORIA

Not everyone has the network Susan does to tap the social and emotional dimensions of healing. However, that does not mean this dimension can't be used effectively by everyone. Gloria demonstrated that to me. She had retired three years earlier from her job making omelets and doing kitchen work at a local golf club. The club, an old one with an established staff, had been her home for forty years. She started working there when she was twenty-five. It paid reasonably and provided benefits, so she stayed. With that income and her husband's, they raised three children—two of whom had gone to college—something she was very proud of because she had not finished high school. She had retired at age sixty-five, and soon after that, her fatigue and muscle pains became progressively worse. She was diagnosed with fibromyalgia and chronic musculoskeletal back pain. She was told to exercise and rest, given painkillers to take "as needed," and sent to physical therapy and acupuncture. These helped some, but her pain levels hovered "around four to five out of ten all the time," she told me on our first visit, "especially in the morning."

"It is pretty bad. Sometimes it takes me an hour to loosen up and have enough energy to get out of the bedroom"—a common situation with fibromyalgia.

Gloria was referred to me by her primary care doctor because she wanted to do better and heard that I prescribed fewer drugs than other doctors. As we went through her healing-oriented assessment, I found very little amiss in her life. She had a comfortable clean house and a "nice husband who works a lot"; she tried to eat right and walk outside every morning. She went to Catholic mass each Sunday and prayed daily—"for others," she mentioned nonchalantly. Her ten-year-old grandchild (she had five grandchildren who lived some distance from her) had come to stay for the summer. He was a "nice boy, very active, and in camp most of the day." A year previously she had gone to an acupuncturist that her health system covered, which helped her back pain for a while, but then her insurance stopped paying for it. "It did not seem to help my fibromyalgia or my tiredness," she said.

When we got to questions about her social and emotional life, I noticed a shift in her voice. "Do you have good friends you spend time with?" I asked.

Her voice softened as if she did not want me to hear. "Well, doctor," she said slowly, "to be honest, ever since my retirement I have missed everybody. I was at the club for forty years, rarely missed a day. I miss it now. But they are all so busy. I don't want to bother them."

Gloria, it turned out, was lonely. And she was not alone in that. Each year more than sixty million people in the United States suffer from chronic loneliness. It is common after retirement when routine interactions and friendships at work are suddenly stopped. Although her medical diagnosis was fibromyalgia, her problem was loneliness. Was it a coincidence that her chronic pain and frequent visits to the doctors began soon after her retirement? While I had no objective test that could prove this connection, I did know that reconnecting her to a meaningful social network would help her heal. But how to do that? We needed to find a group that Gloria could join.

She seemed to read my mind. "I went to one of those chronic pain support groups, but I didn't like it. Everybody was so sick. I felt worse afterward."

Back to the drawing board, I thought.

"Well, Gloria," I said after a pause. "It seems to me that you would benefit from finding a place to go each day to work with others and do things that are meaningful for you. Let's think about how to do that." She agreed.

Gloria ended up volunteering at a church food pantry and eventually running it. Her pain improved by 80% in about six months. From the day she started, she said she felt better, and gradually her energy returned. My guess is that she was largely cured. Her recovery might have been shortened and even more effective had she access to a clinic like Dr. Jeffery Geller's.

DR. GELLER

Dr. Jeffery Geller is one of the world's experts on healing chronic illness through social connection. He does this through group visits conducted at a community health center in Lawrence, Massachusetts—the poorest county in that state. Some of his groups gather for specific illnesses—like for weight loss, diabetes, cardiovascular disease—or chronic pain, like Gloria had. Some of his groups are to change behavior—like for fitness, cooking, or stress management. Many have no theme other than improving health and well-being in general. But Dr. Geller has a different agenda from all of that.

"What I am really treating," says Dr. Geller, when only slightly pressed, "is loneliness. More people get better, and faster, when I focus on helping them with that than if I only treat their disease or try to change their behavior." He went on to tell me how he came to this. "At first I was using group visits so I could treat more patients. The demand at the clinic is high and our reimbursement is low. Paying for individual instruction in wellness and lifestyle was not possible. Many of them need help with the same things—diet, exercise, stress, medication management—so why not do it as a group?"

At first, Dr. Geller explained, setting up disease-focused groups seemed the right approach. But then he realized that, like Gloria, the majority of people with chronic illness didn't like going to a group where everyone seemed sicker or more depressed than they were. In addition, many were also lonely, and that loneliness was preventing them from healing.

"Even if they were not lonely," Geller said, "connecting with others was not a bad thing for anyone. It's like social exercise. Nobody can pay for psychotherapy or gym membership anyway. The patients who come to this clinic are poor, and life has not been filled with opportunity. Many of them don't even have the five-dollar copay we ask for. So I decided to start a bunch of groups based not on my desires or their medical diagnoses, but on their preferences and friendships. If they join a group they like, they stick with it. If, at the same time, they get guidance from me, our health coaches, or each other to help change to healthier behavior, they get better. And best of all," Dr. Geller noted, "participants become empowered to be healthier because they are supported by others and others need them. They feel important again."

And that is exactly what happened. Groups began to form that did not conform to the usual medical categories the health care system was trying to treat—like weight loss, cancer support, pain, or post–heart attack. Instead, groups were formed around friendships. Often these took the form of youth groups, men's or women's groups, or groups of mothers and seniors. Some combined these categories because the members just got along with each other. Says Dr. Geller, "patients who found and attended a group they liked not only made friends, but their health improved faster than in disease-based groups. Now many of the groups are run by other patients—with help from our staff."

Dr. Geller and his staff have set up a way to tap into the healing power of the social and emotional dimension for people with few other resources than their ability to find friends and the common human love that accompanies it. It would have been the perfect solution for Gloria and many like her.

THE CAKE

The tools used and exact path in a healing journey are different for everyone. Yet the basic processes are the same. Bill gave up seeking cures, then realized the childhood source of his pain and eventually found a path to self-care that kept him largely pain-free and functioning. Jeff continued to smoke after joining a group to help him quit—but he eventually succeeded by substituting a healthy behavior for an unhealthy one. Maria jumped right into the behavioral change without preparation and planning—and suffered from it. Later she found a way to connect it to something more fulfilling in her life. That is when it became a long-term solution and lifted her out of sadness and struggle—and improved her diabetes. Susan and Clara began their journeys in a different dimension: the space they lived in. Susan also added tools from the social and emotional dimension of healing. Accessing the love and care of others helped her recover during her most difficult time in the curing of her cancer—when she felt she could not go on. And it came in an unexpected way.

About the tenth week of Susan's weekly chemotherapy, a deep fatigue hit her. The word *fatigue* does not really describe it adequately. It's hard to describe using any language. It's like having a hundred-pound millstone around your neck and being thrown into the bottom of a river. You can move around a little bit, but you can't get back to the surface. The amount of oxygen is low, and the effort it takes to move is huge. You know you can't get back to the surface, so you are just watching and waiting as the world goes by. Sharks and other scary animals seem to be swimming nearby in the murky water. I too felt her fatigue, especially toward the end of the day when there was a lack of will to even speak. It was more than the fatigue we expected and she'd had from the start of chemotherapy. It kicked in most drastically in the middle of chemotherapy and stretched out for several weeks and into the summer.

On this particular Fourth of July, we had four generations of family with us, including my mother and the grandbaby. But I was worried that she would not be able to participate in one of her favorite family holidays—the Fourth of July and especially the making of The Cake.

This was not just any old cake—it was The Cake. It was a cake Susan prepared for the family gathering every year for over thirty-five years. Everyone looked forward to it. It was, of course, a depiction of the American flag. Susan had been making this cake since before we were married. She usually served it after the family dinner when all were gathered to celebrate Independence Day—a ritual revealed right before the fireworks. Originally, The Cake was made from a cake mix, with thick cream cheese frosting, and decorated with blue and red food coloring and sprinkles. Not the picture of healthy food. Over the years she had substituted healthier ingredients such as blueberries for the starry field and strawberries for the red stripes. She also began to make a light whipping cream frosting with healthier fat and less sugar. I tried to encourage her to use whole grains in the cake mix, but that never quite worked, and I must admit it didn't have the same result as the good old Betty Crocker cake mix, so we ended up sticking with the latter.

But on this particular July Fourth, Susan had just received her tenth weekly chemo treatment and was very tired and anemic. She had not cooked for weeks. Still, despite how she was feeling, she decided to make it.

My ninety-year-old mother, who has moderate dementia, had come to visit, along with my sister and her daughter. We had the core family and more—it was the first July Fourth also for our new grandchild. Despite her dementia, my mother responded with tremendous joy when she saw her great-grandbaby, a reaction that was infectious to us all. Perhaps it was this joy, and that all of her family was together, that motivated my wife to make The Cake. Others helped. Susan made the cake part with the Betty Crocker mix, and our daughter prepared the whipped cream frosting and decorated The Cake while the others played with the baby.

After dinner, Susan placed The Cake on the table to an enthusiastic reaction from everyone. My mother, who had never seen The Cake before, reacted with more great joy.

"It's beautiful!" she said. "I'll have a big piece."

My sister, who usually goes sugar-, gluten-, and dairy-free, ate three pieces. My son, normally not a cake fan, had two; and I—remembering the rabbits—had one myself. The kitchen was cleaned up. We went outside and shot off fireworks and shared music together. When my mother left a couple of days later, her final words were, "Thank you for having me. It was such a joy to see the baby." Then, after a pause that made us think she was confused, she turned to Susan and said "And oh, thank you for that cake!" There was an understanding in her eyes, rarely seen any more with her advancing dementia.

The next day we saw a clear change in Susan. She began to make travel plans. She wanted to go to a wedding we'd been invited to; previously she had been noncommittal, but now she looked at the calendar to plan the trip. She started talking politics again—something she loved. She mentioned walking the Camino de Santiago again, and planning a visit to see her mother and family in Florida the next winter. She spoke of taking care of her grandchild more fully next spring. She considered resuming her volunteer work teaching English as a second language. The Cake had become a healing agent and helped turn things around. It didn't change the physical side effects—she still had the fatigue, her red blood cell count and hemoglobin were still low, and her hair kept falling out—but after The Cake was made and served, she recovered something she had lost during the treatment. It was something even more fundamental than her hair, her toenails (which she also lost) and her white blood cells. Her soul was returning—and along with it, the joys of her life.

CHAPTER 8

Finding Meaning

How mind and spirit heal.

From birth to death, we humans are constantly trying to understand and make sense of the world. We are meaning-making machines. But unlike machines, we operate in nonrational ways, most of which occurs outside our awareness—even while we sleep. These attempts at sense-making continuously take in information and compare it to both past experience and the current context, determining how to respond. That response is triggered (or not) depending on subtle judgments we make concerning our safety, the social situation, and our very survival. We absorb and integrate that information from many sources at once—our body, sensory perceptions, relationships, memories, beliefs, and hopes—and use that information to create our universe and trigger biological responses.

Meaning is more like a thought field shifting between people and their environments, and it emerges from multiple interacting judgments rather than a single thought. What we believe and expect drives what we see and how our minds and bodies react. Stress, for example, with all its physical, emotional, and mental consequences, often has less to do with an actual threat than with what we believe the threat to be. Meaning is not simply held in the mind; it is constructed in our body by our culture.

The way to access our healing capacity depends on using tools from any of the dimensions of a person to find and construct meaningful responses. We have talked about three of those dimensions—the external environment, our behavior (including lifestyle and medical treatments), and how we use our emotions and social relationships.

But the most powerful way we have for making healing work is our own automatic assumptions about whether healing is possible; that is, the story we, our family and friends, and culture tell us about the way things are and can be. In this chapter, I describe patients who have broken out of limiting assumptions and experienced dramatic healing. As in other chapters, I will show you how systems science documents how this healing works and can be enhanced in daily life. My patient Jake showed me how simple and powerful this process can be if we take control of it.

JAKE

Jake was on the edge of death—now for the third time. No one knew why. He had been a tobacco farmer all his life—as had his father and grandfather before him. They did not own the farm; they only worked it. He did not smoke, did not drink, and worked hard every day except Sunday. At eleven years old, he was pulled out of school to work the farm when his family needed extra hands and money to survive. That lasted the rest of his life, even as he grew up and started his own family. Farming, family, and church were the anchors of his life. Jake was a mild-mannered and deeply faithful man. A man of simple needs and little talk. Content with his life. His only major venture outside the farm was a short trip to Vietnam in the military. He was drafted and shipped over with an infantry division just before the end of the war. His unit left six months later and he was discharged back home. That was years ago. He had been healthy all his life, as far as he knew. But he rarely visited a doctor. Then, for reasons neither he or his doctors could explain, he ended up in the intensive care unit (ICU)—not once, but three times—each time on the verge of death.

Each ICU admission had the same pattern. Jake developed a fever and began to get short of breath. X-rays revealed a sudden, severe pneumonia—in both lungs. "A whiteout," they called it. As the doctors watched in frustration, the pneumonia spread, eventually covering his entire lung fields and dropping his blood oxygen to dangerously low levels. The first two times that happened they needed to intubate him (insert a breathing tube) and put him on a breathing machine. Sputum and blood cultures did not reveal a cause. No bacteria were found, and viral levels were also inconclusive. The infectious disease specialist we called in assumed it was a virus and said Jake must have an immune problem. The immunology specialist we called in suspected the same, but no specific immune problem was found. Each of the first two times this happened the pneumonia lasted about six weeks—with two weeks on the breathing machine—and then it gradually cleared up. It took Jake about four months after that to fully recover and get back to work. Now, for the third time in as many years, it was happening again.

When I visited Jake in the ICU, the specialists were debating when to intubate him again. "Probably tonight," said the internist in charge of his hospital care. His pneumonia was spreading as before, and his oxygen levels were beginning to drop. The oxygen by mask was barely keeping him in the range needed for survival. Jake's breathing became more labored by the hour, and he was tired. But the internist wanted to delay as long as possible. Being intubated is never a very good idea unless you absolutely need it. I sat by Jake's bed to see how he was doing and explore what he was thinking of all this.

He was circumspect. "Well, Doc," he said between labored breaths, "I guess . . . the Lord . . . has some purpose in it. . . . Maybe . . . I done somethin' . . . bad or maybe . . . he just wants . . . to test my faith. . . . We all have . . . our cross to bear."

Did he have others pulling for him? I asked

"Oh sure, Doc . . . my family . . . and church prayin' . . . for me every day. . . . I prayin', too. . . . most all day. . . . nothin' else to do . . . I guess."

I was struck by how calm he was, even with his labored breathing, on the edge of intubation and possible death. Could he go through this illness again, having been weakened from the last two times? Then, mostly out of desperation, I had an idea. I tried to frame my proposal in a way he might find meaningful.

"Jake, would you be interested in trying something that might help all that prayer you are having?" I had decided to explore working with Jake's deep faith rather than provide long explanations about mind-body effect, placebo research, the immune system, and visualization.

"Sure, Doc," he responded quickly. "I always want . . . to help the Lord . . . in his will . . . I'm sure he . . . wants me healed . . . I'll help . . . if I can."

I presented Jake with my proposal. "Is there any place in your lungs that you feel is clear? Any place you feel the air goes when you breathe in?" I asked.

Jake thought for a while as I held my breath. Perhaps there was no opportunity to try my idea after all. He took a couple of breaths, deeper than the usual labored ones, and concentrated. Finally, he said, "Sure, Doc . . . air goes right here." He pointed to a place on his lower left chest. "When I take . . . a breath . . . it all . . . goes right there." He pointed again to the same place. An opening.

"Great," I said, seeing a window of hope. "Then here is what I want you to do. As you lie here and pray, I want you to try and relax as much as you can and then imagine in your mind that the air is going into that place and that place is expanding—getting bigger. Imagine that area gradually growing, getting larger and larger, clearer and clearer. Imagine all the love of the Lord and all of those prayers from your family and church and all the air coming into your lungs and clearing away the pneumonia you have—healing your lungs."

We did a few practices sessions in which I encouraged him to visit in his mind a place in his church that he loved, and to feel a sense of peace there. And then to imagine the love and power of the Lord was flowing into that small space in his lung. He got it quickly. Then he smiled. "That be easy, Doc . . . that be real easy . . . to do."

The next morning, I arrived at the hospital to visit Jake, fully expecting him to be on the ventilator. The ICU specialist watching him had thought he would not last the night on his own. Most people tire out and decompensate during the night, and Jake had been on the edge of that the day before. But to my surprise, when I walked into his room, he was sitting up in a chair and still just on the oxygen mask. During the night his oxygen levels had held steady. He smiled when he saw me come in.

"How is it going, Jake?" I asked.

He smiled again. "It goin' fine, Doc. . . . Goin' fine. . . . That thing . . . that thing you taught me . . . works real well. The place for air . . . gettin' bigger." He placed his hand over the left lower chest as he had done before but now using his whole hand to show a larger area. "Got no tube . . . last night." He grinned.

In fact, Jake never got intubated again. The next day his oxygen levels continued to improve, and within a week his pneumonia cleared sufficiently that he was discharged. Jake had healed himself—by using his mind and faith.

THE BODY'S MIND

Coincidence? I wondered. Yes, possibly. Much of healing is coincidence—something statisticians call "regression to the mean." If you go in to see a doctor when you are sickest, what usually happens—no matter what you do—is improve. Doctors mistakenly attribute this improvement to the treatments they prescribe. So do patients. But in this case it didn't seem like regression to the mean was an adequate explanation. Jake had had pneumonia before and recovered, so we knew he could. But he was not yet at the peak of this illness when he turned around. He had never recovered in this short a time—and without intubation.

I didn't know for sure if Jake had really healed himself with his mind and faith. Most patients don't care whether the healing they experience is called "regression to the mean" or a miracle—they are just happy to be better. However, I did know there was rigorous research showing that our mind can influence healing for a number of conditions including pain, anxiety and depression, Parkinson's and Alzheimer's disease, high blood pressure, and heart disease. And it can alter immune function—as it appeared to do in Jake's situation. Professor Alia Crum of Stanford, whose research on "Mind over Milkshakes" I described in chapter 6 (see page 124), has demonstrated how our mind-set, which she defines as our "conscious and embodied expectation to heal," infuses all treatments including those involving drugs, food, exercise, and stress. How we individually and culturally think of and frame a treatment is often the largest contributor to whether and how much that treatment works. Mind-set can also influence the amount of pain and rate of recovery from surgery.

I was in high school when President Nixon visited China in 1972, and the reporter James Reston, who accompanied him, described the amazing power of acupuncture to treat pain, including his own after an emergency operation he underwent there. He described doctors doing full-blown open heart surgery on patients without anesthesia—under the palliative influence of acupuncture alone. I saw similar cases of surgery done without anesthesia using hypnosis during my rotations in psychiatry in the United States. We know the role of the mind in healing is huge, but how it operates is still largely a mystery. At the time I met Jake, studies were just emerging exploring the influence of visualization on biology. Most of these studies involve creating specific images in the mind under relaxed conditions, seeking to influence biological processes. We now know that visualization can influence a number of conditions. This includes reduction of pain, bleeding, and infection after surgery, and acceleration of recovery time. Chronic conditions also benefit from visualization, including high blood pressure, chronic pain, depression, and PTSD. Professional athletes routinely use visualization to enhance endurance and performance. Golf and other skill-based games improve through mental practice.

In 2015, Dr. Mimi Guarneri and Rauni King from Scripps Hospital, along with a colleague, Dr. Shamini Jain from Samueli Institute, conducted a study at Camp Pendleton, California, testing whether mental relaxation in the presence of another combined with mental imagery could help Marines with PTSD. All the Marines in the study had been deployed to Iraq or Afghanistan and suffered significant PTSD on their return. All had received standard treatment with medication and counseling. In the study, half of the Marines were given continued standard treatment and half were given a visualization tape to listen to, along with four treatments of a relaxation method called "healing touch," an approach taught to nurses in which they hold their hands over the patient—similar to what I used with Susan during her chemotherapy. After each of the four deep relaxation sessions, the Marines were asked to listen to a visualization CD once a day for twenty minutes. The CD took them to a safe place of their choosing where the relaxation response was reinforced daily. After three weeks, the Marines were tested again for PTSD. There was more than a 25% drop in PTSD scores in those who used the relaxation sessions and visualization tape compared to usual treatment—an improvement as great as any current PTSD treatment we have with medications or psychotherapy. After the relaxation sessions and visualization practice, the average PTSD scores for the group went below what was considered abnormal. The usual care group improved slightly but was still above the cutoff for PTSD.

JOE

What I found most remarkable about this, however, were the stories service members told about the "coincidental" effects visualization had on them. Joe, a thick-skinned Marine who had been deployed four times, recounted how a buddy, killed next to him in a battle, appeared to him during one of his visualization exercises. The appearance was more than an image, he said. His buddy reached out and touched him—"I felt it," said Joe. His buddy then said that he was fine and that he would always love Joe and be watching over him. "Go on with your life," the phantom buddy said, "you have lots of life left to live, and we did good together."

Joe did not tell his physician about this episode, but broke down in tears at his next healing touch session with the nurse. "Now I know everything will be okay," he said to her after the session. Later, Joe's wife noticed how much less agitated he was. Joe had what is called an "exceptional spiritual experience," meaning one that goes beyond the normal experiences of everyday consciousness. People who have such experiences often describe them as profound, overwhelming, indescribable, and even frightening. They are more than just images—they look, sound, and feel completely real. And the body reacts to them as if they were real. As it turns out, lots of people have these experiences—especially when faced with a life-threatening situation and when they cultivate an open, relaxed mind. They frequently occur during the night and wake people from sleep.

Dr. David Hufford, emeritus professor of sociology and medicine at Penn State University, is one of the world's experts on these exceptional experiences. He told me that between 30% and 40% of people around the world have them at some point in their lives, regardless of the culture they live in. Traumatic experiences increase the likelihood of these experiences. In a study Dr. Hufford did of veterans who returned from the wars in Iraq and Afghanistan, he found that more than 60% of those exposed to combat had these experiences.

"That is a very high rate," he said, "almost double the baseline rate in our culture." These experiences are so profound and sometimes frightening that soldiers rarely talk about them. They are afraid of being labeled "crazy" and put into mental health treatment. Dr. Hufford explained, "If these exceptional experiences are labeled negatively—called hallucinations or a mental illness—that can be damaging. If they are acknowledged as real and treated positively, they can be profoundly healing. Many cultures will use these experiences to help heal a person. Modern medicine usually thinks of them as a sign of illness. We need to reframe how health care deals with these experiences."

In Dr. Guarneri's study, she did not ask how often these experiences occurred in the Marines who did the visualization and healing touch relaxation, so we don't know how common experiences like Joe's were in that group. We do know that hostility scores in the group—something very difficult to improve in war-induced PTSD—dropped markedly in those who did the visualization. They had found a tool and a process to tap into the healing power through their minds and spirits.

BEYOND BELIEF

Belief is a powerful tool for healing. But specific mental practices like those Jake and Joe used do not take optimal advantage of the unconscious processes of meaning-making that occur in the everyday rituals of health care delivery. Research on placebo effects, as described in previous chapters, demonstrates that potential. When ritual and belief are combined with repeated social ritual, they can produce profound effects on chronic illness including pain, mental health, and the immune system. At the time I saw Jake, Dr. Robert Ader, a pioneer in the investigation of conditioned learning and immune function, was demonstrating that by repeatedly pairing the use of an inert substance (a placebo) with an immune-suppressing drug, one could teach the immune system to respond to the inert substance even when the drug was withdrawn. He used rats that had a genetically inbred autoimmune condition—their own immune systems were killing their bodies prematurely, like what goes on in lupus or multiple sclerosis. When this autoimmunity was suppressed with a drug called cyclophosphamide, the rats lived longer. Dr. Ader used a simple process of classical conditioning to train the animals' immune systems to lower their harmful activities. He did this by giving the cyclophosphamide along with a sugar solution. After several pairings of the drug and sugar solution, the drug was gradually reduced but the sugar solution was maintained. Animals who continued to get the sugar solution also continued to have a dampened immune system—and lived almost as long as if they had received the actual drug!

Studies now show that the human immune system can also be taught to do this. Drink Kool-Aid and take an immune-modulating drug a few times together, and soon (within three or four sequences) you can withdraw the drug and get the immune modulation effect—nearly 80% of it—from the Kool-Aid alone. (Don't try this at home! Immune-modulating drugs must be carefully monitored, and this conditioning approach requires precise timing and supervision.) But most people already use the benefit of mental conditioning without even knowing it. Take a headache pill with aspirin in it and you will feel better. Do this a few times, and soon just taking a pill (even without aspirin in it) eases the headache. Meaning influences effect.

When people take an effective brand-name drug for a while, they get used to its working. If they switch to a generic or lower-cost version of the drug, they often report it does not work as well. And it truly won't work as well, but not because the chemicals in the drug have stopped working. Studies have shown that, at least for pain and depression, if a person thinks she is getting a "discounted" drug, rather than the full-priced drug, she will report it as less effective. Another example is that when a "new, improved" drug comes along for an illness (based on hype and advertising), the older drug loses some of its effectiveness as people lose confidence in it. Professor Dan Moerman, the anthropologist from the University of Michigan introduced in chapter 2 (see page 22), demonstrated this dramatically by tracking the effects of established drugs proven to work when a supposedly better drug came along. For example, when a new drug called ranitidine got FDA approval for treatment of stomach ulcers, the company marketed it extensively as better than an established drug called cimetidine. Cimetidine was working well—healing ulcers in about 75% of patients who took it and about 20% more than placebo. However, as excitement grew and use of ranitidine gained popularity, the healing rate of the older drug, cimetidine, diminished—dropping to below 50%. The magnitude of the older drug's effects diminished as the collective mind-set was drawn to the new and "better" drug. So, remarkably, a treatment's healing potency depends not only on how well it actually works, but also on a culture's belief in the relative benefit of alternative treatments for those same conditions. No wonder pharmaceutical companies spend billions pushing new drugs when they first get approved. Not only do the sales go up because of the marketing, but the actual effects are increased if the culture believes they are effective. They are building both conscious and unconscious belief. One of my medical school professors used to admonish his students to "use a new treatment as much as possible when it first comes out, before it loses its effectiveness." Now I know why he said that. Our collective mind affects the magnitude of the meaning. The meaning affects the magnitude of healing.

If this works with rats, how much more effective can it be with humans? Humans have such a powerful mind for making meaning that they can produce this same kind of conditioning with their own words and imagination—no Kool-Aid or pills required. Pediatrician

Dr. Karen Olness of Northwest University reported an example of this in a child with an autoimmune disease similar to that of Dr. Ader's rats. The child needed immune-suppressive medications for kidney disease, but they were making her so nauseous that she could not take them anymore. This increased the risk that her disease would flare and threaten her life. Dr. Olness first used a rose fragrance and paired it with the immune-suppressive drugs and nausea-suppressing medications to condition the child's system to react less severely to the immune-suppressing medications. She also taught the child to imagine a rose during these treatments. Soon the side effects of giving the immune-suppressing drugs could be reduced while maintaining the drugs' effectiveness—provided the child imagined the smell and look of a rose when she took them! The child had learned how to control her nausea and immune system with her mind. Like Jake, she used her newfound visualization skills to heal. Children are especially adept at learning to use their minds to heal. A simple visualization CD for children with irritable bowel and stomach pain is more effective and longer lasting than any medication. All the doctor needs to do is give the child the CD and support her in using it.

DANCE OF MINDS

UCLA professor of psychiatry and best-selling author Dr. Daniel Siegel writes about how modern science is revealing a picture of the mind very different from the traditional one currently held by medicine. Rather than think of the mind as emanating from the brain—inside the skull only—he describes the view emerging from whole systems science that the mind operates more as if it resides between individuals, the culture, and the environment. In his book *Mind: A Journey to the Heart of Being Human*, he explains: "Mind is not just what the brain does, not even the social brain. The mind may be something emerging from a higher level of systems functioning than simply what happens inside the skull. This system's basic elements are energy and information flow—and that flow happens inside of us, and between ourselves and others and the world." A growing number of scientists share this view, as more and more evidence accumulates to support it. I am struck by how consistent this view is with the model Dr. Manu drew for me on his whiteboard in rural India as he tried to explain the ancient Ayurveda view of a person. Rather than being separate from others, as our bodies are, the deeper dimensions of our being—in mind and spirit—show that we are all merged together into one inseparable and overlapping mind. Our mind is collective. If this way of understanding the mind is a more accurate description of what we are as humans, then tapping this power of the mind and spirit is essential in order to fully heal and be whole.

Our collective-like mind's influence on healing goes on every day in the clinical encounter. It does not always require long periods of visualization like Jake undertook or the healing touch relaxation given to Joe, the Marine. The meaning response—both good and bad—can come in an instant. The British physician K. B. Thomas demonstrated this in 1987 with a remarkable study entitled "Is there any point to being positive?" He studied two hundred patients who came to the doctor with no specific pathology, only symptoms of illness. This type of patient makes up about half of all visits to a primary care doctor. He divided the two hundred patients into four groups. Two groups got either a positive consultation, in which they were told they had a clear illness that would resolve soon, or a negative consultation, in which they were told that the doctor did not know what they had or if they would get better. Half of each group was then given a placebo pill and the other half nothing. All treatments took the same amount of time.

Two weeks later, the patients were asked by someone new (not the doctor) if they were better and if they needed more treatment. The results showed that 64% of patients who got a positive consultation were better, compared to only 39% of those who got the negative consultation. About 50% in either the placebo or nontreated groups reported being better. In other words, the coincidental healing rate (the "regression to the mean") was about 50%. But a simple shift in the belief and expectations of patients induced by the language and attitude of the doctor could either increase that healing rate by 28% or decrease it by 22%—a total difference of another 50% from the baseline healing rate. The difference in healing rates between those who got a pill and those who did not was only 6%. The shared mind space between doctor and patient significantly enhanced or interfered with the patient's own healing processes—even from a single encounter.

This dance between minds making meaning does not require the doctor to say anything or that it even be consciously perceived by the patient. The late NIH researcher Dr. David D. Price, whose work on placebo I described in chapter 4 (see page 73), demonstrated in several studies that a doctor's belief influences a treatment's effectiveness—even when the patient does not know of that belief. Oral surgeons who had extracted third molars (wisdom teeth) were told that after the extraction their patients would get either a pain killer, a placebo, or naloxone. Naloxone, a drug used to combat narcotic overdose, could increase their pain. The patients were told nothing, but later asked to rate their pain and need for medications. Patients whose surgeons thought their patients had received an effective painkiller reported less pain and had less need for medications, compared to those patients whose surgeons thought their patients had not received an effective pain treatment—either placebo or naloxone. In fact, all patients got placebo. Without any verbal exchanges, patients seemed to read the surgeon's expectations. People surpass rats or rabbits in reading subtle signals and infusing meaning into those signals—even when they don't know they have done so.

This and similar research makes me wonder if it is truly possible to withhold or hide information from a patient or if they read the situation and react on some level no matter what the doctor attempts to do. Indeed, the dance of the mind behaves more like the ebb and flow of energy and information between people and things. Even if we cannot measure it directly, its impact on healing is profound.

NOCEBO

For the most part, patients and physicians are largely oblivious to the healing and the harm that arise from the mind and spiritual dimension. Like the other dimensions of healing, our health care system seems to mostly miss this. We attribute improvements to the specific treatments given rather than to the context and meaning created during the delivery of those treatments. But we do this at our peril. By not acknowledging the more nonlocal view of the human mind described by Dr. Siegel and others, our health care system not only misses a key dimension for healing, but it may be harming us as well. This is seen most clearly in what is called the "nocebo" effect—the negative impact of ritual and belief on health and healing.

For every ritual, belief, conditioning, or social learning process that improves healing, there is the potential for those same processes to harm. In the 1987 study by Dr. Thomas described earlier, patients' recovery rate was cut almost in half by a single negative encounter with their physician. Dr. Price showed how physicians' subtle nonverbal expectations could increase pain. Professor Fabrizio Benedetti, whose research on placebo I described in chapter 2 (see page 25), demonstrated that the pain-relieving effects of our most powerful drugs—such as morphine—can be almost completely negated by delivering the drug with a negative expectation. Morphine works for acute pain, but the ritual and belief surrounding morphine works—or interferes—to an almost equal extent. The endogenous painkillers produced by our mind are just as powerful. Like most physicians trained in the 1980s, I was taught to let the patient know if what I was about to do to them was going to hurt. Before drawing blood, giving a shot, or doing a biopsy, for example, I told them, "This may hurt a little." Then, after the stick, I would try and calm them by saying, "It will get better now" or sometimes, "Now that wasn't so bad, was it?" This happened (and still happens) thousands of times a day in health care. It turns out that by saying this, I was increasing my patient's experience of pain. To add insult to injury, if I tried to reassure them afterward and they were still feeling pain, this made things worse still because my attempt at reassurance was also communicating to them that they should be over it. Now I say nothing to my patients about pain before a procedure. I only describe what I will be doing and then create a mental distraction or have them use a visualization tape or music during the procedure. They can make up their own mind from my description if it will hurt them or not.

The nocebo effect impacts more than pain. And it is also not just transmitted though the clinical encounter. It can be embedded in our cultural beliefs and social communications. Studies by Professor Winfried Rief and colleagues from the University of Marburg, Germany, demonstrate that clinical trials consistently show higher side effects in those receiving placebo when the active drug being tested has higher side effects. These adverse effects are not just from the subjects' baseline symptoms, which they attribute to the drug—although that does happen; the adverse effects produced by giving the placebo actually mimic those of the specific drug being studied. For example, placebo-treated groups in studies of different antidepressants with different side effects will report from two to five times the rate of adverse effects specific to the drug being studied—tricyclic placebos produce tricyclic drug–like side effects, and serotonin-like side effects occur in the placebo groups of the serotonin drug studies. This is often attributed to study subjects being told the potential side effects of a drug before entering a study—part of the process of informed consent. Like Dr. Thomas's patients, these study subjects learn that they might experience specific negative effects—and they do. Unlike Dr. Thomas's patients, however, these side effects continue over the course of the study—often for one to two months—without further communication about the drug. A single encounter with a study coordinator obtaining their informed consent is sufficient to induce negative effects.

The collective mind can influence not only health outcomes, but death outcomes as well. A large study by Dr. David Phillips of the University of California, San Diego, published in the prestigious medical journal *Lancet*, poignantly demonstrates the cultural impact of the meaning response. The study examined the deaths of 28,169 adult Chinese-Americans, and 412,632 randomly selected, matched controls coded "white" on the death certificate. Dr. Phillips showed that: "Chinese-Americans, but not whites, die significantly earlier than normal (1.3–4.9 years) if they have a combination of disease and birth year, which Chinese astrology and [traditional Chinese] medicine consider ill-fated. The more strongly a group is attached to Chinese traditions, the more years of life are lost." He goes on to say, "Our results hold for nearly all major causes of death studied. The reduction in survival cannot be completely explained by a change in the behavior of the Chinese patient, doctor, or death-registrar, but seems to result at least partly from psychosomatic processes." That is, the collective mind.

Chinese astrology assigns one of five elements—fire, earth, metal, water, and wood—to each year (as well as one of the better-known twelve animals), and people born in a metal year, who are expected by the culture to have more lung diseases than people born in other years, actually do have more lung problems—and die earlier than others from lung problems. The same thing is true for lymph problems or immune system problems if people are born in an earth year—thought to be bad luck for the immune system. Major differences in the age at death from lymphatic cancer occurred between those born in earth years and those born in other years. These effects were over and above the impact of other factors, such as smoking, lifestyle, and environmental exposures. Unlike pain, the "side effect" of age at death is a rather hard, objective outcome. The effect was sociocultural—an effect from the collective mind of the culture. The more distant people were generationally from the original Chinese culture, the less this finding held, so that for third-generation Chinese-American people there was no correlation whatsoever—just like non-Chinese Americans.

We do not have to believe in astrology for this to happen; we have only to grow up with a concept that our culture accepts. Stress is often cited as bad for you in Western cultures—thanks to Hans Selye and other scientists of the last century. However, it is also often framed as good for you, as in the phrase "no pain, no gain" used by Joe and his fellow Marines. While both attitudes can harm, people who believe that stress is bad are 43% more likely to die earlier than those who interpret stress as good. Mindset influences mortality.

When Aadi first came to the Ayurvedic hospital to treat his Parkinson's disease, he did not believe in the use of astrology to help him heal. In fact, he had never believed in it, and he told Dr. Manu so each time he came. I think he used the word "poppycock" to describe it. Yet Dr. Manu insisted he get an astrology reading each time anyway.

"He may not personally believe in astrology himself," Manu explained, "but he was raised and lives in a culture that does. He cannot escape its effects, even if they are only psychologically driven. So he might as well try and use information from it to find meaning for his life."

I am not sure whether Aadi ever used that information consciously, but his wife and others in his family commented on how those readings seemed to make sense and described Aadi's life accurately. They, if not he, found them meaningful.

Humans seem to be hardwired to seek out some type of transpersonal or spiritual meaning from illness. This has happened for centuries. When patients arrived at Epidaurus, the ancient Greek center of Hippocrates' medical school, they first consulted with an oracle, who read their spiritual lives to contextualize their illnesses with a deeper meaning before they went on to other treatments. Most indigenous cultures infuse spiritual interpretations and rituals into their diagnoses and treatments. Some of these are clearly harmful—like when a "demon extraction" is substituted for medical treatment in an epileptic. Some can be helpful—like when prayers soothe the anxiety of a patient newly diagnosed with cancer. As with drugs, herbs, lifestyle, and social relationships, our mind-set and spiritual beliefs are simply another tool to use for healing or harm. Short of being hit by a truck or a tornado or an Ebola virus, disease, suffering, and death do not have simple cause-and-effect connections. If we are going to maximize healing from our treatments, we must pay attention to the complex layers of history and traditions, cultural and family influences, and individual beliefs that make meaning in our lives. We need to attend to our collective mind. Until we incorporate an awareness of these forces into health care, they will continue to help or harm us at random, and we will not be able to tap into our full healing potential.

But how can we do that?

PSYKHE

I explore specific mental and spiritual elements of healing with my patients. While there is scientific evidence for the value of each of these elements, the purpose of my exploring these with patients is not to tell them what to believe, but to help them learn how to use their mind and faith to find deeper meaning in their lives. Once we see which elements resonate with them, I look for scientifically validated ways they can enhance those elements' healing power in their lives. This may be a specific mind-body practice, like Jake's visualization, or it may involve helping them link healing behaviors to their spiritual life. I always seek to respect them as they are—with all their wounds and flaws—on a journey to more wholeness and healing.

In ancient times there was no distinction made between what today we call the mind and soul. The Greek word *psykhe,* the root of psyche and psychology, also means "soul, mind, spirit, or the deepest experience people have of themselves." This experience is often "transpersonal" and "transtemporal"—seeming to go beyond the normal boundaries

ELEMENTS OF THE SPIRITUAL AND MENTAL DIMENSION

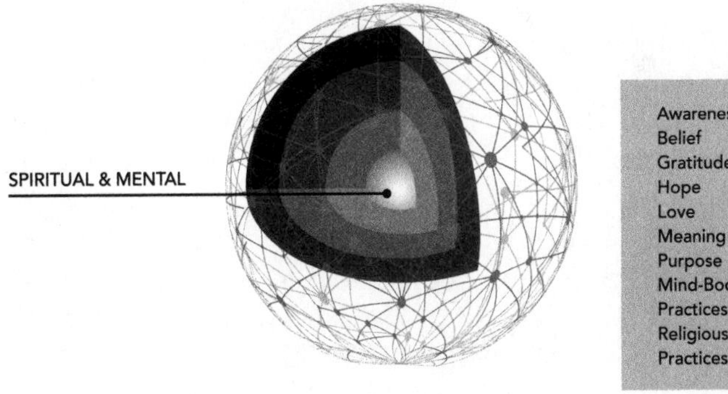

of space and time. This is the dimension of the spirit. While psychologists, clergy, and academics often debate the differences in these terms, I find that when it comes to healing, people use them interchangeably. Those who are atheistic or humanistic will use the terms *mind* or *psyche,* while those with a spiritual or religious preference will add the term *soul* or *spirit.* Whatever they are called, these components provide valuable tools within the inner dimensions of our being for healing. Both disciplines—psychology and religion—tend to be neglected by modern medicine. Thus the role of mind and spirit for healing remains poorly used.

Yet there is substantial evidence that people who engage in spiritual and religious practices stay healthy longer, recover faster, and die with a better quality of life than people who do not. This is, of course, provided those beliefs do not dictate specifically harmful behaviors—such as mutilation, neglect, or violence—or create excessive spiritual (and psychological) distress from guilt, doubt, and dogma. Dr. Harold Koenig, professor of psychiatry at Duke University, has studied, reviewed, and written about the health effects of spiritual and religious practices for decades. In his *Handbook of Religion and Health*, he reviews research showing positive health benefits from participating in faith traditions or spiritual practices. He and others report that the evidence of benefit is particularly strong for mental health conditions such as depression, substance abuse, suicide, dementia, and stress-related disorders. There are also many positive physical health correlations with spiritual and religious practices. Most of the reasons for this make sense. Those who engage in spiritual and religious practices tend to avoid harmful substances (alcohol, tobacco, drugs), engage in social service and support activities, and pray—often in a meditative state—which induces relaxation or catharsis. In addition, some religious beliefs provide soothing explanations for suffering and death accompanied by rituals of forgiveness and reconciliation—further comforting the suffering.

Spiritual-like discussions at the end of life are especially important when we all—regardless of whether we have a faith tradition—seek comfort as we die. Research shows that spiritual rituals and chaplain interactions for those who desire it toward the end of life increase quality of life and satisfaction. As with any medical intervention, negative effects can also occur. Harm is caused by poorly or negatively delivered religious and spiritual beliefs and behaviors, such as blaming the believer for their illness if they remain sick. I have had deeply religious patients admit to me they feel guilty that they have not "prayed deeply enough" if they do not recover. Some religious traditions state that explicitly. Harm also occurs if a religious community on which a person has had lifelong reliance fails to visit and care for the person during serious illness or hospitalization—breaching an unwritten social and moral contract. Whether or not you are religious, if you and your health care professional do not include the mind and spiritual dimension in your conversations—especially toward the end of life—you risk missing out on its use for healing.

THE WOUNDED HEALER

One of the most important effects of a serious illness is its impact not only on the body, but also on the soul (or spirit, or whatever you call your nonphysical inner being). Bodies often heal; souls may not. Sometimes there is a point in an illness when you are not sure if you will ever get better—or if you even want to. It is as if you have lost your will to live. There's no modern medical disease category when a trauma or a stress penetrates your soul. But you feel it nonetheless. You can feel it in some people who suffer from PTSD produced by war, when it is not possible to elicit even a glimmer of hope. You can feel it in the chronic embodied stress of those who have had adverse childhood experiences—when they do not even have a memory of personal power. And you can feel it in the existential threat of a serious disease and its therapy—when a patient asks, "Who am I now?" Soul loss is named in some cultures, especially in Native American and indigenous cultures. They recognize it as a distinct disability separate from any psychological or physical condition. Finding a way back out of such a state is central to recovering one's well-being. Navigating out through that labyrinth is part of the healing journey.

Susan's first cancer changed her view of herself forever. Like many of her colleagues, she had taken a professional life path up to that point—with family in tow. But having cancer at such a young age, along with the triple whammy of surgery, chemotherapy, and radiation, "knocked me out of the path of a normal thirty-five-year-old lawyer," she said. "Even though my body would recover, my spirit had to change. I could never be with my peers or myself in the same way again—pursuing both family and professional careers. After the cure, when they said they got it all, my questions went from 'Why did I get this' to 'Why me?' I realized that I didn't really want to be a lawyer anymore. But then what was I here for, I wondered? Why had I been born?"

For Susan, the illness brought to the forefront what is arguably the most important question in anyone's life: why am I here? Medicine offers chemistry and biology as the answer. People need more than that. They need something more meaningful, something drawn out of the deeper dimensions of who we are—social, emotional, mental, and spiritual. And for most of us, healing requires that we try to answer that question by exploring the mind and spiritual dimensions of our soul.

So here is the irony of healing and what makes it different than curing: the very wound from which we suffer induces the process of healing. To acknowledge and enter that wounding opens the path to wholeness. The priest, writer, and spiritual teacher Henry Nouwen called this "the wounded healer," whereby a person, by accepting and then embracing the fact that he is flawed and wounded, can find a deep peace and joy. He called this the experience of "being beloved"—fully valuing oneself and one's life just as they are. It is an "exceptional spiritual experience" of a different kind. This experience of deep peace and joy can come in a spiritual version, as found by Jake and Joe, or through a different pathway. Aadi found it through Ayurveda, Sergeant Martin through his friends with PTSD, Clara in nature, Mabel with her family, Jeff in running, and Gloria through teaching cooking classes. Each path is unique, yet all lead to the same place of healing and wholeness.

CHAPLAINCY

When my patients seek the spiritual dimension of healing, I may ask if they would like to see a chaplain. Surveys report that most hospitalized patients, and many with serious illness, would like an existential or spiritual discussion with their physician or a visit with a religious professional—but rarely do medical professionals ask patients about their spiritual needs. To help remedy this situation, internist and palliative care physician Dr. Christina Puchalski, founder and director of the George Washington University Institute for Spirituality and Health and author of *Making Health Care Whole: Integrating Spirituality into Patient Care*, trains health care practitioners in how to discuss spirituality in health care. Her yearly course for physicians and other health care professionals teaches them how to integrate patients' spiritual beliefs into their care, address sensitive medical issues that seriously ill patients face, and support health care professionals in providing compassionate care. In other words, it seeks to get health care practitioners and the health care system to take the nonphysical, inner aspects of healing seriously—to recognize and ask patients about the mind and spiritual dimension of their lives.

I am fortunate to be surrounded by people in my family who do look at the spiritual dimension. They have taught me the healing power of attending to the mind and spirit in health care. My father was a chaplain who spent a large part of his career working in hospitals. He was one of the first chaplains to get formal training in hospital chaplaincy—called clinical pastoral education (CPE)—and brought this training into the military. As a young boy, I recall asking him why he, a minister, went to work every day at a hospital, where doctors worked. I thought ministers were supposed to work in churches.

"Why do I work in a hospital?" he replied. "Because that is where a lot of suffering is. I work in a hospital to help alleviate suffering and to heal."

That stuck with me. I wanted to know more. So, before medical school, I decided to do five months of training as a hospital chaplain student. That taught me a lot about healing.

I remember the first patient I was assigned to as a student minister. He was a seventy-three-year-old man dying of metastatic lung cancer and on a morphine drip for pain. He had requested a visit from a chaplain and was willing to see the "student chaplain" first. I was all of twenty-one years old, nervous as a cat, with no idea what I was going to say. When I entered his room, I was relieved to see that he was asleep—apparently sedated by the morphine. Thinking I was off the hook, I sat next to his bed and began to softly read a few prayers. After a few moments, he opened his eyes to look at me. Then he reached his hand over and placed it on my hand and said, "Son, you are going to be okay." Not only was my cover blown, my most basic assumption about healing was flipped on its head—he was healing me! In the spiritual dimension, healing emerges in the space between people—in the collective mind—and its benefits can go either way.

After getting her first breast cancer and recovering from it, my wife also shifted her life focus from being a lawyer to getting a degree in pastoral care. She then worked in a chaplain's counseling center for the military. I was amazed at the stories I heard from her of the spiritual struggles faced by service members and their families. She heard stories with a view of suffering they did not tell me about as a doctor in the clinic. She also told me about healings I had not known were happening to my patients. I looked for the physical causes of their suffering to prescribe a treatment. But with this focus I often totally missed other influences that perpetuated their suffering—influences that my wife was picking up on. The wounding of the cancer and its treatment had awakened her intuitive skills in listening and spiritual care. In recent years our daughter Maeba has enlightened me about the power of the spiritual dimension to heal. After earning her M.Div. degree from Yale Divinity School, she did an additional year of formal CPE training at Yale University Hospital. Prior to becoming a chaplain, she did premedical training and worked in medical research at Johns Hopkins. She also worked in Nepal at a school run by Buddhist nuns and at a clinic in Ethiopia treating children. These experiences and her formal trainings enable her to see the whole person—spiritual, psychological, and physical—and the ways they are linked.

One evening, Maeba was called to visit a man hospitalized for uncontrolled high blood pressure. He was on multiple medications, yet his blood pressure remained dangerously high. After she sat and talked with him for a while, he told her it was the anniversary of the death of his wife, whom he had loved deeply. Maeba prayed with him, holding up the joy of his and his wife's love and the deep sorrow of his loss to clear view. He began to cry, and she sat with him while he mourned. That night his blood pressure returned to normal, and he was discharged the next day. The mechanisms responsible for this are likely explainable. The catharsis of his weeping and the social witness of my daughter likely reduced the stress hormones that were raging through his body and elevating his blood pressure. How often these types of biological healings occur through the spiritual dimension is unknown. Although hospitals with full-time chaplains will chart their visits along with all the other health care professionals, it is rare that those notes are followed or "measured" as drug treatments are. Sources like the *Journal of Pastoral Care & Counseling* are full of case studies like this. How often doctors and nurses read them, much less use these visits in an integrative fashion to heal, is unclear. Thus they remain invisible to most of us health care.

DAVID

Sometimes healing is, as in the Beauty Way, for the collective mind and not just an individual patient. Once Maeba was called to do a baptism of a premature baby born to a drug-addicted mother who, after the birth, walked out of the hospital without a word. The baby was on life support; he was so underdeveloped he could not live on his own. It took social services several days to track the mother down to ask permission to take him off life support after it became apparent he was not going to make it. When they finally got the mother on the phone, she refused to give the baby a name, but did give permission to take him off life support—and then asked that he be baptized. Several of the nurses caring for the abandoned baby were distraught. Not only did he not even have a name, but the mother's only indication of her desire to love the baby—her parting request—was to have the baby baptized. Chaplain Maeba was called in to baptize the baby before he died. The only witnesses were the nurses and one of the doctors who had cared for him and tried to save him. As Maeba prepared the water and the ceremony, she asked the baby's name. The nurses gathered, and, after consulting together, decided to name him David.

The ceremony began. Each caregiver was offered a chance to hold their hands over the water to bless it with their healing touch. "David," Maeba said, "I baptize you in the name of the Father, and of the Son, and of the Holy Spirit," and because of the special circumstances in which she was baptizing a motherless child, she added, "One God: Mother of us all, amen." As the water was placed on the premature infant, the group began to spontaneously weep. This collective catharsis lasted several minutes. The ventilator was then turned off and the baby died. A deep sense of peace emerged, even as everyone grieved David's death. After a silence that under any other circumstances would have seemed long and awkward, but in this context was to be cherished, one of the neonatal ICU nurses commented, "I needed that. For all the little Davids who die here." There was a collective deep breath. She had spoken for all. Despite his short life, his unfortunate circumstances, and his major woundings, David was among the beloved, and it healed them all.

It is not just patients who need mental and spiritual healing. In many ways, the nurse in the neonatal ICU was speaking for all health care—practitioners and patients. Physicians and nurses report the highest rates of burnout of any profession. Nearly half of all physicians have burnout—defined as lack of enthusiasm for work, feeling apathetic, and becoming more callous toward people. The highest rate of burnout is among physicians and nurses in primary care—those at the front lines of health care—where it affects more than 50%. These physicians also have high rates of substance abuse—nearly 15%. Rates of burnout in primary care have risen nearly 20% in the ten years since 2007. As a hospital chaplain, Maeba found that her spiritual care was frequently needed by the staff. This led her to hold a monthly breakfast for the staff of the pediatric ICU.

The causes of burnout are many: excessive workload, clerical burden, inefficiency in our health care system, loss of control over medical decisions, and difficulties in work-life balance. Burnt-out physicians and nurses are not the best healers.

But the primary cause of burnout is, in my opinion, the erosion of meaning. This arises from the lack of opportunity for physicians and nurses to care for themselves and patients in all their dimensions. The imbalanced focus in medicine on the physical aspects of disease, along with the economic and administrative forces dominating medicine, squeeze out the dimensions of healing that they know produce benefit for patients and would allow them to heal the whole person. Those in primary care who see the decline in patients' health and well-being year after year—when they know what could keep them well—bear the heaviest burden. The discouragement of burnout is magnified when they see that the patient's environment, the social and emotional factors, lifestyle and behavior, and the inner dimensions of the mind and spirit also need attention—but they do not have the time or tools to attend to them.

Unfortunately, this discouragement begins in medical school. Medical students in their first year have high levels of altruism and empathy. This empathy drops lower with every year of training, from the time they enter to the time they are licensed four years later. It continues as they get into practice and find that health care is not designed to help patients heal and stay well, and it does not provide the primary tools they need. Our "health care system" is a triple oxymoron—it produces only about 20% of the public's health, it is difficult for those working in it to deliver compassionate care, and it is not an integrated system. No health, no care, and not a system!

Health care needs a new way of thinking and a new design. It needs to shift its economic incentives toward prevention and whole person care, even as the industry profits from doing the opposite. Physicians and nurses need new types of skills and tools for the clinic and hospital. Patients need to expect—even demand—something different from what they are getting from health care. Health care needs to bring healing together with curing. Health care needs a miracle.

MIRACLES

Miracles happen. Most people know this. Many can describe miracles—small or large—that they have seen or experienced in their lives. Miracles in healing are those recoveries that modern science cannot explain. That does not mean they are not explainable. But usually scientists and physicians don't bother to try. They are considered too hard to investigate. Adding the mystery of a miracle to the uncertainties of science makes it even harder. Our research at Walter Reed on how laying on of hands works—through electromagnetic frequencies coming off the hands—explained Susan's boost in energy after I tried it. At least part of why the Marines with PTSD got better with healing touch is explainable—even if from placebo effects. But that does not mean these healings are any less miraculous. In his encyclopedic book *The Future of the Body*, Michael Murphy documents instances of unexplained healing from all over the world—including the meticulous documentation by the Catholic Church of the rare dramatic miracles from visits to Lourdes in France. While more than seven thousand healings from visits to Lourdes have been reported, the church has verified only about seventy as major, unexplained, miraculous healings. These types of miracles are just the dramatic ones that, although they provide evidence that truly mysterious healing can happen, also distract us from the more common and less dramatic miracles seen in health care every day—that is, if we look.

One of the more common "miraculous" events toward the end of life is someone waking up from a coma or sometimes even coming back from the dead to say goodbye to loved ones. My father's death is an example. My father was a Christian minister—Presbyterian. He had served for thirty years in the military and been in three wars—WWII, Korea, and Vietnam. He then spent ten years as a hospital chaplain; ten years as a prison chaplain; five more in service to a poor, rural region in central California; and five more serving the destitute in Las Vegas and San Diego.

He was a man of deep faith who sought to emulate Christ. He believed that God works through people. Once I asked him if he had ever been afraid under fire during the wars. He thought carefully, then told a story about how once bullets passed through the poncho rolled up around his waist. He then said, "No. I was never afraid. I felt Christ next to me."

He and my mother were married nearly sixty years. They had been through the three wars together, moved more than twenty times, and raised four children. They brought their family to Vietnam, Germany, Oklahoma, Texas, California, and New York City—moving almost every two years. They were deeply bonded.

Then, at eighty-six, my dad had a major hemorrhagic (bleeding) stroke and was rapidly dying—falling into a coma within three days. As he lost consciousness, the doctors attempted multiple interventions. They placed intracranial monitors into his head to track the pressure on his brain and catheters to try and drain the blood. "It looks like a crown of thorns," my cousin said. My father had a tube placed down his nose, and they restrained his arms—splayed out to the sides. "Like he is tied to a cross," our son, Chris, said. In this very painful situation and before he went completely unconscious, I asked him if he wanted any pain medication or sedation. He said no. All I could give him was water on a sponge. For me this all evoked the image of Jesus on the cross. Meaning drips thickly over events at the end of life. Gradually, the family came in from all over the country to be with him. He continued to bleed into his head, and the coma became deeper. After about six days, when most people had arrived, he was completely unconscious, not responding even to deep pressure on his sternum. We gathered around him. Our youngest daughter Emily sat at his feet and sang to him for hours. We prayed.

In the evening of the sixth day, my mother came up close and kissed him. Suddenly he woke up and asked, "What happened?" My mother told him he had had a stroke and was in the hospital and the family was all around. They kissed again and each said, "I love you." He then lapsed back into the coma and died the next day. He had come back from a coma to say goodbye to her. A miracle? Perhaps. Explainable? Perhaps. But this kind of happening is not unique. Anyone who has worked in palliative or end-of-life care for a while has witnessed these kinds of miracles. They are more common than the dramatic ones documented in Mr. Murphy's book—and often more meaningful. "It was a miracle for me," my mother recounts, even now, almost ten years later.

Palliative care does not just palliate; it heals—socially, emotionally, mentally, spiritually, and often physically. In a meticulous study published in the *New England Journal of Medicine*, a team led by Dr. Jennifer Temel of the Massachusetts General Hospital randomly divided 150 patients with terminal lung cancer into two groups. One group received standard medical treatment only. The second group was given the option of standard medical treatment plus complete and early palliative care. This care included rapid treatment of pain and distress; psychological, social, and spiritual support, including help with end-of-life decisions; and whole person, integrative care. If the cure-focused treatment was causing more suffering, patients were encouraged to discontinue—the opposite of what usually happens in medicine. Under these circumstances, it was not surprising to find that those in the palliative care group had less pain and less depression and improved quality of life. However, to the surprise of the researchers and the medical profession, when the curative medical treatments were used less often and healing approaches used more often, the patients also lived longer—on average 11.6 months compared to 8.9 months in the curative-only group. It was a small and unexpected miracle. A drug that extended life this long would be rapidly approved. It's still often a struggle to get coverage approved for palliative care.

In America and many other countries, health care does not do dying right. Only about one-third of patients receive formal palliative care, such as the care hospice provides, at the end of life. Few physicians are trained in palliative care, so they don't know what to do once curative treatments are no longer reasonable. Surgeon and author Atul Gawande described this tragedy in his book *Being Mortal*: "This experiment of making mortality a medical experience is just decades old. It is young. And the evidence is, it is failing." The U.S. National Academy of Medicine agrees. In 2014, they published a landmark report, *Death and Dying in America,* recommending that the principles of palliative care be expanded well beyond the end of life and that all physicians be trained in its principles. Those principles include the "frequent assessment of the patient's physical, emotional, social, and spiritual well-being." In other words, healing, as embodied in palliative care, should be part of all health care training.

INTUITION

Mystics describe a state of total unity with the universe, where they see everything connected and have access to all knowledge and wisdom—what they call the mind of God. They also say this knowledge is not unique to them—it is available to all. I learned about this connectivity from my wife, who learned it from her illness and the wounds of her childhood. Susan had always had a spiritual bent and a keen intuition. She went to Yale Divinity School for one year before leaving to go to law school. After being diagnosed with breast cancer the first time at thirty-five years old she returned to spirituality with the hunger of one in mortal crisis and used this dimension to help her decide on treatment and healing. Her father had recently died of lung cancer, and the word *cancer* struck fear into her heart. She thought she would die soon. This drove her into deep introspection and prayer and further cultivated her already skilled intuition. When difficult decisions arose—like whether to do additional chemotherapy for which there was no good scientific evidence of benefit at the time—she would dive into deep thought and prayer until it became clear what to do. This enhanced intuition has served her well. After she was cured, she went back to school to get a pastoral counseling degree and then worked with military couples faced with deployment and war. It is there that we both—I as a doctor and she as a spiritual counselor—saw the kind of "soul loss" that so often impacts service members and veterans, and healing from the soul's restoration. These veterans need spiritual guidance as much or more than medical treatment. Susan has an uncanny ability to know what they need and how to guide them—an intuition she developed out of her own suffering and wounds.

This sixth sense—this intuition—is a way the mind integrates complex information from many sources: from our body, sensory perceptions, relationships, memories, beliefs, and hopes. The response usually occurs below our awareness. Research led by Professor Gerard Hodgkinson, of the Centre for Organizational Strategy, Learning and Change at Leeds University, England, summarized findings from several decades of research on this process. They concluded that intuition is the brain drawing on this tsunami of signals to form a response and decision—but it is a decision made rapidly and unconsciously. That response occurs in the body first—thus the term *gut* feeling. Electrodermal responses—changes in the electrical charge on the skin—usually occur before we are consciously aware of the feeling. All we are usually aware of is a general feeling that something is right or wrong, or that we should turn right or left, go or stop, run or freeze. Often this feeling is right, but not always. Intuition can also mislead. I have had patients who blindly trusted their intuition and abandoned any science- or evidence-based medical treatment, only to suffer and die needlessly. In other words, intuition can be as uncertain as science. Says Professor Hodgkinson, "Humans clearly need both conscious and nonconscious thought processes, but it's likely that neither is intrinsically 'better' than the other." Intuition and science are both imperfect sources of knowledge. Healing requires the integration of both.

For centuries, healers from many cultures have claimed to be able to tap into these spiritual dimensions of healing. But does science show that we interact directly with the collective mind? Is there evidence for spiritual healing? To find out, I led a team in a massive critical summary of the research exploring this type of intuition. I was interested in whether spiritual reality—not just our mental beliefs and social rituals—interacted with material reality. Our goal was to see if there was rigorous evidence—as good as any evidence in modern biological science—that our intentions can interact with the world outside the normal boundaries of time and space: that is, nonlocally. The study was funded by the late Laurance S. Rockefeller three years before he died. It took more than five years to complete and involved dozens of prominent healers and scientists from around the world. We gathered and analyzed hundreds of studies, using state-of-the-art methods for detecting error or bias, and then discussed and synthesized the information in three meetings. The methods and results were published in a book called *Healing, Intention, and Energy Medicine*. We found that, as in other areas of medical research, when scientists tried to isolate the effects of spiritual healing there was uncertainty as to the magnitude of any single outcome. Most results, as in other areas of medicine, showed small effects, difficulty in replication, and bias in publication—all the challenges described by Stanford professor Dr. John Ioannidis in chapter 3 (see page 61) for medical science in general. The best of this research, however, supports the claim by mystics that the connectivity underlying our gut feelings occurs continuously and everywhere. Like electrons, once they touch are always interacting, all living things are always touching. Everything is connected. Susan and many others who, like her, face serious illness, seem to use this mysterious connectivity to navigate the labyrinth of healing through time and space. From this inexplicable connection, the miracles of life arise.

PRAYER

But does this mean that direct spiritual healing—like laying-on-of-hands and prayer—works? It seems it does. And their effects are often about the same magnitude as that of drugs. So far, our understanding of these phenomena remains in the realm of mystery. We do know, however, that the miracles—those unexplained events of healing—probably arise from this mystery and can be tapped if we look for them and use them. Prayer is one tool from the spiritual dimension of healing used by billions. But like other specific approaches to healing, when research attempts to isolate its effects from the other dimensions—the effects shrink and often vanish. Physician and author Dr. Larry Dossey is one of the world's best thinkers and writers about research on healing prayer. He notes the robust but small effects of prayer when studied in randomized controlled trials. In general, he recommends that the spiritual dimensions of healing be left to professional clergy and the physical dimension of healing to

section 3

YOUR HEALING JOURNEY

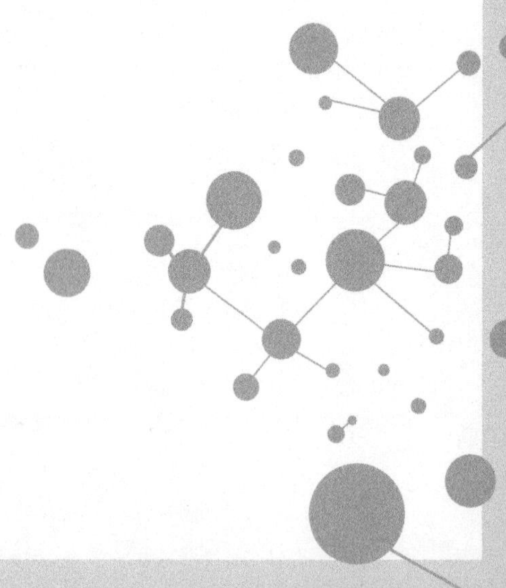

CHAPTER 9

Integrative Health

The balance of curing and healing.

For millennia, the fundamental nature of the therapeutic encounter has remained largely the same: a person who had been functioning normally and without giving a thought to her health now notices that something is wrong—she doesn't feel well. She seeks someone to help, usually a person with specialized knowledge. In various cultures and eras, this "practitioner" may have been called a shaman, a barber, a priest, or a physician. The ill person hopes the practitioner can help restore her previously normal function. Usually the practitioner does an assessment and makes recommendations, often suggests behavioral change, and then does something to the patient—gives her potions or pills, sticks her with needles or manipulates her body structure, cuts her, or conducts some other ritual. The practitioner administers the healing agent.

The details of this transaction and its rationale have varied from culture to culture and over time. Ancient Greek physicians thought they were manipulating "humors" within the body. Ayurvedic practitioners used the idea of consciousness and *doshas* as the basis for applying their treatments. Ancient Chinese practitioners framed their interventions around the manipulation of "chi" or energy. Shamans and priests sought to divine a spiritual malady and drive out demons or evil spirits.

Then, around the turn of the nineteenth century, about 200 years ago, a new idea arose—a radically different way of understanding the human being and its treatment in health and disease. That new understanding was that all things were made up of small physical substances

and parts—chemicals, cells, and other elements that comprise organs and people—and this was best studied with a new approach to knowledge called the scientific process. Modern biomedical science emerged and began breaking the body down into smaller parts and manipulating these, creating theories about how the parts fit together and testing those theories for accuracy. The science of the small and particular—sometimes called "reductionism"—was born. With this came the concept of the human being as a set of mechanical and chemical processes. All biological and psychological processes arose from these chemical interactions, organizing themselves into increasingly complex arrays and manifestations that peaked in the human being. We are, in this view, literately a bag of chemicals elegantly organized to survive and reproduce. Thinking, feeling, and even our very souls are epiphenomena of these chemical interactions. It was a powerful concept.

The value of this thinking soon proved itself in profound and practical ways. The chemical and cellular model of life controlled infectious disease—the number-one killer of humans two hundred years ago. Over time, chemistry produced antiseptics, antibiotics, and analgesic approaches that dramatically alleviated pain and suffering. The physician finally had some tools that were based on more than just magical incantations and historical knowledge. The impact of these discoveries was so dramatic that many of the old ways of thinking—the more holistic views of a person—were discarded. A medical treatment industry grew up around chemistry and physiology and the mechanical manipulation of the body. The pharmaceutical and surgical industries were born. Today, those who have access to this curative approach when they need it are grateful. Those who do not have it want it. The science of the small and particular has been a resounding success—until recently.

By discarding the more holistic, health-promoting, and nonphysical dimensions of what we are as humans, we have lost something essential in health care. While we improved our science and certainty for managing acute disease, we sacrificed what most people value about being alive, and we lost how healing works in chronic illness. Our

improvements in health waned. The costs of medical care soared. The value of the mechanical and reductionist model has reached its limits. But by attending to the whole person and integrating this with the scientific process and curative medicine, we can unleash the power of healing and well-being in ways that humanity has never experienced before. In this chapter, I will describe how you can access healing *and* curing and bring them both into your health care and your life with integrative health. Trevor taught me what can happen when we do not integrate these aspects of healing. Mandy taught me what happens when we do.

TREVOR

Trevor began to pray. He was at the end, as far as he knew. He was now back for his fifth visit to the hospital and waiting for a possible kidney transplant. It looked like the possible kidney would not come through again. This was the third time that year and second time in three months that he had been hospitalized to seek a kidney and it had fallen through. It was now 7 AM and his wife was packing up to go home. He had a strong feeling that if he did go home now he would never return.

Almost two years to the day he had been in this same hospital after a failed kidney transplant; his body had rejected his wife's donated kidney, and it had to be removed. The prospect of going back on dialysis for another long and indeterminate time, with no functioning kidney, and the knowledge that his wife was living with just one kidney, was devastating. He was finally on the top of the transplant list again, and prepped.

"Give me a few more minutes," he implored his wife. "Something will happen."

His wife sighed. "You are so stubborn," she said. "It's time to go home."

She had always been right before. The pattern of past visits was the same. Hospital personnel called late at night and asked them to come in because they might have a match. He and his wife usually got to

the hospital around midnight, which gave him time to be admitted and prepared for surgery. The kidney match would be confirmed about 3 AM. It was now 7 AM—well past any realistic hope that the transplant would proceed. But he insisted on waiting longer. Trevor went back to praying. He had to believe a miracle would occur. That was all he had left.

But deep down he knew that his wife was right. His "stubborn optimism," as she called it, had gotten him into this mess. It was also what had made him who he was—a successful lawyer and one of the most beloved public servants in his community. A community he had risen out of and returned to help. He was the lucky one, the smart one, the successful one, the one who had escaped a life of poverty and incarceration—and returned to help those who had not escaped. He was one of five children born in a small shack on a dirt road; his father picked fruit and his mother cleaned houses. Neither of his parents had been educated beyond the fifth grade. But they both worked hard and disciplined their kids to do the same. With their love and encouragement, Trevor excelled—in sports, in academics, in popularity. With good grades and an athletic body, he landed a football scholarship to an elite college. He graduated and went on to law school, taking honors and then returning to his community as a public defender—helping those he grew up with get justice and giving back to his community and church. He set up community gatherings where successful members of the community met with children to inspire and mentor them.

When he was growing up, his dad would say that Trevor was always "healthy as a horse." Trevor believed that and never thought about his health. Except for vaccinations as a child and some periodic sports physicals, he never went to a doctor. None of his family ever did. They did not have health insurance and could not afford medical care. If he had an earache or sprained his ankle, his mom would patch it up with home remedies. He always recovered.

When he was hired as public defender, he got health insurance, so he went in for a checkup. That was five years after he left college football and regular athletics. These days, he mostly sat in an office. The doctor was alarmed. Trevor's blood pressure was dangerously high. The doctor prescribed two different medications. "If we can't get it down, we will need to put you in the hospital," he said.

Trevor came back a week later, and while his blood pressure was now out of the alarming range, it was still not normal. The doctor prescribed a third medication. He returned three weeks later. His blood pressure was now under control, but he felt terrible. The medications made him tired, interfered with his sexual function, and made it hard to sleep.

"You will adjust," said the doctor. "The most important thing is, your blood pressure is now down. It was dangerously high." He paused, then emphasized, "You know, it is the silent killer."

Indeed, he was right. Worldwide, untreated or undertreated high blood pressure is the most common risk factor for stroke, heart attack, kidney disease, and heart failure. In the United States, more than seventy-five million people (one in every three adults) has it. More than 30% of people with high blood pressure don't know they have it, and only 50% have it under control. Estimates are that more than one thousand people die each day from high blood pressure. Estimated costs are $50 billion per year. The situation is worse in less economically developed countries. The WHO estimates over one billion people worldwide have high blood pressure—most of it undetected and poorly controlled. Lifestyle is a major risk factor—both for getting it and for controlling it. So is genetics. Over their lifetime, most people will require two or more drugs to control it. The doctors had Trevor on three drugs and were satisfied that it was being adequately treated. From the biological perspective, their job was done. But the job was not done. While they were treating Trevor's disease, they had left out, as often happens in health care today, Trevor. It was this neglect of Trevor as a whole person that would eventually hurt him.

Current guidelines for treatment of high blood pressure recommend more than just drugs. The Joint National Committee on Prevention, Detection, Evaluation, and Treatment of High Blood Pressure (JNC 7) also addresses the behavioral dimensions of healing. Lifestyle modifications are recommended no matter what level of high blood pressure a person has. This includes exercise (which Trevor had stopped doing), a low-salt diet (which Trevor had never even thought to consider), not smoking (Trevor did not smoke), or weight gain (which Trevor had experienced since stopping sports). His doctors asked about these things and suggested he start exercising again and go on a low-salt diet. They gave him a handout of foods to avoid and recommended the DASH diet (Dietary Approaches to Stop Hypertension). But, they emphasized, he would always need the medications. The Joint National Committee also recommends close attention to the social and emotional aspects of healing. The section on "Adherence to Regimens" states: "Motivation improves when patients have positive experiences with and trust in their clinicians. Empathy both builds trust and is a potent motivator. Patient attitudes are greatly influenced by cultural differences, beliefs, and previous experiences with the healthcare system. These attitudes must be understood if the clinician is to build trust and increase communication with patients and families." The committee goes on to list other reasons for "nonadherence," including denial of illness, perception of drugs as symbols of ill health, adverse effects of medications, cost of medications, and lack of patient involvement in the care plan.

Unfortunately, Trevor's doctor had missed the class on empathy and trust, and Trevor had many of these reasons for nonadherence in his life—plus his stubborn optimism. He would be okay, he thought. His doctors never learned all this about Trevor. They did not know him well and did not inquire. They were not able to effectively engage him in behavioral change and found out nothing about his social and emotional background. He needed more than lifelong drugs, with their side effects, which were a key reason for nonadherence. The Joint National Committee Guidelines summary for primary care practitioners covers about twenty-five pages. There are eight pages devoted to drug management, but only one page to lifestyle and one page to nonadherence.

Trevor left his visits with physicians both alarmed and skeptical. He had felt fine before. Now he felt terrible. How had he gone from "healthy as a horse" to an impotent invalid in a matter of weeks? Plus, his insurance did not cover the entire cost of drugs. Some were expensive. Wasn't there a better way? He had read that high blood pressure could be controlled by diet and exercise. He had been an athlete. Why couldn't he use this approach? He inquired around in his community for alternative options to drugs. Several of his friends said they had gotten off medications and felt great by exercising and eating better food. They recommended a local practitioner who used "natural" approaches for treatment of disease. She provided the hope Trevor was looking for. Not only was it possible to treat blood pressure naturally, she said, but diet and supplements could actually replace drugs. The side effects of medications could be avoided. She knew of the DASH diet but said that was just a start. She pointed to a "more effective" diet called the "Rice Diet for Hypertension" that would get people totally off drugs. The diet was developed at a clinic only a few hours from where Trevor lived—at Duke University—and had been "proven" to work for more than seventy-five years. He could go to a private center that delivered this diet or—for less cost—she could help him get on a "cleansing" diet and supplements that would do the same thing. She would help him to make it work with his life.

Trevor, optimistic as always, thought this sounded good and began to work with her. He stopped the medications and started the diet and supplements. He immediately felt better. After three weeks on the diet and supplements he went into a drugstore and had his blood pressure checked. It was almost normal. He was back to his old self—or so he thought.

He didn't see another doctor for ten years—until after his feet began to swell.

THE INTEGRATION GAP

The gap in health care between curing the body and the dimensions of healing is not confined to blood pressure. It is a general gap in health care—one that needs closing. In a recent comprehensive review I took of family medicine, I counted the number of recommendations for the use of drugs and other disease treatments compared to other dimensions described in this book—environmental, behavioral, social/emotional, and mind/spirit. Of the 361 health care management recommendations made during the review, 226 referred to drug management, 87 for behavior and lifestyle, 20 concerned complementary and alternative healing methods (mostly to avoid them), 19 addressed social and emotional counseling, and 9 were for mind-body or spiritual practices. In several lectures on chronic pain, for example, nondrug approaches were recommended as a first-line management in all patients. After one lecture on chronic pain that recommended use of complementary and integrative approaches to pain management, questions from the physicians were focused not on evidence for the effectiveness of these approaches, which ones were covered by insurance, and on how to implement the recommendations. The physicians pointed out that they were not well trained in the delivery of nondrug approaches for pain, that patients did not seek out these practices, and that the health care system did not pay for them. While evidence and a number of recommendations to use these healing dimensions is an improvement over review courses I took a decade ago, there is a lack of integration between curing and healing in our delivery systems. This gap between evidence and practice is difficult to bridge.

STANDARD SYSTEM ALLOWS GAP

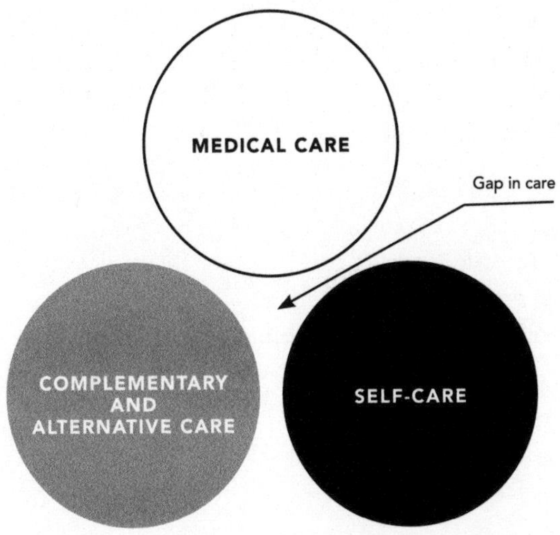

Trevor's doctors treated his numbers but failed to engage him in the lifestyle and social and emotional dimensions required for healing. The alternative practitioner used a diet that can rapidly lower blood pressure in the short run, but has not been shown to be effective in the long run. People cannot stick to it, yet they may think they have eliminated their problem. The herbs and supplements she recommended are not proven to work for high blood pressure. Yet she and Trevor believed in them. The two practitioners—the conventional doctor who addressed Trevor's biology and the alternative practitioner who provided Trevor with what he hoped for—never communicated with each other. Both knew about an effective and proven long-term dietary treatment for high blood pressure—the DASH diet—yet neither could deliver it. Had he followed that diet, Trevor would still have needed drugs, but likely in reduced numbers or doses—and he would have felt better. Despite increasing evidence and recommendations by national organizations to use more behavioral and lifestyle changes, doctors get very little training in nutritional therapy and even less in dealing with the social, emotional, and cultural dimensions of healing. Complementary and alternative practitioners are rarely trained in how to work with serious diseases and have even less training on how to coordinate what they do with physicians. Trevor fell into the gap between evidence-based medicine and person-centered care. The result was fifteen years of "silent" and poorly treated high blood pressure. When he went back to the doctor to see why his legs were swelling, they discovered he had kidney failure produced by poorly controlled high blood pressure. This led to years of kidney dialysis and the abortive attempts to get a transplant.

Trevor needed an integrative health care approach—one that bridged and coordinated the treatments between his biology and the rest of him; between drugs and self-care; between medical treatment and the social and personal determinants of health; between the treatment "agents" and his own "agency"—his inner capacity to heal.

The miracles of modern molecular medicine, with all its success over the last hundred years, have reached a limit when it comes to managing most chronic disease. Extensive research has repeatedly shown that even full access to medical treatments produces only about 15% to 20% of a population's health; the rest depends on lifestyle, environment, and social and personal determinants. This failure to focus on the whole person and delivery systems that address health determinants comes from how medical care is delivered—in silos and directed at discrete parts of people—without empowering them to heal. Modern medicine, so powerful in making miracles around acute disease, is now missing 80% of what's needed for healing chronic disease.

The most recent description of this dilemma was published by leaders at the U.S. National Academy of Medicine in a report called *Vital Directions for Health and Health Care*, edited by Drs. Victor Dzau, Mark McClellan, and Michael McGinnis. They describe how the money spent each year on health care in the United States (the most recent figure then was $3.2 trillion) is no longer providing the value it once did. They find that "an estimated 30% is related to waste, inefficiencies, and excessive price; health disparities are persistent and worsening; and the health and financial burden of chronic illness and disabilities are straining families and communities." They collated expert input in nineteen papers and made four main recommendations: pay for value, empower people, activate communities, and connect care. Had Trevor's physicians been paid to get him better, not to just give him drugs (that is, pay for value); had he been empowered to take responsibility for his health (empower people); had the community he lived in trusted the medical system (activate communities); and had there been an integrated approach between his medical treatment and his more natural approaches (connect care), Trevor would not have been lying in a hospital bed pleading for more time and praying for a donor kidney to appear.

Soon after the publication of *Vital Directions*, Samueli Institute and the Institute for Healthcare Improvement released the Wellbeing in the Nation (WIN) plan, which described how the United States could build an infrastructure to enhance healing in communities across the globe. The report recommends establishing a national well-being index and a community well-being extension service network to facilitate local integration of community well-being efforts. By addressing prevention, health promotion, and well-being, any community and its members can flourish. Both these reports point to local examples. Many communities already have sufficient resources to do this. The integration gap can be filled if we have the will to change our approach and rebalance curing with healing.

FROM SOAP TO HOPE

In the history of medicine, the use of a chemical, cellular science is very new. Our understanding of cell function and the chemistry of cure is only about two centuries old. Oxygen, for example, that essential molecule for survival, was discovered by Joseph Priestley in 1774. The establishment of reductionist science as a basis for medicine is only about a century old—being solidified as the gold standard after the Flexner Report on medical education was published in 1910. The application of this science for human testing in the form of randomized controlled trials (RCTs) is a little more than sixty years old—the first one was done in 1948. The solid establishment of RCTs as the gold standard for what is called evidence-based medicine today is more recent, with a concerted push from academics in Canada and England in the 1970s. The application of technology to further refine and manipulate the body is still more recent. By any metric, the science of medicine is young. So young, in fact, that the downsides and limitations for the prevention and treatment of chronic disease are only now beginning to emerge. As these limitations are more understood, there has been a parallel resurgence of interest in holistic approaches that were dismissed in the last hundred years. As I discovered in my practice, an integrative approach to health was needed—one that merges and coordinates curing and healing. To do that, I had to make a shift from the way I had been taught in medical school and practiced for decades—an approach exclusively focused on finding the disease—to a way of working with patients that enhanced their healing capacity. I had to widen the lens of my practice to reach out of the regular clinic visit to one that touched people in their life-space. I do this by going from what traditional medicine calls a SOAP visit to what I call a HOPE visit. Let me explain.

Most patients don't realize it, but when they visit their physician, he or she already has a specific plan to structure and report on the visit. In almost every visit, a physician will summarize the encounter with something called a SOAP note. SOAP stands for *subjective*, *objective*, *assessment*, and *plan*; it's designed to label the patient with a disease or illness diagnosis and its corresponding treatment.

SOAP is the way that every medical student, resident, and nurse and many other medical care practitioners learn how to organize their thinking around an encounter with a patient. Electronic medical records are built around the SOAP.

Subjective starts with the patient's chief complaint—what he came in for and what he says is bothering him. This complaint is filled in with further questions looking for additional subjective information reported by the patient.

Objective is what the practitioner observes; it includes observations of the body itself and laboratory test results and imaging. While there's no explicit ranking of subjective and objective, most practitioners have a bias toward the objective, giving it more value in the assessment than the subjective or what the patient says.

Assessment is meant to be a succinct summary of what the clinician thinks is the problem and is essentially the diagnosis. This diagnosis is usually attached to a code or a set of terminologies that form the lexicon of all medicine. The assessment is not only how we categorize patients to research them and get new knowledge; it also forms the categories around which we pay the practitioner, and track outcomes for the health care system. Thus it is essential to the livelihood of the health care system and the practitioner.

Finally, the *plan* is what we intend to do about the diagnosis, whether that be the execution of a treatment, the providing of advice, or further assessment and testing. Physicians are taught that the plan needs to align with the assessment and, under ideal circumstances, with at least with the objective part and hopefully, with the subjective part as well. The SOAP note is how we organize the entire experience of the patient visit and follow-up. In most medical encounters, no matter what the patient presents with, they will go out of the office framed in a SOAP. That SOAP is rarely shared with patients; if it is, we rarely ask them whether it makes sense. We don't expect them to know what the diagnostic codes, descriptions, and plans should be or what they mean. Good communication in a clinical encounter entails explaining the assessment and plan in nontechnical terms and the research evidence, with the goal of engaging the patient in clinical decisions. This process is called shared decision making, and it is almost universally espoused as important for every chronic disease decision—yet it is rarely done. Physicians vary considerably in their skill at communicating the assessment and plan to patients, and usually any SOAP discussion remains technical.

The SOAP process happens tens of thousands of time every day around the world; it structures the medical encounter and drives the medical treatment engine. The SOAP note is formulated around a set of basic assumptions that organize all modern medical education, research, and practice. SOAP uses a pathogenic framing: it is about disease and illness, not healing. It is the way modern medicine diagnoses diseases and aligns them with treatment. How much evidence connects the assessment part to the plan part of SOAP determines whether a treatment is judged to be evidence-based or not. This, in turn, structures the way research is done, such as how patients are selected for clinical studies. This then restricts what is allowed in health care. It keeps modern medicine focused on seeking cures. This constant search for cures creates multiple treatments that are "done to" the patient. Because SOAP uses the biomedical, biochemical paradigm, it often misses the dimensions of healing found by and in other parts of patients. The concept of *salutogenesis*—the process of healing—is a concept I and others have expanded on from Aaron Antonovsky, who first coined this term in the 1970s. *Salutogenesis* rarely comes up explicitly in a clinical encounter. Doctors focus on *pathogenesis*—the process of how disease is produced—and how to counteract it. No wonder most clinical encounters are not person-centered or holistic and miss most of healing. We doctors always must fit them into a

SOAP! In the medical profession is it called the "tyranny of the chief complaint"—and we are stuck on it.

Doing a SOAP process with each patient visit is important for disease diagnosis and treatment, but if we are to balance curing with whole person healing, we need more than SOAP. We need an encounter focused specifically on healing. So, to balance the standard medical encounter with healing, I follow up the SOAP process with a HOPE note. HOPE stands for healing-oriented practices and environments, and it addresses dimensions of physical, behavioral, social/emotional, and mind/spirit—and so tap into the 80% of how healing works. It involves a set of questions designed to help the person identify and navigate a unique pathway to healing. The HOPE questions probe how the person is already engaged in healing, and then seeks to match that with good evidence to enhance those activities. It highlights what the person has intuitively discovered and adds the rational elements derived from rigorous research. Since both intuition and science are uncertain by themselves, pairing these different ways of knowing maximizes the benefit for both curative treatments and the person's healing capacity. It optimizes the meaning response. By doing a HOPE, I help patients avoid the gap that Trevor had fallen into.

The story of another patient, Mandy, illustrates how SOAP and HOPE together create integrative health and healing.

MANDY

At forty-five years old, Mandy should have been able to maintain a household—but now she could not. Even before the accident, she had struggled to care for two teenaged boys and a nine-year-old daughter, a husband who worked a lot, and a part-time job. Her life consisted of juggling schedules, meals, household chores, phone calls, and social media. There was no time for self-care. She had worked full-time until fifteen years ago. Then, in what she thought was a relatively minor car accident, she sustained a neck whiplash and shoulder ligament tear on her right side. She gave it time to heal and followed all instructions, including physical therapy and taking anti-inflammatories. But the pain never went away. It became chronic. Soon she had major neck stiffness and intractable pain down her shoulder and right arm. A fifteen-year journey with neuropathic pain had begun.

Over that fifteen-year period, she was diagnosed with multiple other conditions, from depression to anxiety to PTSD to neurosis. She continued to try and maintain as healthy a life as possible: exercising as she could, doing physical therapy, eating well, and cultivating relationships with friends and family. As with many patients in chronic pain, these were challenging activities. Most of her encounters with medical professionals resulted in being prescribed more medications. At one point, she was on more than five medications, including the opioid OxyContin, from which she had difficulty freeing herself. The pain would flare up when she tried to taper off of it. Eventually, with the help of an inpatient pain treatment group, she got off the OxyContin and began taking other, less addictive drugs, such as Neurontin and Lyrica, which partially improved both her neuropathic pain and crying episodes. "Let me warn you, Doc—I cry," she said on her first visit with me, tears already welling up in her eyes. "Sometimes I just cry for no reason—sorry." I waited until she stopped.

Her pain was significant. She rated it between five to seven out of ten on a daily basis. It was accompanied by spasms and stiffness in her neck and right shoulder. Over the fifteen years, she had had many other treatments besides drugs: regular physical therapy, steroid injections, and electrical stimulators and psychotherapy, all from conventional pain clinics or her primary care doctor. Like Trevor, she entered into the parallel world of complementary and alternative medicine, seeing chiropractors, acupuncturists, herbalists, homeopaths, and mind-body practitioners. They all seemed to help a bit, some more than others—temporarily. She found that hot baths and meditation helped the most—when she had the time to do them. Sleep was never in the cards, both because of her busy family—the boys were up late doing homework—and because the pain did not ease at night. She woke frequently and never felt rested. Sometimes she would just go into the bathroom and cry.

She came to me because she heard I might help her enhance her own healing capacity. She had heard I had a different approach and would work to integrate it with her regular medical treatments. So we set up a HOPE visit and began to discuss the dimensions of healing in her life. We explored a list of options that science shows helps people with chronic pain heal. I asked her questions like the following:

1. What gave her the greatest joy and well-being in her life? What was her most meaningful activity?

2. Did she have friends and a supportive family—anyone to cry with, to love, who would nurture and support her?

3. What was her daily behavior like? The medical treatments? Her lifestyle—diet, sleep, exercise? What did she do to relax?

4. What was her home like—the physical environment where she spent most of her time? Did she have a special place to give her an escape from the daily chores and hubbub of the day?

THE ELEMENTS OF WHOLE PERSON HEALING ADDRESSED IN A HOPE VISIT

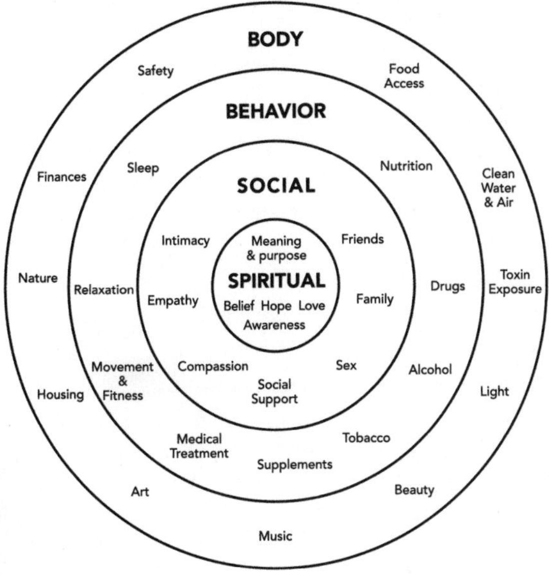

These are the main questions I go through with patients during a HOPE assessment, using a chart like the one you see here. Mandy and I made a map to help her navigate toward a healing path, showing these dimensions and the elements in them that we would explore. With patience and persistence, HOPE can often change the trajectory of illness and restore well-being—even if, as in chronic disease, cure is not possible.

Three things emerged during my dialogue with Mandy. First, many things were right in her life and supported her healing. She had a wonderful family and some good friends. She paid close attention to the food her family ate—lots of fruits and vegetables, fish, whole grains, and minimal sugar. She tried to exercise daily—at least doing her physical therapy each day. But she had challenges in many areas—especially in rest and relaxation. Her schedule, the needs of the household, and her pain made relaxation a challenge. Five years previously, she thought she had been getting better more rapidly, but then was involved in a second car accident. In this one, she struck her head but did not lose consciousness. After evaluating her, the doctors said everything was okay. Soon after that, her crying episodes started. She could not stop thinking of both accidents and that she might never recover. That is when she was diagnosed with PTSD. This was also when the antidepressant medications and counseling were added—providing some relief in her mood but not much for the pain.

I then asked her a question I ask most of my patients: "What do you think is going on?" The timing and setting of this question are key to getting a deep and meaningful response. The purpose of the question is to help patients search their intuition—their heart or gut or soul, depending on how they perceive it. My job is to see if I can match what comes from that intuition with reasonable scientific evidence that might be used to enhance the patient's healing. As it turned out, Mandy's answer held the key to her recovery.

"Well," she said after a slight pause, "it's my brain—there seems to be something wrong with my brain."

"Why do you say that?" I probed and waited.

“Well, I noticed that the first few times I got acupuncture, I had a big relief—like maybe 95% better. Pain down to 1 or 2. But it didn't last. I tried it several times, but after a while it didn't work at all. So I gave up. It was like my brain was trying to heal but could not absorb the treatments. It just wasn't sticking. Like I said, something is wrong with my brain.” Mandy started to cry again. “Sorry, doctor.”

Our integrative health team got together and looked at the situation. Clearly, the acupuncture was producing endogenous opioids—those internal painkillers that all our brains produce. But after the treatments, her levels of those went down and she was no longer responding. The acupuncturist suggested that she had just not had enough treatments. Repeated acupuncture will not only induce endogenous opioids, but eventually also increase the density of opioid receptors in the brain, making the person more responsive to her own brain's painkillers and prolonging the effect. She just needed more treatments.

The neurologist disagreed. If increases in brain receptors were the problem, they should have shown at least some evidence of effect. Mandy had first done twelve weekly acupuncture treatments, and then an additional four acupuncture treatments spaced once a month. That should have been sufficient for acupuncture to “take,” he said. Something else must be going on. He wondered if the head injury she had sustained in her second car accident had caused a problem. I mentioned that her crying episodes—a sign of possible decreased cortical inhibition of her emotions—had begun after the second car accident. This can also happen from brain injury. To see if we could find any evidence for this, we ordered a positron emission tomography (PET) scan.

While neuroimaging technology is advancing by leaps and bounds in medicine, the interpretation of what we see in those images—especially in the brain—is still being worked out. Our interest in this for Mandy was to explore if there was any evidence of brain dysfunction in areas preventing her from responding to the acupuncture. Dr. Daniel Amen is an American psychiatrist who has the most extensive experience in the world in the use of PET scanning to refine our understanding of brain diseases; he has read over twenty-five thousand, including many looking for the effects of subtle brain injury. I had read his book *Change Your Brain, Change Your Life* and wondered if PET imaging would help us in working with Mandy. A PET scan is a rather crude but inexpensive way to look at metabolism in the brain. We hoped that if the PET showed clear changes in the frontal areas of her brain—especially an area of the ventro-medial frontal cortex—this might explain both the crying episodes and the failure of acupuncture to take. It was worth a shot, especially in light of Mandy's own feeling that her brain was not functioning properly.

The PET scan seemed to confirm her feelings and our hypothesis. It demonstrated a reduction in glucose metabolism in the left frontal lobe, not exactly where we had hypothesized, but in an area where some of the executive functions and inhibitory pathways to pain and emotional control might have been damaged. We had no way to know whether this was caused by the car accident or if this explained her ongoing pain and temporary response to opioids and acupuncture. But it seemed to confirm our belief that Mandy needed to try to regrow those areas of the brain. More important, the scan energized Mandy to want to reengage in her own self-care—something she had neglected over the years. The simplest way to regrow the brain is to exercise it. We suggested either biofeedback or an intensive set of relaxation response exercises. Mandy liked that idea, so our next task was to find a method that she enjoyed and could maintain long enough to enhance function in that part of her brain. Mandy decided to try mindfulness meditation.

MIND-BRAIN-BODY

Most of modern biomedicine focuses on treating diseases of the mind—mental and psychosomatic illnesses—by manipulating the brain. But the reverse is also possible. The brain and the rest of the body can be treated through the mind. Mandy needed a way to regrow a part of her brain that had become injured and dysfunctional, even possibly atrophied, by years of pain and treatments to alleviate it. While someday we may be able to regrow parts of brains using stem cells or direct electrical stimulation, those days are not here yet. Our experience with drug and herbal treatments also shows that those methods provide only partial relief in a few and risk producing side effects in many. In the meantime, there are methods to regrow the brain through behavior, social learning, and mind-body practices. Physical exercise can increase neural growth generally. Mandy did some exercise but could not engage in intensive physical training. Also, we could not use exercise to grow the specific areas that seemed to be problematic for her. Biofeedback of brain waves can growth brain areas—often in specific areas. That approach required multiple visits and sophisticated equipment. Virtual reality is another method but is generally not viable for chronic pain. These also cost money and are not easy to incorporate into self-care. We needed an approach Mandy could bring into her daily life. The one that seemed the most practical and meaningful for Mandy was mindfulness meditation training.

For Mandy, this meant creating a process for her to do deep relaxation every day for at least eight weeks. I knew about the research showing that patients who engage in at least eight weeks of mind-body practices such as mindfulness or meditation for thirty minutes a day can grow areas of the frontal lobe that Mandy had lost. She was excited to try this. She had previously tried meditation and found it helped her feel better, and have less anxiety, but she had not kept it up. The challenge now would be integrating it into her daily life. For this, the behavioral medicine and health coach on the team came into play. They worked with her to design—with her family—a process allowing her to engage in thirty minutes of mindfulness meditation every day. She preferred this over the visualization that Jake had done, or heart-rate variability biofeedback—another evidence-based option. The first attempt failed because as long as she was in her house, she felt overwhelmed by responsibilities for her family. She had no place in her house that she could fully relax.

The behaviorist and health coach helped her organize that special place in her house. It turned out to be in her bedroom, where she constructed her own little nurturing corner. The family cooperated to ensure that this place was isolated and not invaded by the rest of them.

In her own little corner, she placed some of her favorite sacred symbols and family mementos that she enjoyed. She decorated it with soft cloth and low light. A CD player was set up to deliver favorite music or nature sounds. It was her own optimal healing environment. A set of reminders to both the family members and herself, sent simultaneously through a cell phone app, allowed her to engage in over thirty minutes of mindfulness and breathing practice every day for more than two months. At that point, a repeat PET scan showed improved neurological function in the frontal lobe. This encouraged her to continue. She also noted that her sleep had improved and her pain had dropped from the usual 5 to 7 on a scale of 1 to 10, to a 4 or 5. It was now time to try acupuncture again.

Research shows that it takes between eight and twelve weeks of acupuncture for opioid receptor density to change in the brain. But this had not previously worked for Mandy. We hoped that now that she had the right neurological foundation, the acupuncture would take. Mandy had used her mind to change her brain. So she began a series of twenty acupuncture treatments using a combination of body and

INTEGRATIVE HEALTH CLOSES THE GAP

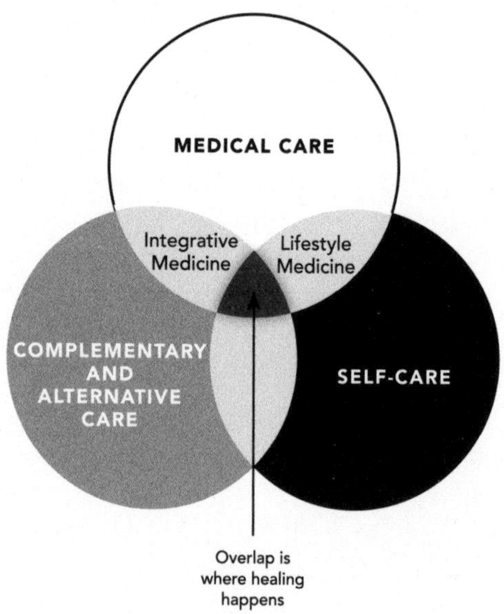

ear points. Gradually, over the next two months, the rebound of pain she had previously experienced after acupuncture began to diminish. Within three months, her pain levels were down to 1 or 2 out of 10, and she could scale back her acupuncture to once every month and eventually once every three months. More important, her quality of life, functional capacity, and ability to tap her own healing capacity increased. She learned that when her pain began to increase, it was often because she had not engaged in sufficient self-care, either by not getting enough sleep or by skipping her mindfulness practices or ignoring increased stress in her life. Her medications were now only a low-dose antidepressant, which, along with her restored frontal lobe, prevented most of the crying, and acetaminophen for an occasional pain flare.

Mandy was the beneficiary of integrative health.

I use the term "integrative medicine" in reference to the merger of conventional medicine—as I was trained in—and complementary and alternative medicine, such as acupuncture, chiropractic, or massage. The term "lifestyle medicine" is used in reference to the merger of conventional medicine and behavior in the form of self-care, such as nutrition, exercise, and stress management. "Integrative health" is at the intersection of all three of these fields with good scientific evidence and patient-centered care as the driving principles for its application. This is what Mandy had at her disposal. This is the future of health care for chronic disease.

A SHIFT TOWARD HOLISM

There is a story that around the year 500 BCE, an enlightened ruler in Tibet did a remarkable thing. He invited master healers from all the major healing traditions of the world to a yearlong conference of learning. Physicians came from corners of the known world, including Greece and the Middle East, North Africa, China, and India. Their purpose was to share the best of their craft and synthesize the most effective treatments known to humanity—in other words, to create a truly integrative approach from the world's healing traditions of the time. What emerged was a remarkable system that informed and infused medical thinking for over a thousand years. It was the integrative medicine of its day.

We need a similar effort to integrate the best healing traditions from around the world today. In an age of instant information and global interaction, patients are already exposed to and using practices from multiple healing traditions and nonconventional systems. In 1993, Dr. David Eisenberg of Harvard published a study in the *Journal of the American Medical Association* showing that over one-third of people in the United States regularly sought out so-called complementary and alternative medicine (CAM) practices and visited alternative healers. A decade later, that number was 40% and climbing. The use of so-called complementary and alternative medicine is even higher in Europe, South America, and Eurasia and up to 80% in the populations of non-Western countries. But rarely do conventional doctors know about these practices. Rarely do patients tell doctors when they are using them, and rarely do doctors ask about or offer them. The gap between curing, healing, and self-care is greater than ever. Patients are the ones saddled with trying to do the proper integration that the profession should be doing. The consequences of this gap can be tragic when people like Trevor, struggling with high blood pressure and eventual kidney failure, seek out more holistic practices but without appropriate scientific input. We need another concerted effort today—like what was done in Tibet a thousand years ago—with the help of modern science and information technology.

Fortunately, there is a shift toward more integration in health care today. The effort is occurring—but with difficulty. In 1948, the WHO came out with a controversial definition of health. The WHO defined health as more than just curing physical disease, but "a state of complete physical, mental, and social well-being and not merely the absence of disease or infirmity." It declared that this definition should be the goal of all health care. However, most of modern medicine went on its reductionist way—looking for finer and finer divisions of the body into the small and particular. The study of DNA was under intense research when WHO published its definition, with the Watson and Crick discovery of its structure published in 1953. The first randomized clinical trial (RCT)—done in the same year as the WHO definition—launched the role of reductionism onto the stage of human testing for medical decision making. As we've discussed, the RCT has become the primary tool for deciding what is good evidence in health care. For the last five decades, this science of the small and particular has continued to dominate biomedical research and clinical practice—being applied everywhere and to everything.

Then, gradually, international groups began to respond to our need for rebalance and more whole person care. In 2001, a landmark report from the Institute of Medicine (now National Academy of Medicine) called *Crossing the Quality Chasm* laid out ten principles for the redesign of health care to provide more patient-centered, holistic care in medicine. The first three recommendations were as follows:

1. Care is based on continuous healing relationships.

2. Care is customized according to patient needs and values.

3. The patient is the source of control.

The report also called for good evidence, shared information, better safety, anticipation of (not just reaction to) patient needs, prevention, and cooperation among clinicians. In other words, team care. In a major effort to live up to these principles, four main primary care associations in the United States—in pediatrics, family medicine, internal medicine, and obstetrics-gynecology—published a joint set of guidelines for the Patient Centered Medical Home in 2007. The idea behind this was to provide care that is the following:

- Patient-centered: takes into account the needs and preferences of the patient and family
- Comprehensive: covers the whole person, including their physical, mental, prevention, wellness, acute and chronic care
- Coordinated: is organized to integrate all elements of health care delivery
- Accessible: includes 24/7 care, with telephone and IT communications

- Committed to quality and safety: ensured thorough continuous improvement

In other words, the call was for medicine to be more responsive to the whole person, be more integrated, and be more focused on prevention and health promotion than our current system. Echoes of *Crossing the Quality Chasm* reverberated throughout the mainstream.

Other groups and other countries too have pushed for more integrative and holistic care. In 2008, the international Institute for Healthcare Improvement (IHI) defined and began to support training for achieving the "Triple Aim" of health care worldwide: (1) improving the patient experience, (2) improving the health of populations, and (3) reducing the per-person cost of health care. The concept of pay for value (rather than for procedure or treatment) emerged from these efforts. The goal was described clearly by visionary leaders such as IHI founder Dr. Don Berwick, who called for an "integrator"—an organization that accepts responsibility for all three aims. Dr. Berwick went on to create the Center for Medicare and Medicaid Innovation, which funded and tested new models of health care, demonstrating how to implement pay for value. Pay for value efforts were already under way in England, Europe, Australia, Singapore, Japan, and other countries. These innovative models are gradually moving more fully toward the type of integrative health care that people like Trevor need to prevent disease and stay healthy, and that Mandy used to heal herself from chronic pain.

But implementing these aspirational principles has been a challenge. Medicine still largely follows individual treatment processes and pays for doing things to a patient rather than supporting healing with a patient. We still spend most of our money and time looking for treatment agents that only incrementally add to overall health, rather than optimizing our own agency for transformational healing. The will is there, but the ways are weak, and the economic drivers are against this when it comes to healing. Recently, the Peterson Foundation funded Stanford's Center for Excellence in Primary Care to find the top 5% of primary care practices that meet the Triple Aim and the patient-centered medical home model, and to describe the characteristics of their success. Not surprisingly, those characteristics were almost identical to those listed in *Crossing the Quality Chasm.* The most effective health care went beyond simply doling out treatments. These practices spent time probing the other dimensions of healing. They addressed the whole person, organized care to make the patient the driver of their own healing, and created teams of caregivers—all processes addressing the behavioral and the social and emotional dimensions of healing. They provide integrative health care at its best.

A NEW WAY TO HEAL

The two missing spheres of integrative health—complementary and alternative practices and lifestyle medicine or self-care—have been growing in research and practice in parallel with the mainstream calls for more person-centered and holistic care. If your physician is interested in learning more about these areas, he or she (and you) can learn more from my description in the next chapter. Many of these resources bring lifestyle and behavioral change into treatment, beyond using them just for the prevention of chronic diseases. Physician pioneer Dr. Dean Ornish has emphasized this point and demonstrated it in rigorous research for decades. In his most recent best-selling book, *The Spectrum,* he brings together the elements of lifestyle medicine to show that we can reverse chronic disease and turn on disease-preventing genes. This is indeed a new way to heal, compared to what most doctors have been learning.

As Trevor and many of my other patients have taught me, behavior is only one dimension needed to tap into the 80% of healing. Almost all patients that I see in my practice know that behavior is important for health. But, as was tragically true for Trevor, having that knowledge is not enough. A recent study published by the Mayo Clinic concluded that only 2.7% of the population engages in the four main behaviors that keep people healthy—not smoking, eating a high vegetable diet, engaging in regular activity, and undertaking adequate stress management. Nor does simply engaging in healthy behaviors address the deeper levels of a person—the social/emotional and mind/spirit dimensions—that are so essential to finding the permanent path to healing. Maria changed her behavior, but wasn't healed until she found a group to teach cooking to. Sergeant Martin was using a treatment—hyperbaric oxygen—proven not to work. Yet by engaging in it with a group of other service members, he improved and healed himself. Had Norma not been enrolled in the clinical study I was running on arthritis, she might never have been motivated enough to move through her pain and return to her volunteer job. For Mabel, as for many seriously ill people and elderly or frail patients, social relationships were the central dimension to her healing and well-being.

We saw in chapter 7 that at least one health care system—the Nuka System of Care in Alaska—could shift their delivery of health care to a relationship and patient-centered paradigm. The success of this system is partially based on anchoring it in Alaskan Native traditions. But the world is increasingly mobile and made up of diverse traditions with multiple cultures and languages. Is it possible to build an integrative healing system flexible enough for our increasingly mobile and multicultural world? To find out, I visited one system that is attempting to do just that.

Dr. Rushika Fernandopulle was born in Sri Lanka, where he found, as I did in Vietnam, that much care still comes from traditional practitioners who use natural substances and conduct ancient rituals—just as Aadi did in the Ayurvedic hospital in nearby India. Infectious disease, lack of sanitation, trauma, and malnutrition were common in Sri Lanka. But Dr. Fernandopulle noticed one thing about people with chronic disease and mental health issues: if they could get clean water and food and had access to the basics of modern medicine, they were happy and generally did well. Their lifestyle and social relationships supported lifelong health. As in the five places in the world identified by author Dan Buettner in his book *Blue Zones*, where people live the longest, healthiest lives, the Sri Lankans had less medicine and less illness than many in Western countries. Traditional practitioners and grandmothers coached people on how to live. There was no gap between the medical space and the life space. The only gap was science.

Then Dr. Fernandopulle came to America and got arguably the best scientific and medical training available at Harvard. Like me, he saw the miracles that modern science could bring to curing. Like me, he had been exposed to both the advantages and the limitations of ancient traditional healing systems. And like me, he saw that for chronic disease, people in the West were not doing better—yet they were paying more. So he set out to try to fill the gaps in the health care system he worked in here. But he found it extremely difficult to change a system that paid for and reinforced only treatment and cure. Like me, he found that the nature of the medical encounter, the payment system, the electronic medical record, and the SOAP note was not designed for healing the whole person. Finally, he gave up trying to change the systems and set out to design and build a new system that could change the nature of health care and fill the gap between curing and healing. He called it Iora, after a small bird in Sri Lanka.

Superficially, the job of an Iora practice is the same as any medical clinic—to prevent and treat illness and disease; to help people get and stay well. However, the second you dig even a little bit deeper, you realize it is indeed very different from typical care. The clinic is filled with specially trained professionals called "health coaches," who work hand in hand with the nurses and doctors to address any area that might impact your health or interfere with your healing. It provides standard treatments like vaccines, medications, minor surgery, and counseling. But it can also provide information on nutrition and behavioral change, stress and social services, and access to financial or legal help, if needed. And it can link you to responsible complementary and alternative practices and integrate that care into the other services. Every member of the health care team and the patient have full access to all information in the health record—which is structured around the patient rather than the payments—and is fully accessible to the patient at all times. The need to worry about the cost of treatment is eliminated, as all care in Iora practices is provided for a flat fee per patient per month (paid for by what Iora calls a sponsor, which could be an insurance health plan or self-insured employer, for instance). Hospital or specialty care is additional, but the Iora team works closely to provide a broader range of care than traditional primary care, improve access, and eliminate unnecessary care (which makes up one-third of medicine), and to facilitate recovery after specialty treatment. Healing and recovery are ever present. Group classes and individual assistance in nutrition and behavioral change are available, and the staff are tuned in to the social/emotional and mental/spiritual lives of the patients. The space is warm and welcoming, without the usual barriers or industrial feel of typical clinics. The health care team knows you. Employees are selected for and trained in listening and empathy. Unlike most clinics in health care, you will not be interrupted within the first sixteen seconds of the encounter. The feel of caring is palpable.

And it heals better. Like the top 5% of primary care practices identified by Stanford, Iora's outcomes are stellar. Data on ten of the clinics open for two years or more shows remarkable results. This includes engagement rates of 85% per year; retention rates of 90% (94% of those engaged); a total medical expense decrease of 14% per year; in-patient admissions and emergency room visits more than 40% below the Medicare fee-for-service average; and a 21% improvement in hypertension outcomes. In addition, Iora has a 90 Net Promoter Score across Medicare markets (this means patients recommend them to others). One hundred percent of patients needing urgent care get a visit within twenty-four hours. Iora's STAR ratings (the Medicare system of quality in five different categories) increase yearly up to 30%.

By the standards of the Triple Aim, the patient-centered medical home, and even the Stanford assessments, Iora meets and exceeds those measures. Equally important, the patients, practitioners, health coaches, and communities enjoy the practice more. Practitioners suffer less burnout, and nurses and physicians feel their skills are well used.

But can this approach be applied in diverse settings with a variety of average people? The answer is that it can. Iora clinics are now up and functioning with good results in areas as diverse as college towns, the Las Vegas strip, and poverty-stricken areas of Queens in New York.

"What is needed now," says Dr. Fernandopulle, "is a health care system that truly wants and will pay for this type of integrated care."

HEALING THROUGH PURPOSE

No matter where we start or how we navigate the elements of healing, it is when we can link them to our purpose in life that deep healing happens. This happens more often when the dimensions of healing are aligned. It also happens more often when good science is brought into the process to enhance it. It can happen dramatically when a person finds those elements that induce their greatest meaning response. Then we go beyond the 20% improvement found in cure-based medicine and tap into the 80% of healing potential that lies dormant in everyone.

In his book *Life on Purpose*, Dr. Victor Strecher, professor of public health at the University of Michigan, has summarized the extensive and startling research showing how a life of meaning and purpose prevents and treats chronic disease, reduces suffering, and even prolongs life. When a person feels that they have an important purpose in life, when their values and actions align—especially when that purpose gives back to others—they simply do and are better in all ways. Purpose has been correlated with reduced weight, better sleep, more friends, better sex, faster recovery, less relapse from addictions, less risk of Alzheimer's disease and dementia, less heart disease, lower health care needs, and lower death rates.

We even know the biology of purpose. It increases growth in the ventriculo-medial prefrontal cortex of the brain—the brain location of one's "sense of self"—and it can even maintain and elongate telomeres—the genes that predict your length of life. That individual sense of purpose, when aligned with our family, community, and work, will enhance the health of others in those areas, too. Companies whose employees feel cared for and are aligned with company goals and mission deliver more profits and last longer than companies that don't. Families and communities with purpose have more vibrancy and happiness, less violence and poverty, better health and well-being. Thus the goal in engaging in the HOPE process is to link your healing dimensions to why you are here in the world—your meaning and purpose in life—and to create a meaning response in mind and body.

Once we understand the dimensions of healing and the individual elements of meaning and purpose in creating health and well-being, it changes our perspective on health care and illuminates the path out of the current health care dilemma of higher costs, less satisfaction, and poorer health. My patients who use this approach find that they are no longer victims of a system not designed for them. This understanding becomes the foundation for true health (not just health care) reform.

What is needed now is a willingness to bring healing back into health care. The most effective way to do that is to bring it deliberately and intentionally into your life. You may not have access to integrative health care in a Nuka- or Iora-like system or get your care from one of the top 5% of patient-centered medical facilities. But this should not matter. Remember, only 20% of health comes from the treatments you get by walking into a doctor's office or visiting a medical clinic. The rest—the 80%—comes from you, from using the dimensions of healing already embedded in your life. By engaging in a HOPE-like process, you can unleash that 80%.

In the next, and final, chapter, I provide a simple set of instructions and accompanying tools for doing a HOPE visit. You and your physician can use those tools to access your healing dimensions. In the appendices, I provide a process that you—even without your physician—can use for your own journey to healing. Take this journey into your life; work through the questions yourself; take what you discover to your physician if she is willing to partner with you on that journey. If your doctor is hesitant, give her this book; when she has finished it, ask for impressions. It is my hope that doctors find these principles and tools useful in their own lives. I have. They might even help to ease their burnout and be more patient-centered in their practices. You can be your doctor's healer!

The oncologist had unintentionally set my wife up to make The Cake, which was so effective in advancing her recovery. We had tried many other treatments to help her with fatigue, anemia, hair loss, and the risk of heart and nerve damage from chemotherapy. These included both conventional medications and alternative supplements of various types. For most of the alternative treatments, there was little evidence. For a few, there was evidence of harm. The oncologist offered several drugs for dealing with the side effects of therapy. Some worked well, especially for nausea and severe white blood count drops, but again, the evidence for many of them was slim, and nothing helped much for her extreme fatigue.

Then, during one oncologist visit just before the July Fourth holiday, Susan described again her tiredness and shortness of breath. The doctor was headed for the door when I asked about Susan's anemia—low red blood counts. She looked at the labs: "Oh, yes, they are low," she said. "You have anemia." She paused for a bit and then said, "You know, that is most likely what is causing your fatigue. But it is nothing to worry about, Susan. It's expected with chemotherapy. It's not in a dangerous range, so we'll keep an eye on it. It's normal for what you are going through. You will start getting better soon—after the chemotherapy."

Susan told me later that on hearing this, a light went on in her mind. This was "normal," and it was up to her to get through it. After that visit, she said to me, "As I understood it, the doctor basically said to just tough it out. That's what I thought. That is what I am doing and will keep doing. Let's really celebrate the Fourth. It's time to be *normal.*"

It was a few days after that Susan mustered the energy to make The Cake. The oncologist, of course, never knew about The Cake or most of the other factors that sustained Susan's healing during the onslaught of the treatment. She didn't have time to. But without The Cake and the hope it engendered in Susan, the healing transformation she had during her cancer treatment might not have occurred. It was a hope the oncologist had given almost as a side comment, thrown out as she put her hand on the door to leave for the next patient. I thought of all the times I had done the same thing with patients. I thought now that it doesn't have to be this way in health care—to focus so much on the treatment and cure that we often miss what induces the healing.

SPIRIT MATTERS

This was the fifth trip to the hospital for Trevor to see if he could get a kidney. When he arrived around midnight, the doctor said that if the possible kidney did not match for him that night, they would discharge him in the morning and start again later in the year. Trevor's wife stayed with him and went to sleep in the chair in his hospital room. In the quiet of the early morning, Trevor reflected on what his wife had said; how his "incorrigible optimism" had gotten him into this mess; how he had not trusted the doctors and believed too much in natural treatments; how he had focused so much on giving back to his community—following his one passion and purpose—that he had neglected himself and his own health. Had there been a system of integrative health to fill the gaps between drugs, diet, and self-care; had the care he received been more person-centered; and had it been better linked to his purpose, he might have avoided years of suffering and expense, prevented the injury his wife endured when she donated her own kidney unsuccessfully, and not had to endure his current almost total dependency on the medical system. Perhaps, he thought quietly to himself, his optimism, his passion, his purpose, his prayer had all been misplaced. He was in a deep despair—hopeless. All he wanted was to be well so he could go back and help his people—young people especially who had been like him. He wanted them to have the opportunity for a full and successful life.

Then he did something he was not supposed to do. He got out of bed without assistance and kneeled to pray. His knees hurt. The IV pole pulled at his arm. He felt dizzy. At the side of the bed he prayed his favorite Bible passage from Isaiah 6:8: "Then I heard the voice of the Lord saying, 'Whom shall I send? And who will go for us?' And I said, 'Here am I. Send me!' " He then got back into bed and thought of the hymn "I Am Here Lord." A deep peace suddenly came over him. At that moment "I knew I was going to get a kidney," said Trevor. He described feeling much more than his usual optimism. It was an overwhelming feeling of release—of giving himself up to whatever God wanted of him and that he was being held in the Lord's loving hands. He fell into a deep sleep—better than he had for weeks.

He awoke at 7 AM to his wife packing, getting him ready to be discharged back home. No call for a kidney had come in during the night. When he was fully awake he sat up and reached down to put on his socks—but something held him up.

"Ready?" his wife said, wondering why he was hesitating. It was long past the time they would have called him had the kidney been a match. But he was not ready. All the things that might happen should he leave now raced through this mind. He would have a dialysis treatment. He would go home and get back to work in his law firm and his community—a passion and purpose he would pursue it until the end. He would go on until it was his time to die, he thought.

"Let's wait a bit," he said to her. They sat in silence, waiting for the doctor to come in to discharge him. He just couldn't bring himself to put his socks on.

When the doctor came in to the room he looked at them with an unusual smile. "Are you ready to go?" the doctor asked, in a strange tone.

"Sure, we are all packed up," said Trevor's wife, ignoring her husband's still bare feet.

"Well, then." The doctor could no longer contain himself; now he was smiling broadly. "You better unpack and get ready for the operating room. We found a kidney. It came in this morning—and it is a match!"

Trevor's wife sat there, stunned. Trevor took a deep breath and broke into a smile to match the doctor's. Finally, he simply said, "Okay then."

He would be healed.

CHAPTER 10

Creating Healing

Your HOPE consultation.

Doctors don't want frustrated, unhappy patients, and patients don't want burnt-out, unhappy doctors. None of us wants to feel like we are victims of the health care system. But all too often, that is what we get. It does not have to be that way.

To understand why this happens and how to improve it, we need to look beyond the individual doctor, to the health care system and the environment. We then see there are many pressures on the health care system that push it away from the delivery of patient-centered and integrative health, especially for chronic and preventive care. When you as the patient are aware of these pressures, you can counteract them by creating healing relationships with health care professionals and your own healing environment. This chapter describes the forces that can help you and your health care team connect with the inherent healing power in you and in everyone. Let's take a moment to summarize the forces operating on the current health care system.

UNDERSTANDING THE FORCES IN HEALTH CARE

Our modern medical system was originally set up to provide acute care. Problems that require immediate intervention, include injury, trauma, infection, heart attack, and stroke, are much better managed than chronic conditions.

Increasingly, most doctors are subspecialists. Except for those trained in primary care or family medicine, most doctors emerge from medical school well equipped to deal with only part of you—your cardiovascular system, or your bones and muscles, or your digestive organs, or your brain and central nervous system, or your endocrine system (glands and hormones). This is fine if your problems are restricted to these systems, but most health problems—especially those caused by stress and lifestyle—affect the whole person, including body, mind, and spirit. Specialists are not trained to look at health problems in this way.

We are fascinated by technology. Technology has produced tremendous advances in health care and will continue to do so. But there is a downside. The more inventive we get with diagnostic and surgical technology, the more we lose touch with the essential humanity of each patient. Patients are hooked up to blood pressure cuffs and monitors, injected with needles that withdraw blood, operated on through robotic arms attached to tiny cameras, and examined through ultrasound, MRI, and CT scans. Doctors can now peer into our brains, our organs, the very cells and genes of our body and obtain objective information about what is going on there. This is useful, of course, for diagnosis and treatment of disease, but the process tends to reduce people to objects, to depersonalize us. We are treated as if we too are machines, in need of repair, rather than living, breathing people with emotions, fears, and desires, in need of healing.

Doctors live with the potential for mistakes and lawsuits. Given the uncertainty in the science of medicine, the risk for error is high. Doctors don't like this, and many overcompensate with unnecessary care in the hope of overcoming that uncertainty. However, that rarely works. More is not better. In fact, the overuse of medical technologies is one of the main causes of harm to patients. In addition, the risk of malpractice suits or discipline from oversight boards leads many doctors to practice so-called "defensive medicine": ordering extra tests, waiting for specialists to "bless" a diagnosis, and focusing on extra paperwork, which also is often not in the best interest of the patient or based on good research evidence.

Doctors have information and work overload. Once, for my birthday, my father gave me a coffee mug inscribed with the words "Cognitive Overload." The message was clear—slow down and relax. Take time to listen, especially with your heart, not just your brain. We are all flooded with waves of information daily, and it is impossible for any one person (or even a group of people) to extract, synthesize, and make good use of all the information that is now available. In addition, many doctors are overworked. They get paid by volume. Fee-for-service payment systems and reduced fees per patient mean less time per patient. In this system, patients do not always get the best care science has identified, because doctors either do not have time to distill important, evidence-based information; do not know about the latest research; or simply do not have enough time to deliver it. In previous chapters, I have described the consequent rising burnout rate of health professionals. Another consequence is medical error, such as prescribing or delivering the wrong dose of medicine or misreading a test result. The Institute of Medicine reports that preventable human errors in hospitals lead to the deaths of nearly one hundred thousand patients every year in the United States, making it nearly the third leading cause of death. Medical error kills more people than highway accidents, breast cancer, or AIDS. Overload is partly the cause of this.

Managed care increasingly dominates our health care system. Attempts to contain the escalating cost of health care puts treatment decisions into the hands of insurance administrators or government regulators rather than doctors and patients. Both patients and their doctors are frustrated that therapies they consider important or useful are not covered by insurance, or covered only minimally—even when there is sound scientific evidence for their use. This further restricts doctor-patient time together, as reimbursements depend on how many patients are seen and how many procedures are performed. When physicians have only fifteen minutes—or sometimes just five—to devote to a patient, conversations are rushed and patient-doctor relationships don't develop. Patients more often leave with a prescription for a drug rather than a recommendation for lifestyle change, let alone delving into the deeper dimensions of healing. This is not a good environment for prevention, the management of chronic illness, or optimal healing.

The hierarchy in health care puts patients last. The standard medical hierarchy goes like this: doctor, nurse, medical assistant, patient. When you enter the hospital or outpatient system, if you are like most patients, you are dis-eased, dis-robed, dis-empowered, and eventually dis-charged. Such a system prevents a collaborative partnership with your doctor and prevents your doctor from being your advocate within the system.

There is an increasing diversity of patients and practitioners. Patients come into the system from a variety of cultural backgrounds and with personal preferences and beliefs about their health. Too often, doctors and other health professionals are not prepared to provide care that is sensitive to their patients' culture, ethnicity, or belief differences. Witness what happened to Trevor because of this disconnect. In many cases, language may also be a barrier to communication. Even in the alternative medicine world, patients should be wary of "turf" battles among different alternative practitioner groups, each claiming, for example, that their approach—be it naturopathy, chiropractic, or acupuncture—is the best for everyone. No single approach works for everyone or even for the same condition in different people.

SYSTEMS WORKING TOWARD INTEGRATIVE HEALTH

That is the bad news. The good news is that health care systems around the world now implement more integrative health care and are seeking to build a more balanced approach to healing chronic illness. I invite you to seek out these practices, ask for them from your physician, health care system, government, and insurance provider, and bring them into your life. What patients like Trevor could not get twenty years ago is increasingly available today—if you look and ask for it. Integrative health care comes in a variety of forms and names.

In the previous chapter, I provided an overview of policy guidelines and health systems seeking to optimize a patient-centered medical home and other integrated or pay-for-value approaches to health care.

I gave several examples, such as the Nuka and Iora systems and the work from the Institute for Healthcare Improvement and Stanford evaluations of the top 5% of primary care in the United States. The Commonwealth Fund reports on such exemplars in integrated care on a regular basis. What most of these systems did not do, however, is integrate complementary and alternative medicine (CAM) approaches into their delivery. Thus, many of them are missing one of the three legs of fully integrative health care: conventional care, complementary care, and self-care. Let me give you a brief overview of groups that are integrating this second leg of integrative health—the Integrative Medicine and Health, traditional, and CAM efforts—around the world.

INTEGRATIVE MEDICINE AND HEALTH

The best global overview of the rise in complementary and alternative approaches to healing is being done by the WHO, whose office of Traditional & Complementary Medicine (T&CM) tracks and advances information, research, and access to non-Western (nonconventional) practices. The use of these practices by patients and physicians is extensive—ranging from between 30% to nearly 90% of the general public in some places. Countries such as Singapore, Japan, China, and Korea provide some or even full coverage of T&CM practices for their populations. Eighty percent of the 129 member countries in the WHO assessment provide acupuncture (originally an approach only in traditional Chinese medicine), including eighteen (14%) with insurance coverage. As of 2012, thirty-nine member countries (30%) had doctoral-level training programs in T&CM, and seventy-three (56%) had government-funded research institutes. The economic output per year in herbal and natural products alone is over $83 billion in China, $7.4 billion in Korea, and $14.8 billion in the United States.

Around the world, the reasons patients give for their use of T&CM are similar to the reasons many of my patients give for seeking complementary and alternative medicine: easier access, dissatisfaction with exclusively conventional care, and a desire for safer and more natural or whole person care. Cost savings were also cited, and there is some data to support this. Reports from WHO and the RAND Corporation (an independent international research group) show lower costs with equal outcomes with some types of T&CM for chronic pain. When integrated into primary care, practices that include T&CM report lower costs for hospitalization and drug use.

The WHO Strategy report and others have found that, as illustrated in Trevor's experience, the two systems of T&CM and conventional medicine often do not integrate with each other—in any country. Usually, T&CM and conventional hospitals and clinics operate separately. A review by RAND researcher Ian Coulter of over seventeen thousand studies on what is called "integrative medicine" around the world showed that only five studies explored full integration between the systems. This means that patients are, unfortunately, caught between these systems and therefore need to become their own integrators. This is challenging, given that the quality of training and products in CAM is often neither regulated nor oriented toward scientific evidence as much as conventional medicine. While some countries, such as Australia, Canada, and certain European countries, closely regulate the quality and use of natural substances such as herbs and supplements, many other countries do not. Supplement and herbal companies can market and sell such products with dubious or inadequate science. The WHO report notes the wide variety and quality of regulations on T&CM compared to conventional medicine worldwide.

While it is not the purpose of this chapter to give a comprehensive summary of global T&CM practices, special mention of a few regions may help readers understand better how to use these systems to achieve their own integrative health. More information is regularly posted on my website at DrWayneJonas.com.

The United States has made outstanding progress in developing integrative medicine in recent years, catalyzed by the NIH, the Office of Alternative Medicine (OAM, which I directed from 1995 to 1999), and then the National Center for Complementary and Integrative Health, which replaced the OAM. This effort facilitated the development of several academic health centers. For those who get their care at academic health centers in the United States, there is a growing group providing integrative medicine and health. The Academic Consortium for Integrative Medicine and Health is made up of over seventy academic health centers and teaching hospitals that provide integrative medicine. In the United States, these include schools such as Harvard, Stanford, Johns Hopkins, Duke, and others, such as the universities of Arizona, Minnesota, Maryland, and California. This effort was supported for several years by a group of private philanthropists, the Bravewell Collaborative. Bravewell, which has since closed, supported not only the academic development of integrative medicine, but also a research network, a movie, and a National Academy of Medicine summit in 2009 called *Integrative Medicine and the Health of the Public*. That summit called for adding the principles of integrative health into health care for more holistic care by incorporating nutrition, mind-body practices, the use of more natural substances, and other complementary treatments into mainstream medical care.

There are many other groups leading the integration of nonconventional medicine into the mainstream. These include the European Society of Integrative Medicine (ESIM) and the International Society for Complementary Medicine Research (ISCMR), which held their tenth and twelfth international congresses, respectively, in 2017. Having followed this field for over three decades, I am struck by how often the philosophies and approaches that begin in these groups get taken up (with or without the same labeling) by mainstream medicine. These groups represent the "stay tuned for what may become the future of prevention and healing." They are the canaries in the coal mine that, instead of alerting to danger in health care, alert to innovations in healing. Most of these organizations seek to better integrate what they do into conventional biomedical health care systems.

One of the pioneers and continued leaders in the area of integrative medical education is Dr. Andrew Weil. His University of Arizona Center for Integrative Medicine has medical education programs and fellowship training—led by Dr. Victoria Maizes—that has taught over 1,500 physicians in the foundations of integrative health, developing a cadre of young doctors with the knowledge and skills for healing.

Look up their graduates for a doctor near you. Dr. Weil is a best-selling author whose multiple books describe how you can incorporate integrative medicine in your life. His most recent title, *Mind Over Meds*, is a well-researched book full of practical suggestions for using lifestyle approaches and natural substances to treat many of the conditions, for which most doctors prescribe drugs. This is an especially timely topic as we try to tackle the epidemic of opioid drug overuse and its damaging effects.

Recently, a remarkable experiment in integrative health was launched at the University of California, Irvine (UCI). An entire health sciences college encompassing the schools of medicine, nursing, pharmacy, and public health was formed under the principles of integrative health. The college was launched through a joint partnership of UCI and Susan and Henry Samueli (who also fund the Samueli Integrative Health Programs that I run). The goal of this new college is to "educate the next generation of health science professionals to transcend current boundaries; foster clinical programs with an increased focus on lifestyle, prevention, wellness and optimal health; and promote discovery of an expanded set of tools and platforms that fosters a systems approach to health, inclusive of all forms of evidenced-based healing—conventional and complementary." This will indeed be a new way for health care professionals to learn how to balance curing and healing—and a way to attend to those factors that make healing work.

Other examples include the Cleveland Clinic, one of the top medical centers in the United States. It has started a program in what is called "functional medicine"—a term coined by Dr. Jeffrey Bland over thirty years ago. It seeks to integrate science-based nutritional and lifestyle modifications with mainstream science for delivery in health care. In his recent book *The Disease Delusion*, Dr. Bland describes how the merger of nutrition with genomic medicine is creating a paradigm shift in healing that uses whole systems science and the ancient concept of food as medicine. The Cleveland Clinic program, directed by Dr. Mark Hyman—author of multiple best-selling books on prevention and health promotion—plans to test this approach for its effectiveness in healing several major diseases. Cleveland Clinic also operates an

Institute for Integrative Health and Wellness that provides a team approach of CAM and mainstream practitioners. Physicians are gaining greater access to training in nutrition and lifestyle change. The Institute for Functional Medicine (IFM) now offers regular seminars and a certification in functional medicine for physicians. When I last visited the IFM training course, I noticed that they were no longer just preaching to the believers in alternative approaches to medicine. Most of the physicians attending the training were from mainstream organizations like the Veterans Health Administration, Kaiser Permanente, and Providence Health. They were looking for the kind of education in nutrition they did not get in medical school or residency.

The Mayo Clinic—also one of the top health care organizations in the world—has invested heavily in creating new models of healing with both its integrative medicine programs, run for years by Dr. Brent Bauer, and its new multistory Healthy Living Center and programs run by Michael Casey, Dr. Don Hensrud, and others. The Healthy Living Center has taken what we now know from research on health promotion and built a program for facilitating health in everyone, whether healthy or ill. It is this type of integration that is applying what we now know about prevention and the optimal treatment of chronic disease. The Mayo Clinic offers training and delivery to other hospitals and health care centers around the world that seek to adopt these approaches.

The final program to know about is the Center for Spirituality and Healing (CSH) at the University of Minnesota. CSH has been led for thirty years by Mary Jo Kreitzer, a PhD nurse who is a pioneer in the creation of visionary approaches to healing and well-being. Her Model of Well-being has influenced countless patients, professionals, companies, health systems, and policy makers in thinking more clearly about how healing works. It has had a profound influence on my thinking over the years. The course and educational tools from CSH are available to patients and professionals (for more information, see my website, DrWayneJonas.com).

Other organizations offer course in integrative health. While it used to be that many of these courses were taught by practitioners far outside the mainstream, they are now becoming mainstream—just part of good healthcare. I will mention just a few. The Academic Collaborative for Integrative Health (ACIH) is a membership organization for complementary schools, including naturopaths, chiropractors (who also have their own academic membership organization), massage therapists, acupuncturists, and midwives. ACIH represents and advocates for these professions. Recently, the Institute for Lifestyle Medicine, founded and led by Harvard Medical School's Dr. Edward Phillips, is bridging the gap between medical treatment and behavior. Dr. Phillips, along with Yale Professor Dr. David Katz and others, helped organize the American College of Lifestyle Medicine (ACLM), which provides education to licensed health care professionals on how to deliver exercise and nutritional prescriptions. For patients like Trevor, these and other organizations provide physicians with opportunities to acquire knowledge and skills allowing them to bridge conventional care and self-care. While the term *integrative health* is now being used by many organizations—including the NIH National Center for Complementary and Integrative Health—true integration is still rare. What you should look for from those claiming to deliver integrative health are practitioners and health care systems that integrate all three key areas for healing—conventional care, complementary medicine, and self-care. More information on these organizations is also available on my website.

For those who get their care in the U.S. military or Veterans Health Administration (VHA), a radical shift toward more holistic, integrative health is occurring. Admiral Mike Mullen, former Chairman of the Joint Chiefs of Staff, launched a program called Total Force Fitness. This framework incorporated all the elements from the dimensions of healing described in this book, but called it "fitness" rather than health. This included behavioral fitness, social and psychological fitness, and even spiritual fitness. The Total Force Fitness framework is now being implemented throughout the military under various names such as the Healthy Base Initiative and Operation LiveWell.

The last two U.S. Army Surgeons General, Lieutenant General Eric Schoomaker and Lieutenant General Patty Horoho, created signature programs in integrative health for pain and performance. The VHA is implementing a personalized health plan program that integrates veteran goals and clinical goals in a holistic manner. Led by Dr. Tracy Gaudet, former director of the Duke Integrative Health Center, and Dr. Ben Kligler, formerly of Beth Israel in New York, it seeks to transform the way the VHA treats patients, from one delivering cure-focused treatments to a system that enhances personalized self-care and healing for every veteran. NATO has also begun to explore use of integrative health in the military in Europe. A recent report by NATO summarized integrative health activities and recommendations in the military in that alliance.

Similar trends toward integrative heath are happening in Europe. While many European countries have long histories of traditional healing—including systems like spa healing, anthroposophical medicine, homeopathy, and herbal treatments—these practices became largely eclipsed with the rise of modern biomedicine early in the twentieth century. A major summary of the current state of complementary medicine was published in 2015 by the European Union (EU). This four-year study, called CAMbrella, described a diversity of CAM practices and regulations in the EU. One challenge in Europe that seems less prominent in many other countries (except perhaps in the United States and Australia) is a strong skeptics movement that challenges CAM, accusing it of being nonscientific. While there is indeed less science in CAM than in conventional care overall, science is challenged to provide certainty in any medical approach, CAM included. We need more and better science in health care all around.

India had a long history of well-developed traditional systems (and some newer CAM systems) before modern Western medicine arrived and quickly dominated national practice and resources. However, the government has recently invested in developing the science and standards for T&CM in India. These systems include Ayurveda, yoga, naturopathy, Unani, Siddha, and homeopathy. Most of these systems are thousands of years old, except for homeopathy, which was exported from Germany in the nineteenth century and then widely adopted around the world. The WHO reports 508 "colleges" in one or more of these systems in India with over 25,000 undergraduate and nearly 2,500 graduate students per year. There is tremendous experience in these systems. However, having visited, examined, and done research on these topics in India, I can say from personal experience that significant improvement in quality is needed before their approaches can be integrated with conventional medicine. Dual-trained physicians like Dr. Manu are still rare. For the time being, they largely remain separate from mainstream conventional medicine and do not provide an integrative health system.

Traditional Chinese medicine (TCM) was the major system in China until the modern era. During and after the Cultural Revolution, TCM was largely ignored and even suppressed. However, China has now made major investments in research and the integration of TCM and modern Western medicine. A 2017 report released by the Chinese government describes the tremendous growth of TCM and an integrated TCM/Western medicine industry in China. They report nearly four thousand TCM hospitals and forty thousand TCM clinics. This includes 446 integrated hospitals and 7,705 integrated clinics, where both TCM and Western medicine are practiced together. There are over twenty-five TCM medical schools and two hundred Western medical schools offering TCM training. They report 11.5% lower outpatient costs and 24% lower inpatient costs in these integrated practices versus conventional Western practices. Over 15% of health care dollars are spent on TCM in the country. The government sees TCM as having an important role in China's socioeconomic influence outside China. The report ends by saying that "The time has come for TCM to experience a renaissance." TCM does seem to be spreading into other countries. Over 183 countries outside China have TCM programs, and 103 countries formally regulate TCM practices, including 18 that pay for acupuncture in health insurance. Acupuncture has largely been accepted as being safe and effective for pain in most countries, including Europe and the United States. However, based on my experience in China, I can say that the quality of clinical TCM research needs improvement before full integration can occur in the West.

WORKING WITH YOUR SYSTEM AND DOCTOR

None of these systems is perfect, but each moves health care in the right direction. Having spent a lot of time in this space, I can say that these systems share a philosophy of healing and self-care, not just curing. As daunting as the list of forces against healing in modern health care sound, you can overcome many of those forces and create healing collaborations that work for you. Start by creating a healing collaboration with your doctor.

Recently, a patient in her late thirties came to me seeking a prescription refill. She was married, worked part-time, and was raising three teenaged boys. She came to see me because her regular doctor was on vacation and she wanted a refill of a muscle relaxant medication for chronic neck pain. She also wanted a prescription for a sleeping pill and an opioid pain medication.

I never automatically refill prescriptions without examining the patient. When I examined her, I found nothing physically wrong with her neck, so I asked her if she had ever had the pain evaluated. She answered, "I know what is causing the neck pain—it is stress." Every time her husband was redeployed to a new military assignment, she would have to sell the house, organize the whole family's move, find new schools for the boys and a new job for herself, and settle into a new community. All of this was giving her, quite literally, a "pain in the neck," she said.

The muscle relaxants gave her some relief, but the pain always flared up at times of major stress. She also commented on what she thought as an unrelated problem: she had to get up in the night to urinate—sometimes as many as six times. Her previous doctor was unable to find any physical reason for this and had prescribed a medication to inhibit her bladder contractions. I explained to her that the number-one cause of frequent urination, when there is no physical explanation, is stress, and that night is a common time for this to occur.

I explained to her that stress stimulates the sympathetic nervous system, which often responds by sending signals to the body that create an urgency to urinate. "All three of the problems you are describing—neck pain, frequent urination, and difficulty sleeping—might well have one cause," I said to her. "It looks like your nervous system is out of balance, with the sympathetic system getting overstimulated. If you could find ways to induce a relaxation response and balance your nervous system, all three of these symptoms might disappear."

She seemed interested, so we talked about some simple ways to induce a relaxation response, including the breathing and relaxation exercises I described in chapter 7 (see page 122) and summarize in the appendices (see page 260). Finally, though, she said with a sigh, "I just don't have the time to myself to do these things." She left with the prescriptions.

About a month later, she was back in my office. "I decided I'd like you to help me induce that relaxation response," she said. I was not sure what motivated her to change her mind, but I was pleased she was ready to take healing into her own hands. We talked about what she might do, and practiced some simple relaxation exercises in the office. To bring that experience more deeply into her life, she decided to take a yoga class three times a week. "I'll tell my family that this is time I need for my health—doctor's orders," she said. She was creating a healing environment for herself by using me as a health collaborator, not just as a pill dispenser. After two months of yoga three days a week, her neck pain, frequent urination, and sleep issues had all resolved.

Find the right doctor for you. If you too are looking for a new doctor who is more of a healing collaborator than a pill dispenser, treat it like a job interview—you want to hire the best health care professional for you and your family. Consider the two reasons to see a doctor: one is to find out if a problem is acute, serious, and needs immediate attention; the other is to find a partner who will help you manage chronic illness and the prevention of disease. There is no other reason to see a doctor.

Acute situations can be handled in either an emergency room, a walk-in clinic, or the same-day unit of a clinic or health plan. But for chronic care and prevention, look for either a primary care doctor, a nurse practitioner, or a physician's assistant (PA) who is licensed to do family medicine, internal medicine, gynecology, or (if you have children) pediatrics. Interview several candidates until you click with one. This is an important relationship, after all, and could become a lifetime—and life-saving—connection. Show candidates the HOPE assessment at the end of this chapter or on my website and see if they will engage with you in that process. Explore to what extent each candidate already asks patients about the healing dimensions. Your goal is to find someone who will develop a collaborative relationship with you for prevention and healing.

There are three key aspects to a good collaborative health relationship: caring, competence, and credibility. Look for this combination in anyone you entrust with your health. Don't be afraid to ask prospective doctors about their education, experience, and special skills. You can also ask about their views on holistic or integrative medicine. If a doctor tells you that all alternative methods are worthless, or that holistic medicine is a waste of time, this may not be the best person for you. However, no matter what a doctor's opinion of complementary and alternative medicine, if he or she is willing to seriously evaluate the medical research for you and not abandon caring for you, he or she can play a valuable role in the collaboration.

I also suggest finding a doctor who works with a team or has access to a network of other kinds of practitioners, including lifestyle experts, health coaches, nutritionists, behaviorists, and other conventional and alternative specialists. These collaborators may be in the community or in the doctor's own health care center or practice. A good indication is if a doctor routinely offers preventive services, integrative medical care, lifestyle and behavioral therapies, and complementary treatments. Ask about the breadth of the candidates' networks. How many practitioners do they regularly work with? Are all practitioners with whom they work licensed by the state? Do they follow up the care their patients receive from these practitioners and regularly collaborate with other providers to find the best combination of care? Do they make recommendations for self-care and provide evidence as part of the treatment decision process? These are all good signs.

As part of your search for a doctor, look at the team with whom he or she works. Prevention and care for chronic conditions require constant communication and teamwork to evaluate changes in your health and the services needed on an ongoing basis. When you visit the office, get a feel for the culture. Do people communicate with each other? Is there a caring, respectful atmosphere? Or do staff members bark commands at each other and appear frenetic, isolated, and disorganized? Those may have burnout and may burn you.

Look also at how the team members treat you. Do they appear competent? Do you trust them? Do you feel cared about and heard? Does a team member, for example, call you prior to or after an office visit to find out any concerns you have? Does the team include you in decision making? Do they prepare you for the best use of the doctor's—and your—time? And, importantly, are they honest with you about what you need—even if it might not be what you want? A colonoscopy is a good example. After the age of fifty, regular colonoscopies and comparable screening tools dramatically reduce the risk of fatal colon cancer, but most people hate to have them done. A good doctor will encourage and remind you to follow recommended prevention and screening guidelines, even if they are unpleasant.

LOOK FOR THE FIVE-P APPROACH

A doctor has five responsibilities in integrative medicine:

1. **Protect.** Your doctor should protect you from dangerous, disproven, or toxic practices.

2. **Permit.** Your doctor should permit practices that may work and have no harmful side effects—such as mind-body practices, acupuncture, or massage.

3. **Promote.** Your doctor should promote proven conventional practices—such as Pap smears, colonoscopies, and vaccinations—and proven alternative practices, such as acupuncture, massage, and yoga for chronic back pain, and exercise, mind-body practices, and nutritional changes for many conditions.

4. **Partner.** Your doctor should include you as a partner in the health care team and should be willing to research and discuss with you the evidence for all three of the integrative health arms—conventional, complementary, and self-care.

5. **Payment.** Paying for preventive care and health promotion is key to optimizing healing. Whether you have employer-provided health insurance or an individual policy, examine your policy or contact the provider to see what it covers. You can ask your employer to investigate health insurance policies that include complementary and integrative medicine, lifestyle medicine, and health coaching. They can purchase insurance supplements that cover these services. If your claim for alternative services is denied by the insurance company, you should either ask your employer's human resources department to pursue it or have your doctor write to the insurer. Often, contractors who specialize in health care coverage have better success than individuals in pursuing claims approval.

If you like your doctor, enhance the relationship. Have a discussion with him or her about becoming more involved in your health care. This might involve asking your doctor to do some research about the effectiveness of treatments that interest you. Ask your doctor to advise you about prevention and lifestyle changes, including nutrition, exercise, and stress management. Ask how to prevent or minimize the effects of chronic illness and learn about any screening tests you should have. Encourage your doctor to see you as a whole person. During your visits, talk about your family, your work, your interests and hobbies, and any areas in your life that are giving you problems, including your relationships with your spouse, children, or coworkers.

Realize that the doctor's time with you may be limited, so go into the meeting prepared and with an agenda for the visit. Before going into an appointment, think about how your lifestyle affects your health. If you are open to lifestyle changes, ask about available resources. (You could ask, for example, "Do you refer patients to health coaches, nutritionists, or acupuncturists?") Be forthcoming with your health goals. Proactively share what you are hoping to do and how you want to feel. Don't wait until the end to provide key information.

Lastly, make the most of your entire health care team in addition to your physician. If your practice has physician's assistants, nurses, or health coaches, they may be able to supplement the time you spend with your physician. Use their services.

A HOPE CONSULTATION

One of the fastest and most direct ways to engage your health care system in helping you access your own healing capacity is to ask your physician to do a HOPE consultation with you.

We know that both before and after a diagnosis, and between states of health and disease, there are specific health-promoting conditions and actions that can prevent, slow, or reverse chronic disease, strengthen overall health, and improve function, quality of life, and overall well-being. Suffering can be reduced with healing no matter what a person's illness or stage of life—provided those behaviors are meaningful to the person and tap into their inherent healing capacity. Those factors and how they connect to the patient personally are explored during a HOPE consultation and are captured in a HOPE note.

The HOPE consultation is done after a complete medical diagnosis and treatment is completed, including a SOAP note. During the HOPE consultation, the practitioner goes over the core domains of healing with the patient and seeks to reframe the orientation from one of disease treatment to one emphasizing self-healing integrated with medical care. After examining the medical diagnosis and learning about the history and the context in which the patient lives, the

HOPE consultation explores the factors that can enhance healing for the individual. These factors are not specific treatments for disease; rather, they focus on activities that complement those treatments to facilitate improvement in symptoms, function, quality of life, happiness, and well-being. Sometimes the disease also resolves during this process. You and your doctor can learn more about how to do a HOPE consultation in the appendix of this book and on my website, DrWayneJonas.com.

THE HOPE OF HEALING

From the minute we are born, we are subjected to the stresses and traumas of life—all of which steadily erode our bodily systems and structures. These onslaughts include fear, anxiety, pain, toxicity in the environment, the need to keep our bodies upright against the force of gravity, the energy it takes to fight off a cold. Even eating and breathing in oxygen causes our cells and tissues to break down.

When you are having a bad day and everything seems to be going wrong, do you sometimes feel that you are battling emotional and physical disintegration? It may be small comfort to know that there is a principle in physics, the second law of thermodynamics, which holds that everything in the universe moves toward entropy—a state of disorder and chaos. Forces of nature *are* constantly acting to dissipate us into the universe, to make us disappear.

But on most days, we do not disintegrate or fall apart—because we also have an inherent capacity to maintain order and repair damage caused by the stresses and traumas of life—to reverse the chaos of the universe and heal. However, when these repair and restoration mechanisms break down, we develop disease or lose our mental, emotional, and/or physical well-being. Of course, there are virulent diseases or traumatic injuries that will initially overwhelm even the most tuned-up repair systems. But by building up and maintaining your inherent healing capacity, you have a better chance of resistance, resilience, and recovery from the onslaughts of life.

I hope that the journey we have taken together through *How Healing Works* will help you find a path filled with courage and hope. You do not have to feel helpless or in despair when things fall apart. The more aware you become of your response to the forces that influence your life, the more you will realize that the conscious decisions you make every moment of every day can change your future for the better. You can influence all the dimensions of your life, surrounding and infusing yourself with the forces of healing.

You can be whole. You can be healed.

APPENDICES

The HOPE Consultation

This guide is designed to help you work with health professionals to enhance your own healing capacity. The purpose is to integrate the usual disease treatment, or pathogenic approach, with a health-promoting or salutogenic approach (Aaron Antonovsky, a professor of medical sociology, coined the term *salutogenesis* for this approach, to contrast it with *pathogenesis,* the process of disease).

Every day, often dozens of times a day, hundreds of thousands of physicians and health care professionals around the world write SOAP notes. This behavior is so automatic and engrained that they rarely even consider the implications—how it molds and directs their thinking about every patient they see. SOAP not only extends pathogenic thinking to what's done to the patient, it also creates a set of cultural expectations, frameworks, and behaviors to which all modern medicine conforms.

Healing requires a different type of assessment—an assessment of those behaviors and interactions that facilitate salutogenic thinking, and framework a set of expectations and action focused fostering our inherent healing capacity. A patient's clinical diagnosis may or may not be relevant to the ways in which healing happens. For example, the components of healing are often generic—meaning a process that facilitates healing for one disease also facilitates it for another disease. Therefore, the assessment and the plan in a SOAP note is usually not directly relevant to health promotion and healing. This is where a HOPE consultation comes in.

The HOPE consultation—the healing-oriented practice and environments visit—consists of a set of questions specifically geared to evaluate aspects of a person's life that facilitates or detracts from healing; that is, it seeks how to enhance the processes of recovery, repair, and the return to wholeness. The goal of the HOPE consultation and HOPE note is to identify those behaviors that stimulate or support healing processes. It involves evaluating a patient in four different dimensions. First is the *inner dimension*—the perceptions, expectations, and awareness held in the mind. Certain types of mental framing around a life can either facilitate and enhance healing, or impair and block it. The second, *interpersonal dimension,* focuses on social relationships and the culture in which we operate. Again, certain types of social connections and relationships, and the nature of those relationships, can either support healing or interfere with it. Third is the *behavioral dimension*—things we do every day to either support and nourish the body's healing capacity or interfere with it and cause further damage. Finally, there is the *external dimension*; that is, the physical environment in which we live. This includes home, work, school, errands, and recreation, including time in nature and exposure to nourishing or toxic elements around them.

The HOPE note provides a focused, intentional, and systematic way of documenting these healing dimensions, per whole systems science, during a patient visit, providing a tool for addressing each dimension and the elements of healing. The natural overlap of the dimensions enables the patient-practitioner conversation to flow. It complements the disease treatment framework provided by the SOAP. In chronic disease, it fills in dimensions often missed by the SOAP—the environmental, behavioral, social/emotional, and mental/spiritual determinants of health. The HOPE consultation can guide both doctor and patient to improve health and well-being—not simply the treatment of disease. As with any intervention, what happens depends upon the

THE OPTIMAL HEALING DIMENSIONS

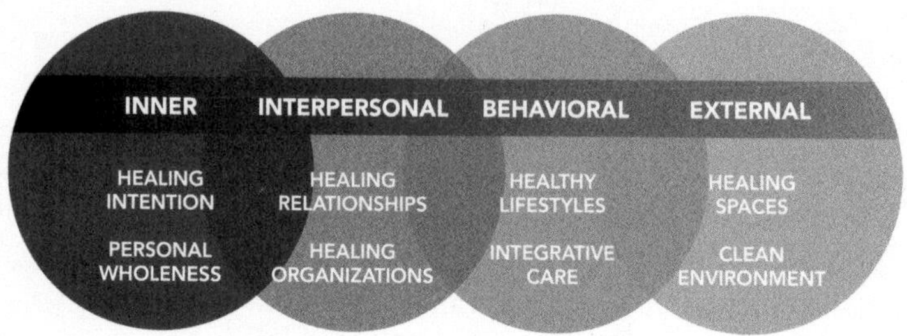

patient's disease and his or her state of health and wellness orientation and readiness. In most patients, the recommendations from a HOPE consultation have a positive impact. It may not cure the disease or improve it significantly, or it may cure the disease or provide major improvement in the illness. In chronic diseases, it can almost always enhance wellness and well-being and improve function, whether the disease is cured or not. However, fully 70% to 80% of what the patient needs from an encounter in the context of a chronic illness is illuminated by the HOPE consultation.

At DrWayneJonas.com, I provide patients and professions with a detailed guide for doing a HOPE consultation. What follows is only a summary of the HOPE elements to familiarize you with the approach. The HOPE consultations four dimensions are: inner, interpersonal, behavioral, and external.

INNER DIMENSION

The inner environment often holds the key to healing and well-being for the patient. This sometimes comes from a spiritual or religious life, or one grounded in meaning and purposeful activities. Often, it involves helping others. It can also be found in a creative pursuit or family activities—any endeavor that brings purpose and meaning beyond the individual. The goal of this part of HOPE is to explore the patient's most profound insight into themselves and see if and how this is connected to their illness, suffering, and healing.

INTERPERSONAL DIMENSION

The social environment is essential to health and healing. Both health and happiness are socially contagious. Social cohesion is not only health enhancing but also essential for sustainable behavioral change in any culture and in any setting. Questions in this part of the HOPE consultation seek to explore the extent of a patient's social connections and support, especially from family and friends.

BEHAVIORAL DIMENSION

Certain behaviors are linked to chronic illness and healing. This section of the HOPE consultation explores what the patient does to help herself or himself heal. Four primary areas are explored; others can be added, as guided by the patient.

Stress management: Research has demonstrated the benefits of achieving a deep relaxation capacity, a mind-body state known to counter the stress response and improve receptivity to personal insight and motivation for lifestyle change. These practices can also enhance health and strengthen personal resilience on their own. In the HOPE consultation, the practitioner explores what the patient does to relax and introduces options such as breathing, visualization, mindfulness and meditation, or biofeedback for regular use.

Physical activity: Physical activity can reduce stress, improve pain and brain function, slow aging and heart disease, and help a person reach and maintain an optimum weight. Fitness, along with proper rest and sleep, maintains functioning and productivity of the whole person throughout the lifespan and in any stage of health or illness. The patient is asked about his or her level of activity, and exercise and methods are offered to assist the patient in attaining an appropriate level of movement.

Sleep: Adequate quantity and quality of sleep improves most symptoms and can reduce stress, relieve pain, improve brain and immune function, slow aging, reduce incidence of heart disease and cancer, and help with achieving an optimum weight. Good sleep helps maintain functioning and productivity of the whole person throughout the lifespan and in any stage of health or illness. The patient is asked about the quantity, quality, and effectiveness of his or her sleep, and the practitioner offers methods to assist in attaining good sleep.

Optimum nutrition and substance use: Ideal weight and optimal physiological function are best supported through proper nutrition and reduced exposure to toxic substances—nicotine, alcohol, drugs, and environmental toxins—that impair function. Food and substance management requires motivation, environmental controls, food selection training, and family, peer, and community involvement. In the HOPE consultation, the patient is asked about use of these substances, about his or her normal diet, and any symptoms of gastrointestinal dysfunction, such as GERD, excessive gas, IBS, or constipation.

Complementary medical care: The patient is asked about his or her use of and/or interest in practices such as acupuncture, traditional or indigenous medicine, naturopathy, or chiropractic, and use of nutritional supplements and herbs. These practices—sometimes referred to as complementary and alternative medicine (CAM)—can facilitate healing if used appropriately or can harm if used inappropriately. They can be integrated with conventional medicine and self-care based on good evidence.

EXTERNAL DIMENSION

A healthy outer environment affects and supports a healthy person. This dimension attends to the physical structures and settings in which the patient lives and how these facilitate healing and minimize adverse impacts on and from the earth. The patient is asked what his or her home and work environment is like and if she has created a special place in which she feels relaxed and truly at home. Attention to architecture and art, time in nature, sound, smell, and light are key elements in producing such an environment. In addition, the HOPE consultation evaluates and attempts to minimize exposure to toxins that can impair healing and produce disease. I recommend a recent book by Dr. Joe Pizzorno, *The Toxin Solution,* to learn more.

Together, these healing-oriented practices and environments spell "HOPE," for individuals and for society.

SAMPLE QUESTIONS FOR A HOPE CONSULTATION

The following questions are used to guide the conversation between the patient and doctor during the HOPE consultation. Other questions can be added and personalized for each patient, personality, readiness, and circumstances.

Inner

- Why do you seek healing? What is your goal and intention?
- Rate your health (1–10) and what changes you expect can happen (1–10).
- Why are you here in life? What is your purpose? What are your most meaningful daily activities?

Interpersonal

- What are your social connections and relationships?
- How is your social support? Do you have family and friends you can discuss your life events and feelings with? Do you have people you have fun with?
- Tell me about yourself. Tell me about your major traumas in the past.
- What makes you feel happy?

Behavioral

- What do you do during the day? What is your lifestyle like?
- What do you do for stress management? How do you relax, reflect, and recreate?

- Do you smoke or drink alcohol or take drugs?
- How's your diet (describe your last breakfast, lunch, and dinner)?
- Do you exercise? If yes, what types and amounts?
- How is your sleep (quality and hours)? Do you wake refreshed?
- How much water, sugary drinks, and tea or coffee do you drink?
- What is your use of complementary and alternative medicine (CAM)—supplements, herbs, use of other CAM practitioners and healers?

External

- What is your home like? Your work environment?
- Is there a place at home where you can go and feel joyful and relaxed?
- What is your exposure to light, noise, clutter, music, colors, or art?
- What contact with nature do you have?
- What are your exposures to toxins, especially heavy metals or EDCs?

See the illustration on page 221 for the map I use to guide patients toward their own healing path.

THE HOPE NOTE

The answers to these questions form the basis for a HOPE note placed in the medical record. From this assessment, a plan for a meaningful response, to enhance what the patient is already doing to heal, is developed together. The goal of the plan is to match additional evidence-based healing methods to the patient's current activities. That match is summarized in a HOPE list for goal setting and tracking.

After the HOPE consultation, I ask my patients to send me their summary of the top three areas they would like to enhance in the first month and a single goal for that month—expressed in terms of actions or symptom improvement. Usually patients need further assistance in accomplishing their goals. Several tools are available to help with this, including:

- A workbook on healing. I give my patients a workbook called *Optimal Healing Environments: Your Healing Journey*, which is also available free from DrWayneJonas.com.
- Health coaching: If appropriate, I connect the patient with a health coach to help them navigate behavioral change, or further testing.
- Health promotion groups: Clinics offer health and well-being groups for general health as well as for specialized populations who need support with managing pain, diabetes, weight loss, cardiovascular problems, and cancer.
- Health analytics: If needed, there are options for science-based testing and artificial intelligence systems to explore specific factors that can increase the probability of health improvements.
- Graphics of the healing dimensions (see page 262) are sometimes provided to help patients visually navigate their many options for healing.

Constructing Your Healing Journey

The following guidelines may seem like simple, even obvious, steps, but they are powerful. Together, they hold the key to 80% of health and healing. As you go through these items, find ones you already enjoy, and then use the ideas and resources in this book to enhance their power. If you find you can incorporate the primary components from each of these dimensions of healing, you will markedly increase the probability of staying well if you are well, or recover if you are under treatment. Working with you doctor or primary care practitioner and a health coach can enhance the effect of these activities.

Many people have told me that they can implement these practices on their own, without professional assistance. The ability to heal is inside you. Making small changes in your day creates large changes over your life. Your hopes, relationships, activities, and places you live and work can spark these healing abilities. As you absorb the ideas described in this book and the summary suggestions in this appendix, note your thoughts, intentions, and expectations. Find the ones that inspire you to live a healthy, vibrant, joyful life with purpose and meaning.

GETTING STARTED

Change is best made in small, thoughtful ways. Start with just one area. As you start to make changes, you'll find that the positive effects will spill into other dimensions of your life.

The following four sets of statements will help you decide where you might want to start. I list the statements in pairs—one pair for each of the four dimensions of healing. Remember that while I have organized these into the four dimensions of HOPE, in reality they are interacting and overlapping dimensions, which is why it doesn't really matter where you start.

First, read the following two statements:

I feel calm and relaxed in my surroundings.

I have a space at work or home for reflection.

If you disagree with these statements, you may want to concentrate on your *physical environment.*

Now consider these two statements:

I avoid behaviors that I know are unhealthy.

I make time for things that bring me joy.

If you disagree with these statements, you may want to focus on the *behavioral dimension.*

Now consider these two statements:

My relationships with others leave me energized.

I feel supported and connected to my family and community.

If you disagree with these statements, you may want to focus on your *social/emotional needs.*

Finally, consider these two statements:

I am fully aware of my body's subtle signs and how they connect to my health.

When I think of my life, I feel hopeful and positive. I like my life.

If you disagree with these statements, you may want to focus on your *mind/spirit connection.*

It does not matter where you begin. Perhaps you want to start with the one you need the most. Or maybe you want to ease in and pick the one that is easiest for you.

Wherever you choose to start, a technique that may help is journaling. This practice can help you heal, grow, become more yourself, and thrive in the following ways:

- Journaling helps bring order to your deepest thoughts and fears.
- Journaling acts as free therapy. It helps you understand the person who knows you best: you.
- You can go back and read what you've written to see how much progress you've made.
- Some find joy in knowing their words help others, so they share their journals. But whether you share your work is up to you.
- Keeping a gratitude journal relieves stress. Exploring what you are thankful for is a powerful reminder of the good in your life.

There are many ways to journal. Grab a notebook, or just pencil your thoughts in the margins of this book. As you turn the pages, know that this is your personal journey to healing. Take it at your own pace. What matters most is that you start!

YOUR PHYSICAL ENVIRONMENT: SURROUNDING YOURSELF WITH BEAUTY AND SIMPLICITY

The places you live, work, play, and receive care affect your ability to find peace, rest, strength, and healing.

Have you ever been somewhere that just makes you feel good and at peace? These healing spaces minimize stress and add joy. They can bring your family and friends together and allow you to be at your best.

Your Home

Of all the places in your life, you probably have the most control over your home. Use this space to support your healing journey. When your home does not bring you joy and peace, you may feel uneasy, disjointed, out of control, unsafe, stressed, and disconnected from yourself and nature.

When you walk in the door after a stressful day at work or school or an appointment, a welcoming home can help return you to a place of peace. Your home's colors, tidiness or clutter, scents, and decor all affect you—continually.

Here are some tips to make your home a place of healing and peace:

- Surround yourself with nature, incorporating natural light, nature views or art, nature sounds, and flowers.
- Decorate with meaning, including photographs of family and friends, meaningful objects, symbols of faith or personal healing, and furniture arranged to encourage interaction.
- Simplify your life by uncluttering and creating quiet spaces for reflection.

Each change in your home is an opportunity to rethink what's in your life. Items that once brought you joy may now make you yearn for the past or evoke feelings of anxiety or anger. Recognize those items and consider replacing them with objects that make you feel good.

A Restful Bedroom

Keeping your bedroom simple, clutter-free, and clean, and ensuring it's dark at night are great ways to help improve your sleep. If streetlights or natural light make your room too bright, purchase inexpensive blackout shades or curtains. Use a clock with a red or blue light, not white or yellow; even better, use a clock that lights up only when you press a button. Surround yourself with comfortable bedding that feels good against your skin. (For more on sleep, see "Recharge at Night," page 280.)

- Color matters. Choose colors to suit your mood. Warm reds, oranges, and yellows energize and stimulate, while cool blue, green, and violet evoke feelings of peace and restfulness.
- Experiment with scents. The sense of smell has a powerful connection to the brain. What you smell can stimulate feelings of well-being, improve your mood, relieve stress, and clear your

mind. What makes you breathe more deeply when you enter a room?

Talk to your care provider about using aromatherapy. Note: If someone in your home is pregnant or has asthma or a chronic lung disease, your doctor may want you to avoid certain essential oils.

- Muffle sounds. Most people now live in loud urban environments. Sounds can be stressful (noise pollution) or soothing. Experiment with playing music to set a mood or to block out noises like street traffic. Carpets, curtains, and soft fabrics absorb sound; hard surfaces amplify them. White noise and simple soft earplugs also help to reduce the decibels.
- Light your day and night. Warm, natural light is soothing, while fluorescent or overhead lighting can be harsh. To create a feeling of warmth and intimacy, try lower, warmer lights. Put ceiling fixtures on a dimmer, especially over a dining table. Wall sconces and side lamps can help. Indirect light is more soothing than direct. Windows and skylights bring in natural light.

On the Road

If you feel like you live in your car or in hotels, make those spaces positive places. Small changes, like keeping the inside of your car trash-free, might make a traffic jam less stressful. Music can sooth and carry you with the traffic rather than against it. Here are a few more ideas for making car rides more pleasant:

- Consider adding an air freshener or car diffuser. Scents of lavender or vanilla relax; orange or eucalyptus scents energize.
- Turn car time into a time of learning or rejuvenation. Books on tape! Podcasts! But don't email or text while driving!
- Take a few minutes to repeat a positive or motivating thought to focus attention and interrupt the stress response.

At the Hospital or Other Care Facility

It's important to make the most of your interactions with the medical care space. This includes taking steps to reduce your anxiety during appointments. When you need to be hospitalized, ask for a single room and a room with a natural view; this has been shown to speed recovery.

Connect with Nature

The restorative quality of nature has been well documented. Take time out to watch a sunset or find a green space to eat lunch in during your day. Working in a community garden or simply enjoying it can help you connect to the earth. If gardening is not an option for you, try walking in a local park or green space. Walk on earth with your bare feet if you are in a safe and sanitary place to do so.

Whether you live in the city, the country, or somewhere in between, be aware of the life around you. You can do this through enjoying artwork that depicts scenes of nature, getting to know local flora and fauna, viewing of green and sky through a window or an online video of waves crashing along the shore.

Track how changes in nature affect your mood, your body, and your energy level. If you find yourself becoming depressed or sad during rainy weekends, try to see the beauty in the raindrops, or reserve an activity you love for rainy days. Or if it's not too cold, go outside and enjoy the feel of the rain.

Set an Environment Self-Care Goal

Wherever you spend your time, make sure that the spaces around you don't add unnecessary stress to your days and nights. Focus on the spaces in which you spend the most time first and then move on to improve the others.

What is one improvement that you can make at home, work, or school today?

HEALTHY BEHAVIOR

Living a healthy life is one of the key things you can do to stay or become well. How you eat, move, relax, and connect to others—all of these play major roles in healing your body, mind, and spirit. The choices you make today matter. And today's choices determine the choices available to you tomorrow.

How to Change

The problem lies not in knowing what you should be doing, but rather in making these changes habitual and meaningful to you. Link the behavior to the meaning and joy in your life. This will prepare you emotionally and mentally to sustain the behavior in the long run.

Before you consider which behaviors are right for you to change now, read the following list on how change happens. These are ten effective ways to make any healthy behavior change stick:

1. **Develop a plan.** Pick one or two small changes that feel manageable and that give you pleasure: two yoga postures, switching from white to whole grain bread, starting tango lessons, going on a picnic, or joining a book club or a volunteer group.

2. **Pick something you can do.** Choose a small, realistic, attainable change. Do that first. Don't pick something you just think you should do. If needed, break it into small parts and do part of it first.

3. **Tell somebody.** Have them ask you about it monthly.

4. **Find a group.** Look for or create social situations that encourage healing behaviors: a walking club, a healthy cooking class, a family or friend to monitor you.

5. **Plan for a slip.** Times when you are not doing the behavior or even intentional slips are important for long-term change. Build in occasional times when you do not do the new behavior.

6. **Know the real reason for making the change.** The most effective reasons for sustained behavior change are intrinsic (I want to feel better) rather than extrinsic (I want to be liked).

7. **It may be hard.** Prepare to be uncomfortable for a while. Change is not easy. Your plan should include how to deal with that.

8. **Be ready.** Sometimes the time is not right to make a change. Maybe today is not the day to start. If so, admit that and take more time to prepare.

9. **Start.** Are you a chronic procrastinator (about 20% of people are) or just procrastinating on this one behavior? If chronic, seek help to deal with that first.

10. **Ask your doctor.** Discuss lifestyle and prevention behaviors with your medical team and ask about any helpful resources your health care services offer—such as behaviorists, health coaches, nutritionists, fitness trainers, or rehabilitation specialists.

EATING, DRINKING, AND COOKING

The rituals of cooking and sharing meals and the effects of eating wholesome food in healthful quantities are profoundly important to prevention, recovery, wellness, and well-being.

Why We Eat

Food is loaded with meaning and emotion. Food is family, tradition, and comfort; sometimes we even use food to self-medicate. When we use food and/or alcohol to fill an emotional void or to quiet or dull negative emotions, this may lead to overeating or unhealthy choices. Some of us overeat or consume alcohol out of stress, anger, depression, anxiety, frustration, or loneliness. Know why you eat, and make eating to fill physical hunger or to enjoy taste—not to dispel sadness or treat pain.

Build a Positive Relationship with Food

As with other relationships in your life, it's important that your relationship with food be a healthy one. This involves some key shifts in thoughts and behaviors:

- Accept that the food rules or family traditions of your past may no longer be needed or helpful for you. For example, give yourself the okay to no longer need to finish everything on your plate.
- Understand that you are a unique person with your own needs and challenges. Learn to trust your hunger and listen to your sense of fullness.
- What you see in magazines, over the internet, and on TV is not always true. If you struggle with a healthy body image, it may help to limit your exposure to unhealthy body images in the media.
- Mind-set matters when it comes to food. Remember the mind over milkshake experiment. Be positive, even in how you talk about food. Thinking of your food as either a diet or bad adds judgment. Changing your language can help. Instead of seeing sweets as bad, see them as a treat.

Eat Mindfully

Too often we eat food without even a thought. It's easy to eat what's in front of you without paying attention to whether you are hungry or when you become full.

Keep these tips in mind:

- Eat slowly. Most meals are consumed in an average of seven to eleven minutes. Fast eating can lead to overeating. The body doesn't have time to cue your brain that you are full. If you struggle with eating speed, try to focus more on enjoying the meal rather than just slowing down.
- Eating includes all the senses—taste, touch, smell, sound, and sight. Paying attention to the multisensory experience of eating is called "eating mindfully." Eating mindfully requires learning your sense of fullness. Be alert to your body's subtle clues rather than waiting for a bellyache. If something is so delicious that

you want to keep eating, try saying, "I can have more later if I'm full. I don't have to eat it now."

- Use a smaller plate. Most people will eat everything on the plate in front of them. Research shows that people automatically cut down on how much they eat if they simply use a smaller plate.

Remember that Food is Your Fuel

Instead of depriving yourself, focus on adding good whole foods. And because vegetables and fruits contain mostly water, eating more of them will increase your hydration levels.

Consider the following when focusing on food:

- Keep a food journal, either on your phone or on paper, to track what you eat throughout the day. We are often not aware of what and how much we eat. Some mobile apps help with this and offer motivation to choose a healthier diet.
- Foods with sugar, high-fructose corn syrup, artificial sweeteners, and unhealthy fats have been linked to heart disease, cancer, and diabetes. High-fiber diets can lessen some of these effects.
- Eating too much and not exercising are the usual causes of obesity, but they are not the only ones. Especially in times of stress, the problem may be not eating enough or not eating the right foods. Some people react to certain foods, like gluten or milk protein. Ask your integrative physician how to determine if there are certain foods you should avoid.
- Your health care provider or a dietitian may be able to help you design a healthy eating plan and set realistic weight goals to keep you healthy.

Drink Water, Always

Water affects weight loss, muscle fatigue, skin health (including fewer wrinkles), kidney and bowel function, and more. Carrying a (refillable) bottle of water with you everywhere you go may help you remember to drink more often. Also, try to drink a glass of water instead of another type of beverage with every snack and meal. Flavored sweet drinks contribute little to better health. Fruit juice should be diluted by at least half.

Recognize Your Patterns and Hurdles

Are you so hungry that you grab a snack on your way home before mealtime? Eat a piece of fruit, a bag of healthy (unbuttered) popcorn, or a handful of (roasted, unsalted) nuts on the way home so you aren't ravenous when you walk in the door.

Are you too tired to make the healthy meal you'd planned, so you find yourself ordering pizza? Try having more easy meals like sandwiches or soup. Make a week's worth of healthy meals and freeze them in small packets to pull out and defrost.

Meal Planning and Mealtimes

Meal planning can be good for your budget, your stress level, and your waistline. Have ingredients on hand for easy pantry or freezer meals if you don't have time to buy fresh ingredients. Know where you can stop for a healthier takeout option if an appointment or workday runs long. Try these meal-planning tips:

- Aim to shop only once a week. Fewer trips to the grocery store and drive-through can save time. Running into the store to pick up an item can lead to overbuying and more stress.
- Eat before you shop for food. If you go to the grocery store hungry, you are likely to buy more than you would if you were full.
- Keep healthy food on hand. It is easier to eat healthy when your pantry, fridge, freezer, and cabinets are well stocked with healthy food. Get rid of what you don't want around.
- Involve your children so they will be more likely to eat healthy and help with meal prep. If they can see the meal plan, it will

cut down on the questions of "What's for dinner?" or "What can I eat?"

- Don't start the plan with all new foods. Begin with a two-week rotation of your favorite recipes. Occasionally add a new recipe.
- Make sure your plan is realistic. If you're accustomed to relying on takeout meals, plan for the occasional takeout.
- Meals planned, prepared, and shared together at home tend to be healthier and more balanced than meals eaten at restaurants or on the go. Meals eaten out are often fried or highly salted. Plus, soda and other sweetened beverages are consumed more often when eating out.
- Meals bring families together. When you can, making time for a family dinner is good for the mind, body, and spirit. Family meals help foster family bonds, feelings of belonging, security, and love. This is especially important during times of change. Eating together builds a sense of tradition that can last a lifetime. A study showed that health promoting genes are turned on before people even eat if they prepare the food together.

Move More

Motion is a lotion. Exercise can help both your body and your mind work more smoothly.

It's important to get least thirty minutes of exercise a day. Ask your doctor to suggest ways to move more. Learn how much exercise is right for you, especially if you are trying to lose weight or have certain physical conditions like heart disease or asthma. Research now shows that it is more important to simply move more often during the day than to do thirty straight minutes of exercise and then sit for the rest of the day.

Look at movement as something to include throughout your day. Your doctor or a physical therapist may give you a list of exercises and stretches you can do whenever you have a few minutes. Can you do leg lifts or ankle circles while waiting or at your desk? I got rid of my sitting desk at the office and now have only a standing and treadmill desk. I do walking meetings whenever possible. Might you park farther from the store to get a few more steps in? Use the stairs instead of the elevator. These activities add up.

Walking provides many of the same health benefits as running and can be done more often with loved ones.

Recharge at Night

Sleep impacts many areas of life—your overall health, pain level, memory, weight control, and even your mood and outlook. Sleep problems can be caused by a host of issues, including light or noise intruding on your bedroom; a mind run amok; breathing problems; medications; pain; depression; stress; substances such as alcohol, caffeine, and nicotine; heart and lung diseases; and even simple inactivity. That's why it's important to talk to your care provider about any issues you are experiencing. Your provider may also help you optimize the hours of sleep that you do get.

Consider these common tips for better sleep:

- Establish a winding-down routine with quiet, soothing activities in the hour before bedtime.
- Go to bed and wake up at the same time each day—even on weekends.
- Maintain a dark, electronics-free bedroom.
- Avoid caffeine, nicotine, alcohol, and sugar for several hours before bed.
- Exercise during the morning or early afternoon.

When these tips aren't enough, it may be time to reach out for professional help.

Make Time for Joy

Even in the most difficult situations, choosing to feel grateful can help you cope. Focusing on gratitude prevents helplessness and hopelessness from taking over.

Instead of worrying about what you can't control, use your mental energy to find moments of joy in ways you can, like these:

- Dream new dreams. You may have had to put past dreams aside, but that doesn't mean you can't come up with new ones. Focus on new goals and dreams that you can work toward.
- Tap into a creative outlet to release emotions and experience the joy of art. Try music, crafting, sewing, drawing, journaling, scrapbooking, birding, or photography.
- Look forward to the future. Maintaining a sense of hopefulness is critical. Finding meaning and purpose in life can lead to happiness. Have something to look forward to. Plan.
- Keep inspiration on hand to help you get through the rough patches. Phone a friend, visit a place of worship, or carry uplifting quotes or readings in your wallet or purse. Inspirational music is literally at everyone's fingertips now with their phone.
- Say yes to things that make you happy. Stay connected with people who recharge your battery and make you feel good.
- Laugh and play. Try a game night at home, play fetch with your pet, do a crossword puzzle, or listen to a comedian on TV. Laughter, humor, and play can reduce stress, boost your energy, and help you connect with others.
- Don't compare your life to others'. Allow your life to be uniquely yours.

Decrease Anxiety

You may not be able to control the stressors in your life, but you can learn skills that will prevent the stressors from controlling you. Be aware of your breathing. Shallow, upper chest breathing is a sign of stress. Taking thirty seconds to do a deep breathing exercise will trigger your body's natural relaxation response. Remember, people who saw stress as strengthening them improved much more than those who saw the same stress as hurting them. Stress, when well handled, can help in healing. Mind-set matters.

Nourish Your Spiritual Self

Focus on love and forgiveness—and start with yourself. If you don't love and forgive yourself, it's hard to inspire, motivate, and encourage others.

Meditation techniques, such as loving-kindness meditation, can help address anger and emotional pain. This practice is used to address feelings such as shame, guilt, fear, chronic pain, a lack of support, and difficulties with other people.

Breathe

Breathing techniques and mobile apps can teach you to use your breath to self-calm. The breath triggers changes in the body's nervous system that help you better manage stress. Deep breathing techniques help reduce feelings of anxiety and stress by blunting the expression of genes turned on during stress and lowers blood pressure.

Put one hand on your chest and another on your stomach. As you inhale and exhale, your abdomen should rise and fall. This is called "belly breathing." If your belly is not involved, your breathing may be too shallow. You can benefit greatly from learning and practicing belly breathing.

Deal with Unhealthy Behaviors

Let's face it, we all do things that we know are not healthy. In fact, allowing ourselves occasional unhealthy behaviors—when we build them into life intentionally—can help us maintain healthy behaviors most of the other times. They are that spot of yang in the yin and vice versa. But it is important that these behaviors don't become your main habits. Once they do, they are hard to break and sometimes require professional help.

Social groups can help—your community center, church, and online support groups. The important thing is to develop awareness of your behaviors and seek help. If you are a very private person, hesitant to share personal issues, that first step you take to seek help is the most difficult. Having someone you trust join with you will make it easier. A group of two is still a community.

Use your healthy relationships to find support to manage unhealthy behaviors before they become a habit. Break bad habits so they do not become addictions. Or turn them into positive addictions. Find healthy habits to fill the void left when ending the bad habits.

Dealing with medical care systems is also a learned behavior. Here are some principles to allow you to keep those encounters focused on healing.

Focus on Prevention

Without proper care, a cough can become pneumonia, a strain can become a fracture, and a muscle pull can become a tear. Early detection of many cancers and heart disease can prevent progression, complications, and death. Maintaining your health care is important to prevent chronic problems and keep you at the top of your game in body, mind, and spirit.

Access Integrative Health Care

Integrative medicine includes the best of conventional medicine, such as procedures and medications, and the best of nonconventional medicine, such as mind-body practices, acupuncture, massage, chiropractic care, energy medicine (like Reiki or healing touch), and supplements.

Integrative health balances this medical and illness treatment with self-care and health creation—fully integrating preventative care and lifestyle with the treatment of disease, illness, and injury. While there are many models for delivering integrative health care, here are a few key clues you can look for in a primary care practice to determine if you are receiving integrative health care:

1. **Team-based:** Integrative health care is best delivered by a team of providers, which can include your physician, physician's assistants, and nurses, as well as other health care professionals with expertise in behavioral change, such as counseling, health coaching, nutrition, massage, acupuncture, or energy medicine.

2. **Transparent:** The team makes available all your health records and test results so that you can track your progress and be an informed part of the decision making about your health and well-being.

3. **Aware:** The team is knowledgeable about you and aware of your health, well-being, and life goals so that they can best support you in your healing journey.

4. **Accessible:** Members of the team are available by phone, text, or email when you have a question or need clarification, so you can stay on track toward your health goals.

Make the Most of an Appointment

Depending on where you are on your healing journey, you may spend considerable time in the hospital or doctor's office. Making the most of health care appointments can help improve care and lessen stress. Consider the following:

- Prepare for the visit: Recognize that it's okay to talk about embarrassing or upsetting symptoms. Write down what needs to be covered during the appointment to ensure you don't forget something important. Bring a list of medications and their use to the appointment.

- During the visit: Advocate for yourself when needed. Clearly express what you need from the doctor. It can be helpful to use a tape recorder for important consults to prevent confusion. Many smartphones have a record function. Taking notes can also help you remember what was said. If you end up confused, ask for a follow-up consult.

- After the visit: Check in with a loved one. How do you think the appointment went? What do you wish had gone differently? Are you missing any important information?

- See chapter 10: Creating Healing (pages 252–259) for an in-depth review of how to work with your doctor and the health care system.

FOCUS ON THE SOCIAL-EMOTIONAL DIMENSION

People are social beings. Relationships provide a sense of belonging, care, and support. Positive relationships can also be good for your health. Love and support reduce stress, boost your immune system, improve quality of life, and prevent feeling lonely or depressed. And they prolong life.

Positive relationships refuel you, especially when your tank is low. These are healing relationships; they are characterized by trust, honesty, compassion, and safety.

By using this checklist, you can decide which relationships are healing and which can be improved. For each relationship, ask yourself if the following statements are true:

- Trust: I feel emotionally and physically safe. I don't have to guard against being hurt.

- Honesty: Both the other person and I can reveal true feelings without harm to either of us.

- Compassion: Both the other person and I have the ability and willingness to understand one another and express kindness.

- Safety: Both the other person and I feel safe with each other—physically and emotionally.

If a relationship leaves you running on fumes, consider options to protect yourself and change the relationship. It is possible to learn skills that improve the relationship's quality and boost its ability to heal. If not, get out of the relationship.

Communicating Is Key

Honest and open communication is key to the healing relationships you are working to build. It can be important to voice feelings or fears that seem unthinkable. When they go unspoken, they can lead to angry outbursts, withdrawal, resentment, and guilt trips that drive a wedge into the relationship.

Most communication has little to do with what you say. Your stance, posture, breathing, and even your muscle tightness all relay a message—as do the tone, speed, and volume of your voice.

Here are some tips for speaking your mind mindfully:

- Relax and breathe.
- Go into difficult conversations with a goal. Example goals include the following: Be honest and direct; express feelings and thoughts; find common ground; create harmony.
- Ask if it's a good time to talk, so you begin the conversation on the right foot.
- Treat the individual with dignity, respect, and courtesy.

Focus on active listening. When you listen, focus on both verbal and nonverbal messages. Here are some tips for active listening:

- Maintain appropriate eye contact for your culture.
- Paraphrase and repeat to confirm that you understand what the other person is saying. Don't jump to conclusions.
- Ask questions to clarify.

- Try not to think about what you are going to say next; it's more important to be attentive, even if it means there is a pause before you talk. Pause and take a breath before you talk.
- Affirm the other person's comments and offer encouragement by nodding, saying yes, or using phrases such as "Tell me more" or "I understand."
- Listen for disclaimers and qualifiers (maybe, but, mostly, usually, probably), as they are typically followed by new information.
- Avoid distractions, such as TV, pets, or other people, so you don't have to compete for attention.
- The more you can encourage the other person to talk, especially in high-stress situations, the more you can understand what they are trying to share with you.

Focus on "I" communication. "I" messages (rather than "you" messages) are the foundation of positive communication. "You" messages may make the other person feel uncomfortable and attacked. They may make the person stop listening, withdraw, or fight back—none of which resolve the question or concern. "I" messages achieve the following:

- Help you take ownership of your own thoughts and feelings.
- Make you explore what you think and feel.
- Increase your chances of being heard.
- Help keep conversations positive.

For example:

"I feel overwhelmed and need help with the chores." (I message) versus "You never help around the house."

Set Goals for Success

Each family or individual defines success differently. Paying attention to goals and celebrating achievements may be helpful on your journey. It is powerful to say, "We hit the goal we were reaching for!" Goals may be small or incremental, but they lead to feelings of pride and motivation for the next step. The recovery process is a careful balance of accepting reality and working toward change.

Some symptoms, conditions, and circumstances lessen with time and treatment. But for others, learning to cope with what is there is a more helpful approach. When recovery isn't possible, shift your focus to discovery. You and your partner may discover steps, self-care strategies, and behaviors that reduce daily challenges and improve quality of life.

Your medical team—especially the behaviorist—may provide advice about what is practical to make sure your expectations are realistic.

Go Ahead and Vent

Venting your emotions is appropriate at times to release tension rather than bottling it up inside. However, there are some ways and places to vent that are more helpful than others. See if any of these work for you:

- Write. Get out a piece of paper and write for ten minutes without stopping. You can even pretend that you are talking with another person or another part of yourself. See what that person has to say, in your own words.

- Talk. When venting to a person, be sure to do so with someone you trust and with whom you are on good terms. Choose someone who is supportive and helpful rather than enabling negative emotions. Tell the person that you just need to vent first, and ask if it is okay.

- Exercise. Physical activity can release chemicals in the brain that relieve stress and tension. Consider yoga, qigong, and tai chi as well as other personal self-care practices.

- Breathe. Since it's impossible to be stressed and relaxed at the same time, use breathing techniques to calm down.

Set Boundaries

Part of maintaining healthy relationships involves setting boundaries—an important part of self-care. A boundary controls how much access others have to your heart, time, and energies. It is a protective fence you build around yourself that allows you to monitor the impact others have on you.

Leaving yourself too open can leave you bruised and battered by the comments, moods, and opinions of others. But staying too closed can leave you isolated and locked inside yourself. Finding the right balance takes time. Set boundaries in your own time frame, and only when you are ready. Counselors can help you with protecting your heart, freeing yourself from the need to please others, and saying no when appropriate.

Learning to establish healthy boundaries can help you in all your relationships, whether with your family, friends, neighbors, or coworkers.

Create Healing Groups and Get Involved

You are part of many groups that influence your life: school, workplace, church, community organizations. Being involved in healthy groups with healing qualities supports your health and well-being. These types of healing groups allow you to participate in making decisions that affect you. They promote open and honest communication, create a climate of trust and personal responsibility, and inspire a sense of belonging. They are fun!

Are you actively involved in an organization? Getting involved is critical if you want the organization to develop a healing culture. Opportunities such as PTA, clubs, committees, and volunteer activities are ways to inspire change. As a part of these groups, set a good example for others. Build healing relationships with your coworkers. This can provide you with opportunities to practice your own self-care and to share with others ways to support greater personal well-being—in family, school, and work environments and in other social situations.

Foster a Culture of Healing

Groups that foster a culture of healing have the following in common:

- Respect for individuals, including their inner lives
- A system of values that is present at all levels
- Honest and open communication
- A climate of trust
- A focus on learning rather than blame
- Opportunities for self-care, like exercise and yoga

Do the groups that you belong to help you to heal or impede you?

Lead or Follow

Ask yourself: Am I a good leader? Am I a good follower? Good leaders and good followers walk their talk. They work on improving their communication skills, they treat others as they would like to be treated, and they are good team players. Examine your role in the groups that you are a part of and explore shifting them toward a healing culture. The best way to do this is to lead by example.

Set a Social/Emotional Dimension Self-Care Goal

Part of any relationship includes dealing with the moods and feelings of others. Self-care is important because it can be easier to deal with the emotions of others when you are taking good care of yourself. Once you are in a strong and healthy place, you will be better able to cocreate a healthy relationship.

What is one thing you can do to improve a relationship in your life today?

YOUR MIND-SPIRIT CONNECTIONS

Who you are at the deepest level includes the thoughts, feelings, and wishes that come from your mind. It also includes your spiritual life and having a sense of meaning or purpose.

The healing that arises from an experience of personal wholeness happens only when the mind, body, and spirit are in balance. A weakness or imbalance in one of these can negatively affect the others. For example, severe emotional stress can cause high blood pressure and other illnesses in an otherwise healthy body. Likewise, a physical illness or injury can cause depression in a usually healthy mind.

Two elements are key to your healing journey:

- Developing an intention and expectation for healing
- Feeling the wholeness that comes from mind, body, and spirit practices

Develop Healing Intention

Healing intention is a conscious choice to improve your health or the health of another. It includes belief in improved well-being and the hope that a goal can be reached. Belief and hope set the stage for healing to occur. As we saw from the research on placebo, belief itself is a powerful healer.

If you don't truly believe that you can be healed, or if some part of you is holding onto the disease or condition, you might disrupt or limit your own healing on a subconscious level. Don't underestimate yourself! By developing healing intention, you set the stage for healing to occur.

Developing healing intention includes awareness, intention, and reflection.

Build Your Self-Awareness

Awareness addresses the question: "How do I feel?" It helps you learn what your body is telling you and to connect to what you think about to who you are.

You can become aware of your body's subtle signals, such as changes in energy level or mood. Bring these feelings to your conscious mind. This allows you to change behaviors that don't contribute to your health and learn new skills to change your automatic responses. Physical symptoms are often messages from your body telling you how it is doing and what it needs.

Some turn to active practices like walking, yoga, or repeating a centering word. Others use religious prayer, rituals, and services. You can also just take a few moments to be quiet or to meditate.

This awareness of how the mind, body, and spirit work together gives you the information you need to guide you on a healing path.

Once you know how you feel, it's essential to know what you want. For those whose lives have diverged from what they had planned, this can be a challenge. But it's key to rebuild this knowledge so you can create new goals and plans that may be different, but are also meaningful and fulfilling.

On a spiritual level, once you connect with your inner self, you can direct your intention to bring this sense of peace and healing in your life.

Take Time to Reflect

The story you tell yourself about your life is powerful. It creates a mind-set that impacts your physical response to any stimulus or situation. This self-story can be a way to help you grasp the themes of your life and find meaning in them. When your sense of meaning in life is altered, it can lead to feelings of distress. Regaining that sense of purpose—even in suffering, or despite suffering—is vital for health and well-being.

Meaning and purpose help you deal with loss and grief, create hope and dispel despair, and find joy and stop sadness. They allow you to accept a new normal, find a sense of well-being within it, and control your outlook.

Journaling, creative writing, art therapy, and peer mentoring may be helpful as you reflect on questions of who you are and what role your illness has played in your life. Also important to your self-story are the questions: What is my purpose? How do I fit into my family, my community, my life? What are my values or spiritual beliefs?

For many, spirituality, faith, and religion are central parts of who they are. They can influence how you cope with trauma, fear, or loss. They may help you find happiness and meaning within rather than from external influences such as wealth, belongings, work, fame, or fancy food, which may leave you feeling empty, lost, and alone.

Experience Personal Wholeness

Personal wholeness is the feeling of well-being that occurs when your body, mind, and spirit are aligned and moving in harmony and balance.

Think about a time when you felt most authentic, most whole, most complete and happy. Perhaps you were doing something that you felt was important and meaningful. It could include reaching a major milestone or completing a difficult task. It could also be something from daily life, like cooking a tasty meal or teaching a child to ride a bike. When the experience of complete wholeness arises, a healing presence or unity occurs.

Activities that connect your physical body with your nonphysical mind and spirit help to integrate your biological responses with your psychological responses. From these practices, you can experience a sense of wholeness that enhances recovery and resilience.

Add a Mind-Body Practice to Your Toolbox

The same mind-body practices that help you develop a sense of self can counteract stress and its harmful effects. The most important thing to know about mind-body practices is that there is no single right way. These practices go through cycles of popularity. However, all have the same intended effect of breaking the train of everyday thoughts and inducing deep relaxation. What doesn't work for someone else may work for you.

Consider these factors when picking a mind-body practice:

- Physical energy: Do you enjoy being physically active? If yes, consider a moving meditation like tai chi, qigong, yoga, walking, and running, or an active meditation like art therapy or journaling. If no, consider breathing techniques, meditation, or mindfulness-based stress reduction, loving-kindness meditation, or progressive muscle relaxation.
- Self-based or practitioner-based: Practices such as acupuncture, chiropractic or osteopathic manipulation, massage, and other bodywork require making time to see an outside practitioner. For some, that time out can be relaxing, while others may find it stressful. Some practices require nothing more than your attention and a few seconds (breathing, mantra repetition). And there are various others that, once learned, can be practiced on your own, such as acupressure, Reiki, yoga, or tai chi.
- Time: Consider what fits into your schedule. Do you have thirty seconds? Five minutes? An hour? There is a mind-body practice for every time frame.
- Belief and conviction: Choose a practice and terminology that fits into your belief system. Whether it's making time for prayer, meditation, or quiet reflection, you are practicing self-care. It is not important to be convinced that the practice will work for you. However, it is important to stay open and to do it. Approach it in a spirit of experimentation. Check it out.

Schedule this time regularly. Just knowing that you have time set aside just for you can be helpful.

Think Positive

Positive thinking is a mind-set that turns anxiety into opportunity. It builds healthy self-esteem and self-value. Remember the experiments of Stanford Professor Crum showing that how one framed stress—either as resilience building or draining—produced the dominant effect that stress had on a person. These skills can keep you from doubting yourself during the ups and downs of life:

- Start each day with the intent to learn something new.
- Give yourself permission to be wrong.
- Start with "thanks" or a gratitude practice.

Self-talk is the stream of thoughts running through your head from the moment you wake up until you fall asleep. If your thoughts are mostly negative, it's more difficult to cope with stressful situations.

Instead of expecting the worst outcome of any situation, focus on the best. When you deal with life's difficulties in a positive and productive way, you'll reap health benefits including a longer life span, greater resistance to illness, and better mental and physical well-being.

Live in the Moment

Notice how much of your day you spend thinking about the past or the future. Thoughts of the past can keep you from being present and making the most of this day—distracting you from the present joy.

Many people think of mindfulness as being in a calm, Zen state. And it can be. But more realistically, it's about being present to your best self. Mindfulness means being aware of what your mind is up to in each moment but not getting caught up in or controlled by your thoughts. It can help to remind yourself: "My thoughts do not control me."

Trust Your Inner Guidance

How often do you ignore what your gut is telling you? You may think, "I should call a friend for support," but decide not to because it's late. Or you may think, "I wish I could reschedule those plans," but attend to them anyway and regret it later.

Over time, as you become mindful of your thoughts and feelings, you will begin to trust your inner guidance. You may notice that when you follow your instinct, you feel better. On the other hand, when you fall back into old patterns of holding back and doing what you think you should, you feel worse.

PAUSE AND TAKE A STEP BACK

Now that you've seen how the four dimensions of your life can affect your self-healing abilities, pause and take a step back. See where your journey began and where it has taken you.

You have seen that self-care means:

- Surrounding yourself with healing spaces (physical environment)
- Making healthy life choices (behavioral dimension)
- Maintaining strong social connections (social/emotional needs)
- Building a strong sense of identity (mind/spirit-connection)

I hope this book has inspired you to begin your healing journey. Perhaps you've already taken your first steps. When you've had time to make some progress, I invite you to return to consider these questions and observations, and reflect on how far you've come and what you've learned. If you have kept a journal, go back and read your first few entries. Have you learned anything about yourself or others along the way?

Note how a change in one area of your life impacts other areas. If you resolved conflicts with others, how did that make you feel about yourself? If you started taking walks, how did it affect your sleep or stress levels or pain?

You might have noticed that some of the changes you made affected those around you in a positive way. By looking deeply into your life and relationships with others, you can work toward peace and healing. That peace and healing will spread to those around you.

Amplify your healing by sharing your experiences with others along the path of life. As I learned from my first patient as a student chaplain before medical school—a 74-year-old man dying of lung cancer—the healer and healee share one goal and one mutually beneficial process. The healing process benefits both and all others with whom they are connected. And that, on the greater human scale, is how healing works.

Additional Reading on Integrative Health

The Cochrane Collaboration: cochrane.org
A respected international online resource for evidence about health care practices. They have an integrative medicine (CAM) section.

The National Institutes of Health (NIH) National Center for Complementary and Integrative Health: nccih.nih.gov
A good source for information on complementary and integrative practices.

Natural Medicines: naturalmedicines.therapeuticresearch.com
A good source of information on natural products—their effectiveness, safety, and quality.

Choosing Wisely: choosingwisely.org/
A good source of information on what you and your doctor should *not* be doing and what does not work.

NOTES

INTRODUCTION

The concepts and data in this book have been drawn from hundreds of readings and references—mostly from the peer-reviewed medical literature. However, because of space limitations, I have selected key references for readers, choosing to include those that illustrate the main points made in each chapter, support some of the lesser-known facts, or provide readers with information and concepts that meaningfully supplement the text. For readers interested in more references on specific topics such as placebo, optimal healing environments, evidence-based medicine, whole systems science, complementary and integrative medicine, the HOPE note, or healing in general, please go to my website: DrWayneJonas.com.

CHAPTER 1: THE PARADOX OF HEALING

One of the most striking observations about healing practices is their tremendous diversity of models, beliefs, practices, and traditions around the world, from spiritual healing to herbal treatments, physical manipulation, surgery, and drugs. Theories of disease are equally diverse, ranging from spirits to consciousness to energy to chemicals. Despite this diversity, all claim to work, and observational studies often support those claims. For further reading about this, I suggest a classic in medical anthropology by Arthur Kleinman and a clear comparative review of different healing systems by Stanley Krippner. These can be found at:

Kleinman, Arthur. *Patients and Healers in the Context of Culture.* Berkeley: University of California Press, 1980.

Krippner, S. "Common Aspects of Traditional Healing Systems Across Cultures," in *Essentials of Complementary and Alternative Medicine.* Jonas, W. B. and J. S. Levin (eds.). Philadelphia: Lippincott Williams & Wilkins, 1999.

I was startled by Norma's response to the placebo. However, this is common in patients—and research studies. Some useful information sources mentioned in this chapter are the following:

Many treatments that have produced 60% to 80% improvement when delivered under normal practice conditions are found later to work no better than placebo when studied in randomized controlled studies. For a good summary, see Roberts, A. H., D. G. Kewman, L. Mercier, and M. Hovell (1993)."The power of nonspecific effects in healing: Implications for psychosocial and biological treatments." *Clinical Psychology Review* 13(5): 375–391.

At the time I was treating Bill, the best data showed that acupuncture was no more effective than placebo acupuncture. That was true until Andrew Vickers and colleagues from Sloan Kettering collected individual data from all the top studies in the world and pooled this data for analysis. This proved that the effects from acupuncture were not all due to placebo—something still not known by most physicians. See Vickers, A. J., A. M. Cronin, A. C. Maschino, et al. (2012). "Acupuncture for chronic pain: Individual patient data meta-analysis." *Archives of Internal Medicine* 172(19): 1444–1453; and, Vickers, A. J. and K. Linde (2014). "Acupuncture for chronic pain." *Journal of the American Medical Association* 311(9): 955–956.

It is hard for people to imagine that most of the effects from surgery might be due to factors other than the surgery, so studies are rarely done to test those other factors. In chronic pain, data shows that 87% of the effect of surgery is coming from factors other than the surgery itself. For summaries of surgery studies and why it heals see Beecher, H. K. (1961). "Surgery as placebo. A quantitative study of bias." *Journal of the American Medical Association* 176: 1102–1107; and, Johnson, A. G. (1994). "Surgery as a placebo." *The Lancet* 344(8930): 1140–1142; and, Jonas, W. B., C. Crawford, L. Colloca, T. J. Kaptchuk, B. Moseley, F. G. Miller, L. Kriston, K. Linde, and K. Meissner (2015). "To what extent are surgery and invasive procedures effective beyond a placebo response: A systematic review with meta-analysis of randomized, sham controlled trials." BMJ Open: e009655. doi:10.1136/bmjopen-2015-009655; Jonas, W. B., C. C. Crawford, K. Meissner, and L. Colloca. "The Wound that Heals: Placebo, Pain and Surgery," *Placebo and Pain*. L. Colloca, M. A. Flaten, and K. Meissner (eds.). Boston: Elsevier, 2013; 227–233.

People with brain injury like Sergeant Martin get better during hyperbaric oxygen treatments, but not from the oxygen. See Miller, R., L. K. Weaver, N. Bahraini, et al. (2015). "Effects of hyperbaric oxygen on symptoms and quality of life among service members with persistent post-concussion symptoms: A randomized clinical trial." *Journal of the American Medical Association Internal Medicine* 175(1): 43–52; and, Hoge, C. W. and W. B. Jonas, (2015). "The Ritual of Hyperbaric Oxygen and Lessons for the Treatment of Persistent Post-concussion Symptoms in Military Personnel." *Journal of the American Medical Association Internal Medicine* 175(1): 53–54; and, Crawford, C., L. Teo, E. M. Yang, C. Isbister, and K. Berry (2016). "Is Hyperbaric Oxygen Therapy Effective for Traumatic Brain Injury? A Rapid Evidence Assessment of the Literature and Recommendations for the Field." *Journal of Head Trauma Rehabilitation* (Open Access) doi:10.1097/HTR.0000000000000256.

CHAPTER 2: HOW WE HEAL

Over the last twenty to thirty years, researchers and practitioners have been repeatedly surprised at how large the improvement is in groups who are not getting an active treatment. Research on this effect—often called the "placebo effect" or "placebo response"—has grown tremendously. The best source of information on this sleeping giant in medicine is the database that is supported and maintained by the Society for Interdisciplinary Placebo Studies (SIPS). You can access this database (updated monthly) at: jips.online/.

A nice single summary of key research findings on the placebo response and its implications for healing can be found in the special journal issue: Meissner, K., N. Niko Kohls, and C. Luana (June 27, 2011). "Introduction to placebo effects in medicine: mechanisms and clinical implications." *Philosophical Transactions of the Royal Society of London Biological Sciences* 366(1572): 1783–1789.

Other selected references readers may find of interest mentioned in this chapter include (in the order they are described):

Jonas, W. B., C. P. Rapoza, and W. F. Blair (1996). "The effect of niacinamide on osteoarthritis: A pilot study." *Inflammation Research* 45(7): 330–334.

Franklin, B., Majault, L. Roy, Sallin, J. S. Bailly, D'Arcet, de Bory, J. I. Guillotin, and A. Lavoisier (2002). "Report of the commissioners charged by the king with the examination of animal magnetism." *International Journal of Clinical and Experimental Hypnosis* 50(4): 332–363. A summary of Franklin's investigation of Mesmerism—using blinded methods.

Beecher, H. K. (1955). "The powerful placebo." *Journal of the American Medical Association* 159(17): 1602–1606. Posited that placebo accounts for about one-third of all outcomes.

Moerman, D. E. (2000). "Cultural Variations in the Placebo Effect: Ulcers, Anxiety, and Blood Pressure." *Medical Anthropology Quarterly* 14(1): 51–72. Showed that placebo responses varied from 0% to 100% for the same treatment depending on the context, and not one-third, as Beecher claimed.

Kaptchuk, T. J., et. al. (2008). "Components of placebo effect: a randomized controlled trial in patients with irritable bowel syndrome." *The British Medical Journal* 336(7651): 999–1003. Elegant study showing how the ritual delivers much of the placebo response.

Kaptchuk, T. J., E. Friedlander, J. M. Kelley, M. N. Sanchez, E. Kokkotou, J. P. Singer, M. Kowalczykowski, F. G. Miller, I. Kirsch, and A. J. Lembo (2010). "Placebos without deception: a randomized controlled trial in irritable bowel syndrome." *PLoS One* 5(12): e15591. One of the first studies to show that telling people they were getting placebos did not significantly reduce their response.

Carvalho, C., J. M. Caetano, L. Cunha, P. Rebouta, T. J. Kaptchuk, and I. Kirsch (2016). "Open-label placebo treatment in chronic low back pain: a randomized controlled trial." *Pain* 157(12): 2766. Confirmation of the above and showing clinically significant improvement for a major public health problem (back pain) from the placebo response—even when patients knew they were taking placebo.

For information about how placebo works in the brain, see the following three articles: Benedetti, F., H. S. Mayberg, T. D. Wager, C. S. Stohler, and J. K. Zubieta (2005). "Neurobiological mechanisms of the placebo effect." *Journal of Neuroscience* 25(45): 10390–10402; and, Amanzio, M., et al. (2001). "Response variability to analgesics: a role for non-specific activation of endogenous opioids." *Pain* 90(3): 205–215; and, Wager, T. D. and L. Y. Atlas (2015). "The neuroscience of placebo effects: connecting context, learning and health." *National Review of Neuroscience* 16(7): 403–418. I also highly recommend the book by Professor Fabrizio Benedetti of the University of Turin, Italy, who is one of the world's most renowned researchers on placebo. See Benedetti, Fabrizio. *Placebo Effects.* London: Oxford University Press, 2014.

It is not the placebo (the fake pill or treatment) that produces healing; it is the meaning that the ritual of treatment produces. See Moerman, D. E. and W. B. Jonas (March 19, 2002). "Deconstructing the placebo effect and finding the meaning response." *Annals of Internal Medicine* 136(6): 471–476; and Jonas, W. B. (June 27, 2011). "Reframing placebo in research and practice." *Philosophical Transactions of the Royal Society of London Biological Sciences.* 366(1572): 1896–1904.

There are now good sources for evidence summaries comparing treatments. These sources include the Cochrane Collaboration database, which can be found at cochrane.org. While Cochrane is an important site for finding evidence summaries from randomized controlled studies, they rarely do comparative reviews across treatments. Some good sources for comparative evidence reviews across treatments like the ones I did for Bill are *BMJ Clinical Evidence Updates* at clinicalevidence.bmj.com/x/set/static/cms/citations-updates.html; and *The Agency for Healthcare Research and Quality EPC Evidence-Based Reports* at www.ahrq.gov/research/findings/evidence-based-reports/index.html. Make sure your doctor has consulted one or more of these sources before he or she prescribes a treatment.

Personal engagement with the deeper aspect of yourself (especially social and emotional traumas) is profoundly healing. See, for example: Pennebaker, J. W. *Opening Up: The Healing Power of Expressing Emotions.* New York: Guildford Press, 1997; and, Smyth, J. M., A. A. Stone, A. Hurewitz, and A. Kaell (1999). "Effects of writing about stressful experiences on symptom reduction in patients with asthma or rheumatoid arthritis: a randomized trial." *Journal of the American Medical Association* 281(14): 1304–1309.

Nondrug approaches to healing are gradually gaining evidence and mainstream emphasis, especially for pain. See, for example: Qaseem, A., T. J. Wilt, R. M. McLean, and M. A. Forciea (2017). "Noninvasive Treatments for Acute, Subacute, and Chronic Low Back Pain: A Clinical Practice Guideline from the American College of Physicians." *Annals of Internal Medicine* 166(7): 514–530; and, Jonas, W. B., E. Schoomaker, K. Berry, and C. Buckenmaier III (2016). "A Time for Massage." *Pain Medicine* 17(8): 1389–1390. doi:10.1093/pm/pnw086. Published online May 9, 2016; and, Crawford, C., C. Lee, C. Buckenmaier, E. Schoomaker, R. Petri, W. B. Jonas, and the Active Self-Care Therapies for Pain (PACT) Working Group (April 2014). "The Current State of the Science for Active Self-Care Complementary and Integrative Medicine Therapies in the Management of Chronic Pain Symptoms: Lessons Learned, Directions for the Future." *Pain Medicine* 15: S104–S113. doi:10.1111/pme.12406.

CHAPTER 3: HOW SCIENCE MISSES HEALING

There is an ongoing debate in biomedical research about the role of what is called "reductionist" science, using approaches such as randomized, placebo-controlled trials (RCTs) as the primary type of evidence needed before accepting, using, and paying for treatments in practice. The importance of RCTs is clear, but their limitations are becoming more evident. Medical science is seeking better ways to collect evidence. For a good overall framing of the debate, see Federoff, H. J. and L. O. Gostin (2009). "Evolving from Reductionism to Holism: Is There a Future for Systems Medicine?" *Journal of Internal Medicine* 302(9): 994–996. See also notes for chapter 4 on systems science.

Other selected citations readers may find of interest mentioned in this chapter include the following (in the order they are described):

Ayurveda is one of the oldest systems of healing in the world. The following chapter gives an excellent overview by one of the world's leading practitioners. Lad, V. D. "Ayurvedic Medicine," in Jonas, W. B. and J. S. Levin (eds.) *Essentials of Complementary and Alternative Medicine.* Philadelphia: Lippincott Williams & Wilkins, 1999; also see Chopra, A. and V. V. Doiphode (2002). "Ayurvedic medicine. Core concepts, therapeutic principles, and current relevance." *Medical Clinics of North America* 86(1):75–89. Recent research at University of California, San Diego, and Chopra Center hints at the mechanisms that might explain Aadi's recovery. See Mills, P. J., et al. (2016). "The Self-Directed Biological Transformation Initiative and Well-Being." *The Journal of Alternative and Complementary Medicine* 22(8): 627–634.

Information on the global use of complementary, traditional, and integrative practices comes from the World Health Organization's Office of Traditional Medicine at who.int/medicines/areas/traditional/en. The WHO defines traditional medicine as "the sum total of the knowledge, skills, and practices based on the theories, beliefs, and experiences indigenous to different cultures, whether explicable or not, used in the maintenance of health as well as in the prevention, diagnosis, improvement, or treatment of physical and mental illness."

Cousins, Norman. *Anatomy of an Illness as Perceived by the Patient: Reflections on Healing and Regeneration.* New York: W. W. Norton & Co., 1979. One of the most clear and touching descriptions of how one man constructed his own healing journey.

The three-armed study led by Professor Jonathan Davidson of Duke, which showed that an herb, a proven drug, and placebo all worked the same for depression, can be found in Hypericum Depression Trial Study Group (2002). "Effect of hypericum perforatum (St. John's Wort) in major depressive disorder: A randomized controlled trial." *Journal of Internal Medicine* 287(14): 1807–1814. My commentary on how both professionals and the public missed the key issue for healing that this study revealed can be found in: Jonas, W. B. (2002). "St. John's Wort and depression." *Journal of Internal Medicine* 288: 446.

Little known to most people, replicability of scientific findings is a major problem in biology, psychology, and medicine. Most findings cannot be independently replicated. For a discussion and data on this issue see the following: Ioannidis, J. P. A. (2005). "Why most published research findings are false." *PLoS Med* 2(8): e124; and, Ioannidis, J. P. (2017). "Acknowledging and Overcoming Non-reproducibility in Basic and Preclinical Research." *Journal of Internal Medicine* 317(10): 1019–1020; and, Wallach, J. D., P. G. Sullivan, J. F. Trepanowski, K. L. Sainani, E. W. Steyerberg, and J. P. Ioannidis (2017). "Evaluation of Evidence of Statistical Support and Corroboration of Subgroup Claims in Randomized Clinical Trials." *Journal of Internal Medicine* 177(4): 554–560; and, Prasad, V., A. Cifu, and J. P. A. Ioannidis (2012). "Reversals of Established Medical Practices: Evidence to Abandon Ship." *Journal of Internal Medicine* 307(1): 37–38. Several groups are trying to address this issue. See a summary of those efforts in Yong, E. (August 27, 2015). "How Reliable are Psychology Studies?" *The Atlantic*.

Partly because of the above, the overuse of unproven treatments and treatments proven not to work is large—likely one-third of everything done in medicine. To remedy this, guidelines for stopping treatments that are often used but known to harm or not help can be found at choosingwisely.org/about-us. I suggest reviewing any treatments you are doing with your doctor using this site to see what you can stop doing.

For a nice summary of the decline effect and problems with scientific validity see Lehrer, J. (December 13, 2010). "The truth wears off: Is there something wrong with the scientific method?" *The New Yorker*. For even more detail on why this happens, see the book by Richard Harris, science reporter for PBS, called *Rigor Mortis: How Sloppy Science Creates Worthless Cures, Crushes Hope, and Wastes Billions*. New York: Basic Books, 2017.

The information for the statin graphic in this chapter comes from Redberg, R. F. and M. H. Katz (2016). "Statins for Primary Prevention: The Debate Is Intense, but the Data Are Weak." *Journal of Internal Medicine* 316(19): 1979–1981.

Evidence-based medicine is not as accurate as most people think. Pulitzer Prize–winning author Siddhartha Mukherjee eloquently describes the uncertainty of science and the challenge of using science for making decisions in medicine. See Mukherjee, Siddhartha. *The Laws of Medicine: Field Notes from an Uncertain Science*. New York: Simon and Schuster, 2015.

CHAPTER 4: A SCIENCE FOR HEALING

There is a need to build better science and information models to address the limitations of the reductionist approach described in chapter 3. In the 1960s, this was called the "biopsychosocial" model of medicine and became the foundation for the specialty of family medicine—the specialty I practice. More recently, what I call "whole systems science" is being fed by large-scale efforts for using "big data" sets drawn from daily health care delivery and linking this data with the basic biomarkers of disease and health—at cellular, chemical, and genetic levels—and then linking that to people's activities, experiences, and long-term health outcomes. It is a big task. The largest ongoing scientific effort in this is the one-million person study by the National Institutes of Health called the Precision Medicine Initiative. See allofus.nih.gov/. For summaries of whole systems and complexity science in primary care, complementary medicine, and implementation science, see the following three references:

On primary care: Sturmberg, J. P., C. M. Martin, and D. A. Katerndahl (2014). "Systems and Complexity Thinking in the General Practice Literature: An Integrative, Historical Narrative Review." *Annals of Family Medicine* 66–74.

On complementary medicine: Verhoef, M., M. Koithan, I. R. Bell, J. Ives, and W. B. Jonas (2012). "Whole Complementary and Alternative Medical Systems and Complexity: Creating

Collaborative Relationships." *Forschende Komplementärmedizin* 19(Suppl 1): 3–6. This entire issue is about the application of whole systems science to complementary medicine.

On health care delivery: Leykum, L. K., H. J. Lanham, J. A. Pugh, M. Parchman, R. A. Anderson, B. F. Crabtree, P. A. Nutting, W. L. Miller, K. C. Stange, and R. R. McDanie (2014). "Manifestations and implications of uncertainty for improving healthcare systems: an analysis of observational and interventional studies grounded in complexity science." *Implementation Science* 9(165): 2–13.

Other selected references of interest include (in the order topics are addressed):

Price, D. D. (2015). "Unconscious and conscious mediation of analgesia and hyperalgesia." *Proceedings of the National Academy of Sciences of the United States of America* 112(25): 7624–7625. What your doctor believes influences your healing response.

Frank, Jerome and Julia Frank. *Persuasion & Healing.* Baltimore: Johns Hopkins University Press, 1961. A classic on the influence of healers on those seeking treatment.

Walach, H. and Jonas W. B. (2004). "Placebo research: The evidence base for harnessing self-healing capacities." *The Journal of Alternative and Complementary Medicine* 10(Suppl 1): S103–S112. Outlines a roadmap for healing by examining placebo research.

de Craen, A. J., D. E. Moerman, S. H. Heisterkamp, G. N. Tytgat, J. G. Tijssen, and J. Kleijnen (1999). "Placebo effect in the treatment of duodenal ulcer." *British Journal of Clinical Pharmacology* 48(6): 853–860. Outcomes vary for the same treatment depending on where the treatment is delivered (home or hospital), the number of pills (two or four per day), and the color of the pills.

Ader, R. and N. Cohen (1975). "Behaviorally conditioned immunosuppression." *Psychosomatic Medicine* 37(4): 333–340. Professor Ader's breakthrough work showed that animals could learn how to alter their own immune system and live longer. This has also now been shown in humans.

The idea that small doses of toxins (or any stimulant) can induce healing is extensively documented in science but not widely known or applied in medicine. The best source of information on this is the International Dose-Response Society led by Edward Calabrese and colleagues at the University of Massachusetts, Amherst. See the peer-reviewed journal *Dose-Response* at dose-response.org for access to this extensive scientific field. Professor Calabrese's database is an encyclopedic source of scientific information showing how toxic substances from oxygen to stressful behaviors such as fasting and exercise can induce protective and reparative responses that lead to healing. See the three articles below for summaries on general mechanisms and how this works in exercise and fasting.

On the biological mechanisms: Calabrese, E. J. (2013). "Hormetic mechanisms." *Critical Reviews in Toxicology* 43(7): 580–606.

On exercise: Ji, L. L., J. R. Dickman, C. Kang, and R. Koenig (2010). "Exercise-induced hormesis may help healthy aging." *Dose-Response* 8: 73–79.

On fasting: Mattson, M. P. and R. Wan (2005). "Beneficial effects of intermittent fasting and caloric restriction on the cardiovascular and cerebrovascular systems." *The Journal of Nutritional Biochemistry* 16(3): 129–137.

Since most of us are overstimulated psychologically, removal of that stimulation through relaxation allows healing on the clinical, physiological, and genetic levels: See the classic work by Benson, Herbert and Miriam Z. Klipper. *The Relaxation Response*. New York: HarperCollins, 1992. Also see Dusek, J. A., H. H. Otu, A. L. Wohlhueter, M. Bhasin, L. F. Zerbini, M. G. Joseph, H. Benson, and T. A. Libermann (2008). "Genomic counter-stress changes induced by the relaxation response." *PloS One* 3(7): e2576; and, Bhasin, M. K.,

J. A. Dusek, B. H. Chang, M. G. Joseph, J. W. Denninger, G. L. Fricchione, H. Benson, and T. A. Libermann (2013). "Relaxation response induces temporal transcriptome changes in energy metabolism, insulin secretion and inflammatory pathways." *PLoS One* 8(5): e62817.

CHAPTER 5: COMING HOME

Detecting disease early is a double-edged sword. The benefits of early detection depend primarily on whether there is a safe and effective treatment for the diseases found. This is nowhere more evident than in cancer, where new technologies are finding the disease earlier and earlier. While it is usually good to catch cancer early, what if our body would have normally taken care of an early cancer on its own? Then treatment might do more harm than good. Even as Susan went through one of the harshest treatments for breast cancer there is—three types of chemotherapy, major surgery, antihormonal therapy—the debate heated up about overtreatment and harm from the type of treatments she was getting. See the following opinion and two studies about this ongoing debate:

Narod, S. A., J. Iqbal, and V. Giannakeas (2015). "Breast cancer mortality after a diagnosis of ductal carcinoma in situ." *Journal of the American Medical Association Oncology* 1(7): 888–896. See also Winer, E. (May 17, 2017). "Breast Cancer: When is Less Treatment Better?" Dana-Farber Cancer Institute, blog.dana-farber.org/insight/2016/10/eric-winer-less-breast-cancer-treatment. And see also Welch, H. G., P. C. Prorok, A. J. O'Malley, and B. S. Kramer (2016). "Breast-Cancer Tumor Size, Overdiagnosis, and Mammography Screening Effectiveness." *New England Journal of Medicine* 375: 1438–1447. Also of concern for Susan was whether treatment might increase the spread of cancer. See Karagiannis, G. S., J. M. Pastoriza, Y. Wang, A. S. Harney, D. Entenberg, J. Pignatelli, V. P. Sharma, E. A. Xue, E. Cheng, T. M. D'Alfonso, J. G. Jones, J. Anampa, T. E. Rohan, J. A. Sparano, J. S. Condeelis, and M. H. Oktay (2017). "Neoadjuvant chemotherapy induces breast cancer metastasis through a TMEM-mediated mechanism." *Science Translational Medicine* 9(397).

Other selected references readers may find of interest mentioned in this chapter include (in the order topics are described):

Sternberg, Esther M. *Healing Spaces: The Science of Place and Well-being.* Cambridge, MA: Harvard University Press, 2009. Already a classic on how space affects our biology and health.

Ulrich, Roger (1984). "View through a window may influence recovery." *Science* 4647: 224–225. If you have to go into the hospital, make sure you can see natural views from the window.

Park, B. J., Y. Tsunetsugu, T. Kasetani, T. Kagawa, and Y. Miyazaki (2010). "The physiological effects of Shinrin-yoku (taking in the forest atmosphere or forest bathing): evidence from field experiments in 24 forests across Japan." *Environmental Health and Preventive Medicine* 15(1): 18. A traditional Japanese healing method now opening to the light of science.

Schweitzer, M., L. Gilpin, and S. Frampton (2004). "Healing spaces: elements of environmental design that make an impact on health." *The Journal of Alternative Complementary Medicine* 10(Suppl 1): S71–83.

Louv, Richard. *Last Child in the Woods: Saving Our Children from Nature-Deficit Disorder.* New York: Algonquin Books, 2008. Children need immersion in nature.

The model and components of an optimal healing environment (OHE) were developed by Samueli Institute over a decade and have been researched and described in several articles and books. Some of the main ones are the following:

Jonas, W. B. and R. A. Chez (2004). "Toward optimal healing environments in health care." *The Journal of Alternative Complementary Medicine* 10(Suppl 1): S1–S6. The entire issue is on OHE in various specialties.

Sakallaris, B. R., L. MacAllister, M. Voss, K. Smith, and W. B. Jonas (May 2015). "Optimal healing environments." *Global Advances in Health and Medicine* 4(3):40–45. doi:10.7453/gahmj.2015.043. An update on healing environments.

Christianson, J., M. Finch, B. Findlay, C. Goertz, and W. B. Jonas. *Reinventing the Patient Experience: Strategies for Hospital Leaders.* Chicago: Health Administration Press, 2007. Case studies of seven different hospitals and how they created optimal healing environments.

Kashman, Scott and Joan Odorizzi. *Transforming Healthcare: Healthy Team, Healthy Business.* Cape Coral, FL: Book in a Box. An in-depth study of how one hospital went from a "D" rating to "top of class" by following the optimal healing environment model.

CHAPTER 6: ACTING RIGHT

The importance of a healthy lifestyle is perhaps the most emphasized and familiar aspect of health and healing to readers. We are, in fact, bombarded with self-help books and advice saying don't smoke, don't stress, drink moderately, exercise daily, and eat healthier food. For ongoing information about the therapeutic aspects of lifestyle, follow the American College of Lifestyle Medicine, which tracks and summarizes this literature constantly at lifestylemedicine.org. I summarize the essence of this literature in this chapter and in the appendices. The main purpose of this chapter is to show that sustainable healthy behavior is more complicated than just knowing the facts. Behavior must be infused with meaning and the right mind-set to be optimally effective.

Selected references readers may find of interest mentioned in this chapter include (in the order topics are described):

Loprinzi, P. D., A. Branscum, J. Hanks, and E. Smit (2016). "Healthy Lifestyle Characteristics and Their Joint Association with Cardiovascular Disease Biomarkers in U.S. Adults." *Mayo Clinic Proceedings* 91(4): 432–442. Less than 3% of the population follows even the top four recommendations for a healthy lifestyle.

Mehta, N. and M. Myrskylä (2017). "The Population Health Benefits of a Healthy Lifestyle: Life Expectancy Increased and Onset of Disability Delayed." *Health Affairs* 36(8): 1495–1502. A nice summary of the key healthy behaviors for population health.

Bradley, E., M. Canavan, E. Rogan, K. Talbert-Slagle, C. Ndumele, L. Taylor, and L. Curry (2016). "Variation in Health Outcomes: The Role of Spending on Social Services, Public Health and Healthcare, 2000–2009." *Health Affairs* 35(3): 760–768. How priorities in spending that enable healthy behavior compared to health care treatments differentially impact actual health.

Squires, D. and C. Anderson (2015). "U.S. Health Care from a Global Perspective: Spending, Use of Services, Prices, and Health in 13 Countries." The Commonwealth Fund. Includes comparisons across developed countries.

Multiple foundations and nations are seeking better ways to deliver health. Here are only a few of the more developed and documented approaches to moving from health care to health and well-being:

Chatterjee, A., S. Kubendran, J. King, and R. DeVol (2014). "Checkup Time: Chronic Disease and Wellness in America—Measuring the Economic Burden in a Changing Nation." Milken Institute. milkeninstitute.org/publications/view/618.

Robert Wood Johnson Foundation (2013). "Return on Investments in Public Health: Saving Lives and Money." rwjf.org/content/dam/farm/reports/issue_briefs/2013/rwjf72446.

National Prevention Council (2011). "National Prevention Strategy." Washington, D.C., U.S. Department of Health and Human Services. Office of the Surgeon General.

National Center for Chronic Disease Prevention and Health Promotion (2009). "The Power of Prevention: Chronic Disease . . . the Public Health Challenge of the 21st Century." Centers for Disease Control and Prevention. See cdc.gov/chronicdisease/pdf/2009-power-of-prevention.pdf.

The Vitality Institute (2014). "Investing in Prevention: A National Imperative." thevitality-institute.org/site/wp-content/uploads/2014/06/Vitality_Recommendations2014.pdf.

Scottish Government (2016). "Creating a Healthier Scotland." scdc.org.uk/news/article/creating-healthier-scotland-summary-report.

Singapore is one of the most progressive and effective health promotion cities in the world and includes traditional and integrative health care delivery. See hpb.gov.sg/article/singapore-comes-together-to-celebrate-20-years-of-healthy-lifestyle.

You don't see what you don't measure. One of the most comprehensive ways to measure well-being in a country has been done in Canada, and it is paying off. Outcomes are better and costs of health care are significantly lower than its neighbor to the south. See uwaterloo.ca/canadian-index-wellbeing/ for how they measure health and well-being.

For a summary of the impact of the community health movement in the United States see Norris, T. (2013). "Healthy Communities at Twenty-Five." *National Civic Review* 102: 4–9.

For plans for advancing nonconventional medicine globally, see "WHO Traditional Medicine Strategy: 2014–2013." World Health Organization. See who.int/medicines/publications/traditional/trm_strategy14_23/en.

WHO plans for addressing chronic disease in general is well summarized in Alwan, A. (2011). "Global Status Report on Noncommunicable Diseases 2010." World Health Organization. See www.who.int/nmh/publications/wha_resolution53_14/en.

The United Nations is also working to address community health globally. See Beaglehole, R., R. Bonita, G. Alleyne, R. Horton, L. Li, P. Lincoln, J. C. Mbanya, M. McKee, R. Moodie, S. Nishtar, P. Piot, K. S. Reddy, and D. Stuckler (2011). "UN High-Level Meeting on Non-Communicable Diseases: addressing four questions." *The Lancet* 378(9789): 449–455.

Other key sources of lifestyle and healing information as mentioned in the chapter are the following:

Metzl, Jordan. *The Exercise Cure: A Doctor's All-Natural, No-Pill Prescription for Better Health and Longer Life*. Emmaus, PA: Rodale, 2013. Exercise induces healing and keeps us functional and alive.

Johnston, B. C., S. Kanters, K. Bandayrel, et al. (2014). "Comparison of weight loss among named diet programs in overweight and obese adults: A meta-analysis." *Journal of the American Medical Association* 312(9): 923–933. It is more important to pay attention that your diet is primarily whole foods and not full of additives or toxins—and that you believe it is healthy—than to worry about its exact composition. This study showed that all the current commercial diets were basically the same when it comes to weight loss.

Studies by Stanford Professor Alia Crum have examined the impact of mind-set on the impact of lifestyle and behavior on health. Mind-set influences all aspect[s] of lifestyle and healthy behavior. See Crum, A. J. and E. J. Langer (2007). "Mind-set matters: exercise and the placebo effect." *Psychological Science* 18(2): 165–171; and, Crum, Alia J., et al. (2011). "Mind over milkshakes: mindsets, not just nutrients, determine ghrelin response." *Health Psychology* 30(4): 424l; and, Crum, Alia, et al. (2017). "De-stressing stress: The power of mindsets and the art of stressing mindfully." *The Wiley Blackwell Handbook of Mindfulness*, 948–963; and, Crum, A. J., K. A. Leibowitz, and A. Verghese (2017). "Making mindset matter." *British Medical Journal* 356: j674.

Do gene changes come from the food we eat or the social environment of the eating? See Ordovas, J. M. (2008). "Genotype-phenotype associations: modulation by diet and obesity." *Obesity* 16(Suppl 3): S40–S46. doi:10.1038/oby.2008.515.

Giordano J. and W. B. Jonas (2007). "Asclepius and hygieia in dialectic: Philosophical, ethical and educational foundations of an integrative medicine." *Integrative Medicine Insights* 2: 53–60. A description of the ancient Greek Hippocratic school of medicine and how it addressed all the dimensions of healing.

Jonas, W. B., P. Deuster, F. O'Connor, and C. Macedonia (2010). "Total Force Fitness for the 21st Century: A New Paradigm." *Military Medicine* (Suppl). 175(8). The United States military's framework for whole systems health and well-being.

Mission: Readiness, Military Leaders for Kids. Report: "Too Fat to Fight: Retired Military Leaders Want Junk Food Out of America's Schools." Washington, D.C., Mission: Readiness, 2010. Obesity is a threat to national security.

For current training in healthy cooking for health professionals, see the Harvard program Healthy Kitchens, Healthy Lives at hms.harvard.edu/news/harvard-medical-school-and-culinary-institute-america-launch-healthy-kitchens-healthy-lives-4-20-07.

For information on complementary, lifestyle, and integrative approaches in cancer, see the Society for Integrative Oncology at integrativeonc.org; and, also the book by Block, Keith I. *Life Over Cancer.* New York: Bantam/Random House, 2009. Dr. Block's book is the best and most comprehensive overview on evidence-based integrative oncology available for patients.

Pletcher, M. J. and C. E. McCulloch (2017). "The Challenges of Generating Evidence to Support Precision Medicine." *Journal of the American Medical Association Internal Medicine* 177(4): 561–562. The NIH needs you to join their whole systems science initiative called Precision Medicine.

Topol, Eric. *The Patient Will See You Now: The Future of Medicine Is in Your Hands.* New York: Basic Books, 2016. How technology is democratizing health care and putting patients in charge of their health.

CHAPTER 7: LOVING DEEPLY

We often think of love and fear as solely psychological—all in the mind—and as having little impact on the body. This is not true, but the myth persists in the modern mind. When we finally break this misperception, it will crack open whole new dimensions for healing. I use this remarkable but little known experiment on rabbits to show how, despite the objective demonstration that love is as powerful as cholesterol-lowering drugs in preventing heart disease, we have largely ignored the former and made an industry of the latter.

Selected references readers may find of interest mentioned in this chapter include the following:

Nerem, R. M., M. J. Levesque, and J. F. Cornhill (1980). "Social environment as a factor in diet-induced atherosclerosis." *Science* 208(4451): 1475–1476. The formal "love your rabbit" experiment described in the chapter.

Titler, M. G., G. A. Jensen, J. M. Dochterman, X-J M. Xie, D. Reed, and L. L. Shever (April 2008). "Cost of Hospital Care for Older Adults with Heart Failure: Medical, Pharmaceutical, and Nursing Costs." *Health Services Research Journal* 43(2): 635–655. Heart failure is costly, and the costs are rising.

Berwick, D. M., T. W. Nolan, and J. Whittington (2008). "The triple aim: care, health, and cost." *Health Affairs* (Millwood) 27(3): 759–769. The triple aim—simultaneously improving health outcomes, and the quality of patient experience and lowering costs—has become the mantra for value in health care.

Christakis, Nicholas. A. and James H. Fowler. *Connected: The Surprising Power of Our Social Networks and How They Shape Our Lives*. New York: Little Brown, 2009. Research shows that your friend, their friends, and their friends all have an impact on your health and healing capacity.

Cacioppo, John T. and William Patrick. *Loneliness: Human Nature and the Need for Social Connection*. New York: W.W. Norton & Company, 2008. One of the best overviews of the science of loneliness and its impact on health.

Farmer, I. P., P. S. Meyer, D. J. Ramsey, D. C. Goff, M. L. Wear, D. R. Labarthe, and M. Z. Nichaman (1996). "Higher levels of social support predict greater survival following acute myocardial infarction: The Corpus Christi Heart Project." *Behavioral Medicine* 22(2): 59–66.

How does the physical presence of a person affect the other? The studies on how electromagnetic waves of the heart impact the electromagnetic waves of the brain of persons standing next to each other can be found in McCraty, Rollin. *The Science of the Heart*. Boulder Creek, CA: HeartMath Institute, 2015. Available at heartmath.org.

Two studies we conducted at Walter Reed Army Institute of Research demonstrated that electromagnetic waves coming off the hands of a healer can increase the energy molecules of cells. See Kiang, J. G., J. A. Ives, and W. B. Jonas (2005). "External bioenergy-induced increases in intracellular free calcium concentrations are mediated by Na+/Ca 2+ exchanger and L-type calcium channel." *Molecular and Cellular Biochemistry* 271(1): 51–59; and, Kiang, J. G., D. Marotta, M. Wirkus, and Jonas, W. B. (2002). "External Bioenergy Increases Intracellular Free Calcium Concentration and Reduces Cellular Response to Heat Stress." *Journal of Investigative Medicine* 50(1): 38–45. This might be the mechanism for the ancient method of laying-on of hands. More research is needed.

Kemper, K. J. *Authentic Healing: A Practical Guide for Caregivers*. Minneapolis, MN: Two Harbors Press, 2016. In this book, Dr. Kemper, professor of pediatrics at The Ohio State University College of Medicine, describes how to use bioenergy healing in day-to-day practice.

Pennebaker, J. W. *Opening Up: The Healing Power of Expressing Emotions*. New York: Guildford Press, 1997. (Second edition published in 2012.) This book summarizes decades of research showing that by engaging past areas of deep personal and emotional trauma, such as through therapeutic writing, the brain, immune system, physiological function, and even health care needs improve.

Even a single episode of therapeutic writing improves pain (in rheumatoid arthritis) and lung function (in asthma). See Smyth, J. M., A. A. Stone, A. Hurewitz, and A. Kaell (1999). "Effects of writing about stressful experiences on symptom reduction in patients with asthma or rheumatoid arthritis: a randomized trial." *Journal of the American Medical Association* 281(14): 1304–1309.

Facing your past traumatic experiences in the presence of loving persons can heal the effects of past trauma in veterans who have gone to war. See Bobrow, Joseph. *Waking Up from War: A Better Way Home for Veterans and Nations*. Durham, NC: Pitchstone Publishing, 2015. And about those who have not gone to war but experienced trauma nonetheless, see van de Kolk, Bessel. *The Body Keeps the Score: Brain, Mind, and Body in the Healing of Trauma*. New York: Penguin, 2014. New discoveries in the healing of trauma are helping to us to understand the fundamental dynamics of healing in general.

Griffiths, R. R., M. W. Johnson, M. A. Carducci, A. Umbricht, W. A. Richards, B. D. Richards, M. P. Cosimano, and M. A. Klinedinst (2016). "Psilocybin produces substantial and sustained decreases in depression and anxiety in patients with life-threatening cancer: A randomized double-blind trial." *Journal of Psychopharmacology* 30(12): 1181–1197. It appears that psychoactive drugs can open people to their fears, which if then reexperienced in a positive manner can permanently heal anxiety, depression, and other emotional ills. Research is ongoing to see if this approach will also work for veterans with refractory PTSD. I predict it will work.

For a description of the social approach to healing individuals in the Navajo Beauty Way and other similar ceremonies, see gonativeamericanconcepts.wordpress.com/the-blessing-way/ and gonativeamerica.com/10-NavajoBeautyway.html.

Moerman, D. E. *Meaning, Medicine, and the 'Placebo Effect'*. Cambridge, MA: Cambridge University Press, 2002. The definitive summary of how meaning and context work across cultures to explain the placebo response.

For a description on how relationship-centered care improved the health of a community of people and became a demonstration model for using the social and emotional dimensions of healing health care, see Gottlieb, K. (2013). "The Nuka System of Care: improving health through ownership and relationships." *International Journal of Circumpolar Health* 72(1): 211–218; and, Driscoll, D. L., V. Hiratsuka, J. M. Johnston, S. Norman, K. M. Reilly, J. Shaw, and D. Dillard (2013). "Process and outcomes of patient-centered medical care with Alaska Native people at South Central Foundation." *The Annals of Family Medicine* 11(Suppl 1): S41–S49.

Group care not only can address loneliness but also facilitate behavioral change and impact health care costs. For a description of the approach taken by Dr. Jeffery Geller, see Geller, J., P. Janson, E. McGovern, and A. Valdini (1999). "Loneliness as a predictor of hospital emergency department use." *Journal of Family Practice* 48(10): 801–807; and, Geller, J. S., A. Orkaby, and G. D. Cleghorn (2011). "Impact of a group medical visit program on Latino health–related quality of life." *EXPLORE: The Journal of Science and Healing* 7(2): 94–99.

CHAPTER 8: FINDING MEANING

It is difficult for scientists and physicians to believe that the subtle and largely immeasurable aspects of our mind and spirit are important for healing. But they are. They need to be considered and used in health care. I have spent a considerable part of my research career exploring this area, seeking to increase the scientific rigor and amount of evidence in the mental and spiritual dimensions of healing. Of course, more research is needed. While the role of mind-body practices, mindfulness, and mind-set is increasingly accepted in medicine, the subtler spiritual aspects of our lives is still largely taboo in medicine.

One of the most thoughtful writers in this area is Dr. Larry Dossey, whose books explore these areas. I recommend starting with his classic, *Healing Words: Power of Prayer and the Practice of Medicine* (San Francisco: Harper Collins, 1993), and also his *Healing Beyond the Body: Medicine and the Infinite Reach of the Mind* (Boulder, CO: Shambhala Publications, 2003).

Daniel Benor's *Healing Research* (Munich: Helix Verlag, 1993) contains a detailed summary of research. A criteria-based, critical evaluation of these areas can be found in Jonas, W. B. and C. C. Crawford (eds.). *Healing, Intention and Energy Medicine: Science, Methodology and Clinical Implications.* London: Churchill Livingston, 2003.

For extensive summaries of the health effects from religious and spiritual practices, see Koenig, H., D. King, and V. B. Carson, *Handbook of Religion and Health, 2nd Edition*. New York: Oxford University Press, 2012; especially for nurses, see Carson, V. B. and H. Koenig *Spiritual Dimensions of Nursing Practice*. West Conshohoken, PA: Templeton Foundation

Press, 2008; and especially for physicians, see Puchalski, C. and B. Ferrell *Making Health Care Whole: Integrating Spirituality into Patient Care.* West Conshohoken, PA: Templeton Foundation Press, 2011. Professor Puchalski conducts an annual training at George Washington University on spiritual issues in medicine.

Other selected references readers may find of interest mentioned in this chapter include (in order of their description):

Classics in the use of guided imagery for healing are the books by Jeanne Achtenberg (*Imagery in Healing*, Boston: Shambhala, 1985) and Carl Simonton (*The Healing Journey*, New York: Bantam, 1992) and Belleruth Naprastek (*Staying Well with Guided Imagery*, New York: Warner, 1994).

Newer, practical sites for getting both information and downloads of guided imagery for use in life can be obtained from the Academy for Guided Imagery (acadgi.com) and the website of Dr. Naprastek at healthjourneys.com. I have been involved in clinical studies with veterans using the work of Dr. Naprastek and found it useful and effective.

The remarkable effects of imagery and healing touch when used with Marines for PTSD can be found in Jain, S., G. F. McMahon, P. Hasen, M. P. Kozub, V. Porter, R. King, and E. M. Guarneri (2012). "Healing Touch with Guided Imagery for PTSD in returning active duty military: a randomized controlled trial." *Military Medicine* 177(9): 1015–1021.

Veterans deployed to war have almost twice the rate of exceptional and spiritual experiences than the general population. See Hufford, David. "Spiritual experiences in Veterans deployed to Iraq and Afghanistan." Personal communication; and, Hufford, D. J., M. J. Fritts, and J. E. Rhodes (2010). "Spiritual fitness." *Military Medicine* 175(8S): 73–87.

We can teach the body to respond in specific ways to inert substances or other signals through the process of classical conditioning. For examples of this, see the classic study of immune suppression in rats by Ader, R. and N. Cohen (1975). "Behaviorally conditioned immunosuppression." *Psychosomatic Medicine* 37(4): 333–340; and, in humans by Goebel, M. U., et al. (2002). "Behavioral conditioning of immunosuppression is possible in humans." *Federation of American Studies for Experimental Biology Journal* 16:1869–1873; and, in other conditions, see Kroes, M. C. W., J. E. Dunsmoor, W. E. Mackey, M. McClay, and E. A. Phelps (2017). "Context conditioning in humans using commercially available immersive Virtual Reality." *Scientific Reports* 7:8640. doi:/10.1038/s41598-017-08184-7; and, Colloca, L., L. Lopiano, M. Lanotte and F. Benedetti (2004). "Overt versus covert treatment for pain, anxiety, and Parkinson's disease." *The Lancet Neurology* 3: 679–684.

Branding (the label on the pill) and price (expensive or cheap) make a difference in the effectiveness of treatments. See Margo, C. E. (1999). "The Placebo Effect." *Survey of Ophthalmology* 44: 31–44, for an example of branding; and, Waber, R. L., B. Shiv, Z. Carmon, and D. Ariely (2008). "Commercial features of placebo and therapeutics." *Journal of the American Medical Association* 299(9): 1016–7 for an example of how price impacts effectiveness. Drug companies know about these effects. How much of the fluctuation in branding and drug prices is to impact their perceived effectiveness rather than because of their real effects?

Moerman, D. E. *Meaning, Medicine, and the 'Placebo Effect'*. Cambridge, MA: Cambridge University Press, 2002. The definitive summary of how meaning and context work across cultures to explain the placebo response.

For a detailed description of the use of conditioned immunosuppression in an eleven-year-old child with a life-threatening disease by Dr. Karen Olness, professor of pediatrics at Case Western Reserve, see Marchant, J. "You can train your body into thinking it's had medicine." *Mosaic: The Science of Life*. mosaicscience.com/story/medicine-without-the-medicine-how-to-train-your-immune-system-placebo.

Siegel, Daniel J. *Mind: A Journey to The Heart of Being Human*. New York: W.W. Norton & Company, 2016. A visionary book by a University of California, Los Angeles, psychiatrist on how the mind works, both inside and outside the body.

For a study on how expectations can be established during a single clinical visit and profoundly affect outcomes in primary care, see Thomas, K. B. (1987). "General practice consultations: is there any point in being positive?" *British Medical Journal* (Clinical Research Edition) 294(6581): 1200–1202.

Gracely, R. H. (1979). "Physicians expectations for pain relief." *Society for Neuroscience Abstracts* 5: 609; also in Levine, J., N. Gordon, and H. Fields (1978). "The mechanism of placebo analgesia." *The Lancet* 312(8091): 654–657. It matters what your physician believes will work, not just what you believe. Ask your doctor about his or her belief in a treatment.

Lang, E. V., O. Hatisopoulou, T. Koch, K. Berbaum, S. Lutgendorf, E. Kettenmann, L. Henrietta, T. J. Kaptchuk (2005). "Can words hurt? Patient-provider interactions during invasive procedures." *Pain* 114: 303–309. Don't let your doctor say "This will hurt," because it will if he does.

Schedlowski, M., P. Enck, W. Rief, and U. Bingel (2015). "Neuro-bio-behavioral mechanisms of placebo and nocebo responses: implications for clinical trials and clinical practice." *Pharmacological Reviews* 67(3): 697–730. The side effects of drugs increase the more we expect them to.

The study on death in China, related to astrology, is found in Phillips, D. P., T. E. Ruth, and L. M. Wagner (1993). "Psychology and survival." *The Lancet* 342(8880): 1142–1145.

A spiritual view of healing through and because of trauma: Nouwen, Henri J. M. *The Wounded Healer: Ministry in Contemporary Society*. New York: Image/Doubleday Books, 1979.

Shanafelt, T. D., L. N. Dyrbye, and C. P. West (2017). "Addressing Physician Burnout: The Way Forward." *Journal of the American Medical Association* 317(9): 901–902. Up to 50% of doctors are burnt out and say they have lost their passion for medical practice and empathy for patients.

Murphy, Robin. *The Future of the Body: Explorations into the Further Evolution of Human Nature.* New York: Tarcher/Putnam, 1992. Mr. Murphy has provided an encyclopedic review of our body's remarkable ability to heal.

Temel, J. S., J. A. Greer, A. Muzikansky, E. R. Gallagher, S. Admane, V. A. Jackson, et al. (2010). "Early palliative care for patients with metastatic non–small-cell lung cancer." *New England Journal of Medicine* 363(8): 733–742. By providing less treatment and more comfort and caring for patients with advanced lung cancer, they felt better and lived longer.

Doctors and our health care system do not deal well with death and dying. See Institute of Medicine. *Dying in America: Improving Quality and Honoring Individual Preferences Near the End of Life*. Washington, D. C.: National Academies Press, 2015 and Gawande, Atul. *Being Mortal: Medicine and What Matters in the End.* New York: Metropolitan Books, 2014. Dr. Gawande writes about the need to extend healing into times of death and dying. I write about the need to extend healing into routine medical care at all times.

For studies on the value and limitation of intuition, see the extensive work by Professor Gerard Hodgkinson and his team of the Centre for Organizational Strategy, Learning and Change at Leeds University, England. Their findings are summarized at leeds.ac.uk/news/article/367/go_with_your_gut__intuition_is_more_than_just_a_hunch_says_leeds_research.

For a rigorous evaluation, using three types of validity, of the research done on mind and spirit for healing, see Jonas, W. B. and C.C. Crawford (eds.). *Healing, Intention and Energy Medicine: Science, Methodology and Clinical Implications*. London: Churchill Livingston, 2003.

For a review and statistical comparison of the outcomes of prayer-like (psychic intention) activity, showing that the effects are similar to that of aspirin in preventing heart disease, see the 1995 study "An Assessment of the Evidence for Psychic Functioning" by Professor Jessica Utts, who chairs the Department of Statistics, University of California, Irvine, and is the past president of the American Statistical Association. Find the study online at citeseerx.ist.psu.edu/viewdoc/download?doi=10.1.1.40.8219&rep=rep1&type=pdf.

CHAPTER 9: INTEGRATIVE HEALTH

Leaders in medical education and practice regularly call for more holistic, humanistic, personalized care. Unfortunately, technology, economics, politics, or tradition often subvert these recommendations. Then, calls for more healing reassert themselves under various names—biopsychosocial, patient-centered, relationship-centered, personalized, humanistic, proactive, holistic, or sharing medicine, for example. Integrative health is the most recent and comprehensive attempt to return healing to health care. We cannot afford a health care system that does not value health, healing, and well-being. If I were to recommend just one book about these dynamics, it would be Kenneth Ludmerer's *A Time to Heal* (New York: Oxford University Press, 1999), which is an encyclopedic history of the forces and dynamics facing a more holistic, humanistic, caring medical system.

Hypertension, like Trevor had, is one of the most important individual and public health conditions in the world. It is treatable, and its complications, which are myriad and include heart disease, stroke, and kidney failure, are top causes of death and disability. For a summary, see the World Health Organization (2013). "A global brief on hypertension: silent killer, global public health crisis: World Health Day 2013." who.int/cardiovascular_diseases/publications/global_brief_hypertension/en.

At the time that Trevor went to the doctor, the major guidelines for treating and managing hypertension were in The Seventh Report of the Joint National Committee on Prevention, Detection, Evaluation, and Treatment of High Blood Pressure (JNC7). See nhlbi.nih.gov/files/docs/guidelines/jnc7full.pdf. The more recent guidelines (called JNC8) have even less detail on integration of the social and nondrug approaches to hypertension, saying it is "beyond the scope" of the recommendations. Without integration of these dimensions into practice, however, more patients like Trevor may fall through the gap.

Other references of interest mentioned in this chapter include the following:

Steinberg, D., G. G. Bennett, and L. Svetkey (2017). "The DASH diet, 20 years later." *Journal of the American Medical Association* 317(15): 1529–1530.

Trevor's "natural medicine" practitioner may have been influenced by a popular book on the Rice Diet. See Rosati, Kitty Gurkin and Robert Rosati. *The Rice Diet Solution: The World-famous Low-sodium, Good-carb, Detox Diet for Quick and Lasting Weight Loss.* New York: Simon and Schuster, 2006. However, what Trevor did not understand was that the original diet, developed by Duke physician Walter Kempner in 1939, was for a very different type of patient than he was. See Klemmer, P., et al. (2014). "Who and what drove Walter Kempner? The rice diet revisited." *Hypertension* 64(4): 684–688.

For summaries of the factors that contribute most to population health and how our health care systems can better address those factors and close the gap see: Kindig, D. A., B. C. Booske, and P. L. Remington (2010). "Mobilizing Action Toward Community Health (MATCH): metrics, incentives, and partnerships for population health." *Preventing Chronic Disease* 7(4): A68; and, Dzau, V. J., M. B. McClellan, J. M. McGinnis, S. P. Burke, M. J. Coye, A. Diaz, T. A. Daschle, W. H. Frist, M. Gaines, M. A. Hamburg, J. E. Henney, S. Kumanyika, M. O. Leavitt, R. M. Parker, L. G. Sandy, L. D. Schaeffer, G. D. Steele, P. Thompson, and E. Zerhouni (2017). "Vital Directions for Health and Health Care: Priorities from a National Academy of Medicine Initiative." *Journal of the American Medical Association* 317(14):

1461–1470; and, Samueli Institute's *"Wellbeing in the Nation: A Plan to Strengthen and Sustain our Nation's Wellbeing, Community by Community"* available at wellbeinginthenation.org.

For information about evidence-based medicine and why it has become so important, see Belsey, Jonathan and Tony Snell (1997). "What is evidence-based medicine?" *Hayward Medical Communications*; and, Jaeschke, R. and G. H. Guyatt (October 1999). "What is evidence-based medicine?" *Seminars in Medical Practice* 2(3): 3–7.

The term *salutogenesis* meaning "the generation of health" was first coined by psychologist Aaron Antonovsky. See Antonovsky, Aaron. *Unraveling the Mystery of Health*. San Francisco: Jossey-Bass, 1987. I have expanded the use of the term salutogenesis beyond psychology into medicine and use it to complement the concept of *pathogenesis* meaning "the generation of disease." See Jonas, W. B., R. A. Chez, K. Smith, B. Sakallaris, and C. Crawford (2014). "Salutogenesis: The Defining Concept for a New Healthcare System." *Global Advances in Health Medicine* 3: 82–91.

Hölzel, Britta K., et al. (2011). "Mindfulness practice leads to increases in regional brain gray matter density." *Psychiatry Research: Neuroimaging* 191(1): 36–43. This research is what made us think that Mandy would benefit from an eight-week session of mindfulness before we resumed acupuncture treatment for her chronic pain.

While the story about the origins of Tibetan medicine as an intentional synthesis from multiple traditions did not likely occur exactly like this, the story does speak to the fact that Tibetan medicine is a tradition that intentionally draws from the multiple healing approaches from India, China, and the Middle East—and, more recently, the West.

For serial data on the growing popularity and use of complementary and alternative medicine in the United States, see Eisenberg, D. M., R. B. Davis, S. L. Ettner, S. Appel, S. Wilkey, M. Van Rompay, R. C. Kessler (1998). "Trends in alternative medicine use in the United State 1990–1997: Results of a follow-up national survey." *Journal of the American Medical Association* 280(18): 1569–1575; and, Nahin, R. L., P. M. Barnes, B. J. Stussman, and B. Bloom (2009). "Costs of complementary and alternative medicine (CAM) and frequency of visits to CAM practitioners: United States, 2007." *National Health Statistics Reports* 18: 1–14; and, Clarke, T. C., L. I. Black, B. J. Stussman, P. M. Barnes, and R. L. Nahin (2015). "Trends in the Use of Complementary Health Approaches Among Adults: United States, 2002–2012." *National Health Statistics Reports* 79:1–16.

World Health Organization (1948). "Definition of health" see who.int/suggestions/faq/en/; also, see "Constitution of WHO: principles." who.int/about/mission/en.

Institute of Medicine. *Crossing the Quality Chasm: A New Health System for the 21st Century*. Washington, D.C.: National Academy of Sciences Press, 2001. A landmark study in which person-centered care is clearly defined and called for.

Ornish, Dean. *The Spectrum: A Scientifically Proven Program to Feel Better, Live Longer, Lose Weight, and Gain Health.* New York: Ballantine Books, 2008. Dr. Ornish is a pioneer in health promotion and lifestyle medicine and this is his most holistic view yet.

Buettner, Dan. *The Blue Zones: 9 Lessons for Living Longer from the People Who've Lived the Longest.* Washington, D.C.: National Geographic Books, 2012. Readers are often surprised by how simple actions can have a significant influence on well-being and mentality.

For information on Iora Health System, see iorahealth.com. Team-based, patient-centered care in action.

For a report on the top-five percent of primary care clinics, see Petersen Health Foundation (2013). "America's Most Valuable Care: Primary Care Snapshots." petersonhealthcare.org/

identification-uncovering-americas-most-valuable-care/primary-care-snapshots.

Strecher, Victor J. *Life on Purpose: How Living for What Matters Most Changes Everything*. San Francisco: HarperCollins, 2016. Summarizes data on how meaning creates health and healing and how to bring purpose into your life. Developer of the JOOL app for purpose in life.

CHAPTER 10: CREATING HEALING

There are a number of health care leaders and systems redesigning the way health care and healing is delivered along the lines of integrative health. I describe some of them in this chapter; see the following for more information.

Burnt-out providers can't heal. Yet the problem of burnout is growing (and now estimated at nearly 50% in primary care physicians and nurses). See Shanafelt, T. D., L. N. Dyrbye, and C. P. West (2017). "Addressing Physician Burnout: The Way Forward." *Journal of the American Medical Association* 317(9): 901–902; and, Dyrbye, L. N., T. D. Shanafelt, C. A. Sinsky, P. F. Cipriano, J. Bhatt, A. Ommaya, C. P. West, and D. Meyers (2017). "Burnout among health-care professionals: A call to explore and address this underrecognized threat to safe, high-quality care." *NAM Perspectives*. Discussion Paper, National Academy of Medicine, Washington, D.C. nam.edu/Burnout-Among-Health-Care-Professionals.

The Commonwealth Fund's link to "exemplars" in health care: commonwealthfund.org/grants-and-fellowships/grants/2012/jul/exemplars-of-local-health-care-delivery-reform.

The World Health Organization has an office of traditional medicine that tracks its use and advances research and application globally. See World Health Organization (2005). "National policy on traditional medicine and regulation of herbal medicines: Report of a WHO global survey" at apps.who.int/iris/bitstream/10665/43229/1/9241593237.pdf; and, World Health Organization (2014). "WHO Traditional Medicine Strategy 2014–2023. Geneva; 2013" at who.int/medicines/publications/traditional/trm_strategy14_23/en.

Herman, Patricia M., et al. (2012). "Are complementary therapies and integrative care cost-effective? A systematic review of economic evaluations." *BMJ Open* 2(5): e001046. Does adding complementary medicine save money? Apparently so, if done appropriately.

Khorsan, R., I. D. Coulter, C. Crawford, and A. F. Hsiao (2011). "Systematic review of integrative health-care research: randomized control trials, clinical controlled trials, and meta-analysis." *Evidence-Based Complementary and Alternative Medicine* 2011(pii): 636134. Most research evaluates CAM practices with little exploration of the true integration of conventional and CAM practices.

National Academy of Medicine. *Integrative Medicine and the Health of the Public: A Summary of February 2009 Summit.* Washington, D.C.: The National Academies Press, 2009. The United States National Academy of Medicine calls for more integration in 2009. This echoed a White House Commission report from nearly a decade earlier. See Dean, Karen L. (2001). "White House Commission on Complementary and Alternative Medicine Policy Town Hall Meeting: Practitioners and Patients Speak Up." *Alternative & Complementary Therapies* 7(2): 108–111.

Information on medical and health education schools with integrative health activities can be found at The Academic Consortium for Integrative Health and Medicine, imconsortium.org.

For integrative medical information in Europe, see The European Society of Integrative Medicine (ESIM) at european-society-integrative-medicine.org.

Information on research in complementary and integrative medicine globally can be obtained from the International Society for Complementary Medicine Research (ISCMR) at iscmr.org.

University of Arizona Center for Integrative Medicine, founded by Dr. Andrew Weil (integrativemedicine.arizona.edu/), is one of the first and premier university centers for integrative medicine. They have taught over 1,500 health care providers and are expanding their services. This is one of the first places physicians go for training when they want to do more integrative medicine.

Weil, Andrew. *Mind Over Meds*. Boston: Little, Brown and Company, 2017. The latest book by a pioneer in natural medicine who popularized the term *integrative medicine*.

Information on the Susan and Henry Samueli College of Health Sciences and University of California, Irvine can be found at uci.edu. This unique college will consist of four schools—medicine, nursing, pharmacy, and public (or population) health—all oriented toward providing education in integrative health at a major public university.

Cleveland Clinic has two major efforts on integrative health. They are Integrative Health and Wellness Institute at my.clevelandclinic.org/departments/wellness/integrative, and the Center for Functional Medicine at my.clevelandclinic.org/departments/functional-medicine.

Bland, Jeffrey. *The Disease Delusion*. New York: HarperCollins, 2014. The latest book by a pioneer of applied nutritional therapy, using systems science approaches. Dr. Bland coined the term *functional medicine*.

Information and training in functional medicine can be obtained from the Institute for Functional Medicine at ifm.org.

The Mayo Clinic also two major efforts in integrative health housed in their Center for Integrative Health (mayoclinic.org/departments-centers/integrative-medicine-health) and their Healthy Living Center (healthyliving.mayoclinic.org/the-mayo-clinic-difference.php).

Tools for self-care and integrative health can be found at the Center for Spirituality and Healing at the University of Minnesota. See csh.umn.edu. Led by nurse researcher Dr. Mary Jo Kreitzer, many of these tools are free or available at minimal cost to the public.

Also available to the public at minimal cost are tools for self-care and integrative health developed by pediatrician Dr. Kathi Kemper at The Ohio State University College of Medicine. I recommend her courses on herbs and dietary supplements (herbs-supplements.osu.edu) and, in mind-body skills training for resilience (mind-bodyhealth.osu.edu). For parents, Dr. Kemper has written the definitive guide to holistic health for children, *The Holistic Pediatrician* (San Francisco: HarperCollins, 2016), originally published in 1996.

The Academic Collaborative for Integrative Health (ACIH) is an association of higher education schools in the complementary health professions—acupuncture, massage, naturopathy, and midwifery. They can be found at integrativehealth.org.

Information on chiropractic medicine education and practice can be found at two sites: the World Federation of Chiropractic, an advocate for a broad role in health care rather than solely spinal manipulation (wfc.org) and the World Chiropractic Alliance, a chiropractic medicine organization primarily advocating for spinal manipulation (worldchiropracticalliance.org). Chiropractic medical education is overseen by the Councils on Chiropractic Education International, but each country regulates their educational and licensing requirements. In the United States, this is the Council on Chiropractic Education (cce-usa.org).

Information on integration of conventional medicine and lifestyle can be obtained from the Institute for Lifestyle Medicine (instituteoflifestylemedicine.org).

ACKNOWLEDGMENTS

So many people deserve thanks for assisting with this work that it would take another book to acknowledge them.

I need to start with my wife, Susan, who let me tell her story of multiple cancer survivals, including the most recent. She keeps me connected to the spirit. She is also my first editor and best critic!

Our children are now my teachers. Our son, Chris, and daughter-in-law, Marzia, and their beautiful child, show me how to thrive. Our daughter Maeba is always taking me deeper into life, and our other daughter Emily "E. J." shows me how to always love learning. Thanks to you all.

My father, Henry, and mother, Joan, still show me their wisdom. I hope I have transmitted a bit of that through this book.

The insights in this book would not have happened without the friendship and long-standing support of Henry and Susan Samueli. Their vision for evidence-based, integrative health has been steadfast. I am confident their impact has only begun. Thanks also to Mike Schulman, who leads the Samueli office, and Gerald Solomon, who heads the Samueli Foundation.

My colleague and coworker Doug Cavarocchi saw the value of this book long before I did and made it happen. He found our agent, Jim Levine, who has been instrumental in molding its message and contributing his passion and expertise continuously. He also found our publisher, Lorena Jones, who has taken a gamble on this vision of the future of health care. She and her team understand the urgency of the message and necessity for its widespread distribution. My co worker Jennifer Dorr helped write the practical appendices and continues to contribute to my website (DrWayneJonas.com). Thanks also to Lexie Robinson, who has supported the production at every turn.

My former colleagues at Samueli Institute have helped shape the movement from health care to health. Joan Walter is a get-it-done professional with tremendous integrity and commitment to healing. Ron Chez taught me how to take healing into the mainstream. John Ives brought insights to the science. Thanks also to Kevin Berry, Bonnie Sakallaris, Mac Beckner, Katherine Smith, Dawn Bellanti, Barbara Findley, Alex York, Shamini Jain, Raheleh Khorsan, Kelly Gourdin, Linda Honig, Viviane Enslein, Courtney Lee, Chris Baur, Brian Thiel, and David Eisenberg, who all still carry the work of healing forward in research, action, and writing. A special call-out to Cindy Crawford, who learned evidence-based medicine from me and then took it to the new heights used in this book and elsewhere.

There are many leaders in health care, research, health policy, and practice from whom I have learned and drawn on for this book. A heartfelt thanks to Daniel Amen, Cathy Baase, Brent Bauer, Berkeley and Elinor Bedell, Iris Bell, Brian and Susan Berman, Herb Benson, Don Berwick, Clem Bezold, Keith Block, Robert Bonakdar, Josie Briggs, Ed Calabrese, Barrie Cassileth, Richard Carmona, Vint Cerf, Bill Chatfield, Margaret Chesney, Christine Choate, Deepak Chopra, Gail Christopher, Luana Colloca, Ian Coulter, Regan Crump, Jonathan Davidson, Larry and Barbie Dossey, Bob Duggan, Howard Federoff, Mimi Guarneri, Tracy Gaudet, Mary Guerrera, Paul Funk, Jeff Geller, Bill and Penny George, Jim Giordano, Andrea Gordon, Jim Gordon, Stephen Groft, Patrick Hanaway, Adi Haramati, Larry Hardaway, Tom Harkin, Mark Hyman, Kurt and Lori Henry, George Isham, Charlotte Rose Kerr, Ruth Kirschstein, Ben Kligler, Fredi Kronenberg, David Jones, Sam Jones, Kathi Kemper, Mary Jo Kreitzer, Linnea Larson, Jeff Levi, George Lewith, Klaus Linde, Michael Lerner, Victoria Maizes, Shaista Malik, Robert Marsten, Barbara Mikulski, Will Miller, Jim Moran, Mike and Deb Mullen, Richard Neimtzow, Bill Novelli, Fran O'Connor, Dean Ornish, Mehmet Oz, Jonathan Peck, Joe Pizzorno, Bill and Frances Purkert, David Rakel, Henri Roca, Stefan Schmidt, Stephen Schmidt, Eric and Audrey Schoomaker, Eric and Patty Shinseki, Esther Sternberg, Soma Stout, Gene Thin Elk, John Umhau, Harald Walach, John Weeks, Andy Weil, Jeffrey White, David Williams, Jim Zimble, and many others. Thanks also to the people of the Bayview Marriott in Newport Beach, California, where about half of this book was written.

And, finally, thanks to all my patients. You are the true healers. When we sit together and see together, we all heal together.

INDEX

E

F

G

N

O

P

R